... be recalled

...e that you ...ot
...erwise you will be

D0414766

Heart Valve Disease

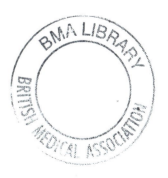

Heart Valve Disease

A Guide to Patient Management after Surgery

Editors

Eric G Butchart FRCS FETCS FESC
Senior Consultant Surgeon
Department of Cardiothoracic Surgery
University Hospital of Wales
Cardiff
UK

Christa Gohlke-Bärwolf MD FESC
Senior Cardiologist
Heart Center
Bad Krozingen
Germany

Manuel J Antunes MD PhD DSc
Professor of Cardiothoracic Surgery
University Hospital
Coimbra
Portugal

Roger JC Hall MD FRCP FESC
Professor of Cardiology
School of Medicine, Health Policy and Practice
Norfolk & Norwich Hospital
Norwich
UK

Foreword by
Shahbudin H Rahimtoola MB FRCP MACP MACC DSc (Hon)

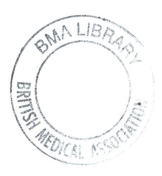

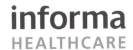

informa
HEALTHCARE

© 2006 Informa Healthcare, an imprint of Informa UK Limited

First published in the United Kingdom in 2006 by Informa Healthcare,
an imprint of Informa UK Limited,
2 Park Square, Milton Park, Abingdon, Oxon OX14 4RN

Tel: +44 (0)20 7017 6000
Fax: +44 (0)20 7017 6699
E-mail: info.medicine@tandf.co.uk
Website: www.tandf.co.uk/medicine

Although every effort has been made to ensure that all owners of copyright material have
been acknowledged in this publication, we would be glad to acknowledge in subsequent
reprints or editions any omissions brought to our attention.

Although every effort has been made to ensure that drug doses and other information are
presented accurately in this publication, the ultimate responsibility rests with the prescribing
physician. Neither the publishers nor the authors can be held responsible for errors or for
any consequences arising from the use of information contained herein. For detailed
prescribing information or instructions on the use of any product or procedure discussed
herein, please consult the prescribing information or instructional material issued by the
manufacturer.

A CIP record for this book is available from the British Library.

Library of Congress Cataloging-in-Publication Data
Data available on application

ISBN-10 1 84214 308 5
ISBN-13 978 1 84214 308 7

Distributed in North and South America by
Taylor & Francis
6000 Broken Sound Parkway, NW (Suite 300)
Boca Raton, FL 33487, USA

Within Continental USA
Tel: 1 (800) 272 7737; Fax: 1 (800) 374 3401
Outside Continental USA
Tel: (561) 994 0555; Fax: (561) 361 6018
E-mail: orders@crcpress.com

Distributed in the rest of the world by
Thomson Publishing Services
Cheriton House
North Way
Andover, Hampshire SP10 5BE, UK
Tel: +44 (0)1264 332424
E-mail: tps.tandfsalesorder@thomson.com

Composition by Scribe Design Ltd, Ashford, Kent, UK
Printed and bound by CPI Bath

Contents

Contributors

Dawn L Adamson MB BS
Specialist Registrar in Cardiology
Hammersmith Hospital and Queen Charlottes
Maternity Hospital
London
UK

Benito Almirante MD
Consultant Infectious Diseases
Hospital Universitari Vall d'Hebron
Barcelona
Spain

Manuel J Antunes MD PhD DSc
Professor of Cardiothoracic Surgery
University Hospital
Coimbra
Portugal

Helmut Baumgartner MD
Professor of Cardiology
Director, Adult Congenital and Acquired
Valvular Heart Disease Program
Medical University of Vienna
Vienna
Austria

Hans H Björnstad MD
Consultant Cardiologist
Department of Heart Disease
Haukeland University Hospital
Bergen
Norway

Eric G Butchart FRCS FETCS FESC
Senior Consultant Surgeon
Department of Cardiothoracic Surgery
University Hospital of Wales
Cardiff
UK

Bertrand Cormier MD
Consultant Cardiologist
Institut Hospitalier Jacques Cartier
Massy
France

Raffaele De Caterina MD PhD
Director, University Cardiology Division
'G. d'Annunzio' University of Chieti
Chieti
Italy

Donald B Doty MD
Adjunct Professor of Surgery
Division of Cardiothoracic Surgery
University of Utah School of Medicine
LDS Hospital
Salt Lake City, UT
USA

John R Doty MD
Adjunct Professor of Surgery
Division of Cardiothoracic Surgery
University of Utah School of Medicine
LDS Hospital
Salt Lake City, UT
USA

Christa Gohlke-Bärwolf FESC MD
Senior Cardiologist
Heart Center
Bad Krozingen
Germany

Gary L Grunkemeier PhD
Director. Medical Data Research Center
Providence Health System
Portland, OR
USA

Roger JC Hall MD FRCP FESC
Professor of Cardiology
School of Medicine, Health Policy and Practice
Norfolk and Norwich Hospital
Norwich
UK

Eric Jacobsohn MBChB MHPE FRCPC
Associate Professor of Anesthesiology and
Cardiothoracic Surgery
Director of Cardiothoracic Critical Care
Chief, Cardiothoracic Anesthesiology
Washington University School of Medicine
St Louis, MO
USA

Bernard Iung MD
Professor of Cardiology
Groupe Hôpitalier Bichat-Claude Bernard
Paris
France

Edward L Kaplan MD
Professor of Pediatrics
University of Minnesota Children's Hospital
University of Minnesota Medical School
Minneapolis, MN
USA

Olivier Nallet MD
Consultant Cardiologist
Centre Hospitalier Intercommunal 'Le Raincy
Montfermeil'
Montfermeil
France

Catherine M Otto MD
Professor of Medicine
Division of Cardiology
University of Washington
Seattle, WA
USA

Pathmaja Paramsothy MD
Acting Assistant Professor of Medicine
Division of Cardiology
University of Washington
Seattle, WA
USA

Peter Pastuszko MD
Assistant Professor of Thoracic &
Cardiovascular Surgery
The University of Oklahoma Health Sciences
Center
Oklahoma City, OK
USA

Bernard D Prendergast DM MRCP
Consultant Cardiologist
Department of Cardiology
Wythenshawe Hospital
Manchester
UK

Giulia Renda MD
Research Associate
Institute of Cardiology
'G. d'Annunzio' University of Chieti
Chieti
Italy

Raphael Rosenhek MD
Associate Professor
Department of Cardiology
Vienna General Hospital
Medical University of Vienna
Vienna
Austria

Frank Rosemeier MD MRCP(UK) DipPEC(SA)
Fellow, Critical Care Medicine
Department of Anesthesiology
Johns Hopkins School of Medicine
Baltimore, MD
USA

Manola Soccio MD PhD
Research Associate
Institute of Cardiology
'G. d'Annunzio' University of Chieti
Chieti
Italy

Thomas L Spray MD
Alice Langdon Warner Endowed Chair in
Pediatric Cardiothoracic Surgery
Chief, Division of Cardiothoracic Surgery
Children's Hospital
Philadelphia, PA
USA

Pilar Tornos MD FESC
Consultant Cardiologist
Hospital Universitario Vall d'Hebron
Barcelona
Spain

Alec Vahanian MD
Professor of Cardiology
Hôpital Bichat
Paris
France

YingXing Wu MD
Research Fellow
Medical Data Research Center
Providence Health System
Portland, OR
USA

Foreword

Heart valve surgery is the second most common form of cardiac surgery after coronary artery bypass graft surgery. The frequency with which it is performed has risen because the age of the population, in whom the prevalence of valvular disease (for example, calcific artic stenosis), has increased while the number of coronary artery surgical procedures is either steady or is decreasing. About 30 years ago, it was emphasized that valve replacement is not a cure but results in the patient exchanging one form of heart disease for another. Thus, knowledge of the problems patients encounter, and how they should be managed by physicians involved in the care of such patients, is of critical importance.

Physicians taking care of such patients may encounter many diverse problems, specifically, abnormal function of the prosthetic valve, antithrombotic management, thrombosis/embolism, pregnancy, specific types of surgery, subsequent non-cardiac surgery and the special and unique needs of children. This book provides a detailed and comprehensive discussion of all of the important issues, and such a book is very much needed.

It is not possible in a Foreword to describe all aspects of a book in detail; therefore, my comments should not be construed as an indication that the chapters mentioned here are the only important parts of the book. Chapter 1 discusses, in detail, the complex post-operative problems that are encountered and their management. For example, it is useful that the authors describe the importance of aggressive glucose control, which has been shown to reduce 1-year mortality. Chapter 2 discusses rehabilitation, which is often overlooked as part of formal treatment, even though it has been shown to improve patient outcome, especially with regard to function and the sense of well-being and normality. Echocardiography/Doppler is the single most useful non-invasive test and is comprehensively covered in Chapters 4 and 5. The problem of valve prosthesis–patient mismatch is also covered. A frequently used criterion indicating a normally functioning prosthesis is 'normal gradient' or 'gradient in the normal range' and the values in the literature are well described, however, this can be seriously flawed. For example, the gradient across the aortic valve is determined by stroke volume and systolic ejection time, both of which are dependent on left ventricular loading conditions and contractility. Thus, it is extremely important to calculate valve area (effective orifice area). To determine whether the valve area is appropriate for a particular patient, the valve area should be corrected for body size and should also be measured 6–12 months after valve replacement. Unfortunately, such data is frequently not available in published series.

An erudite and comprehensive review of antithrombotic therapy, which has proved to be one of the most pressing problems in clinical practice, is provided in Chapter 8 which cites 224 references. The authors also discuss an appropriate use of caution when administering drugs that influence antithrombotic therapy: more specifically, some of the cardiovascular drugs that increase INR, which include Simvastatin, Amiodarone, Propaferone and Quinidine. The prevention, diagnosis and treatment of prosthetic valve endocarditis is covered in Chapters 12 and 13. Chapters 14 and 15 discuss the management of the patient during subsequent pregnancy.

Rheumatic fever prophylaxis is particularly important in developing countries and this subject receives detailed coverage in Chapter 17. The book concludes with a very useful guide to the interpretation of the prosthetic valve literature.

Shahbudin H Rahimtoola
MB FRCP MACP MACC DSc (Hon)

Distinguished Professor
University of Southern California
Griffith Professor of Cardiology
Professor of Medicine
Keck School of Medicine at USC
Los Angeles, CA
USA

1

Intensive care unit management of complex postoperative problems

Frank Rosemeier and Eric Jacobsohn

Introduction

Extubation in the operating room or soon thereafter is now well-established after cardiac surgery, and in many patients, routine admission to the intensive therapy unit (ITU) may be avoided.[1,2] Because of these and other developments in perioperative care, coupled with the use of less-invasive surgical techniques, many cardiac surgical patients may now have a routine postoperative care. However, with medical therapy and the increasing use of percutaneous approaches to coronary artery disease, as well as increasing longevity of the population, many patients who now present for cardiac surgery are extremely high risk, and therefore may have a complex perioperative course. Perioperative mortality remains significant in these patients, especially those patients having complex valve procedures, double valve replacements, combined valve and coronary artery surgery and thoracoabdominal aortic surgery. The development of postoperative complications such as prolonged mechanical ventilation, renal failure, stroke and reoperation for bleeding, significantly increase mortality.[3] Various multivariate scoring systems have been developed to try to predict the complex postoperative course after cardiac surgery patients, and thereby try to intervene early to prevent these problems. More recently, sophisticated measurements such as angiotensin-converting enzyme gene polymorphism analysis, as well as the use of elevated immediate postoperative cardiac troponin-T and natriuretic peptide levels, have been shown to be useful biomarkers to identify cardiac surgical patients with potentially prolonged ITU[4] admission.

A complete discussion of all the complications and management after complex cardiac surgery is beyond the scope of this chapter, but we will highlight some of the important developments in ITU care that are pertinent to the care of these patients.

Postoperative shock and low cardiac output syndromes

Low cardiac output states and shock lead to inadequate tissue perfusion and multiorgan system dysfunction, and increase perioperative mortality. The approach to a shocked patient after cardiac surgery should follow basic principles of the differential diagnosis of hypotension and shock (Table 1.1). In many cases, there will be a combination of aetiologies. The cornerstone of diagnosis remains the clinical picture, coupled with information obtained from invasive haemodynamic monitoring and laboratory values. Although the pulmonary artery catheter (PAC) remains a useful tool in the management of patients after heart surgery, a compelling body of evidence is developing that the use of PAC in critically ill patients may not improve outcome.[5–7] However, none of these studies has focused exclusively on the cardiac surgical patient population. Another major limitation of these studies is that in none of the studies has there been a control in place to assess the competence of those performing and interpreting the PAC data. This is critical, as there is strong evidence that PAC knowledge is lacking in the ITU community at large,[8–10] even in those people who believe that they are experienced in PAC data interpretation. Therefore, the effect of the PAC on outcome in cardiac surgery patients remains uncertain. Furthermore, cardiac output determination using a haemodilution technique in the setting of severe tricuspid regurgitation and/or right ventricular failure may potentially be misleading,[11,12] requiring the use of alternative methods for haemodynamic monitoring (Table 1.2).[13] Of these techniques, transoesophageal echocardiography (TOE) is well studied, but the use of continuous monitoring of ITU patients with echocardiography is not yet a reality. TOE is extremely useful in the early diagnosis and management of haemodynamic instability in ITU

Table 1.1 Differential diagnosis of shock in the postcardiotomy patient

Hypovolaemic shock
- Haemorrhagic: occult (chest, abdomen, retroperitoneal)/observed
- Non-haemorrhagic

Cardiogenic shock
- Myocardial failure: (systolic and/or diastolic; RV and/or LV)
  - Ischaemia/infarction/preservation injury/ischaemia-reperfusion injury
  - Myopathy: restrictive/obstructive/infiltrative/hypertrophic/drug-induced
  - Metabolic: $\uparrow PO_4^{2-}$, $\downarrow Ca^{2+}$, $\uparrow H^+$
  - $\uparrow$Afterload (drugs, hypothermia, late IABP deflation and early IABP inflation)
  - LV: $\uparrow$BP, HOCM, AS
  - RV: PHT, PE, HPV, PEEP
  - $\uparrow P_a$, ARDS, $\downarrow Po_2$, $\uparrow H^+$, $\uparrow CO_2$
  - Myocardial rupture (septum or free wall)
  - Myocardial contusion
- Valvular
  - Acute valvular insufficiency (pre-existing, perioperative exaggeration of existing problem or new aetiology)
  - Valvular stenosis/obstruction
  - Thrombus, undiagnosed myxoma, SAM, mechanical valve problems
- Conduction
  - Brady- or tachydysrhythmias
- Pericardial tamponade

Distributive shock ('vasodilated shock')
- Sepsis
- SIRS: postoperative pancreatitis, post-CPB SIRS
- Acute adrenal insufficiency
- Anaphylaxis
- Thiamine deficiency

Obstructive shock
- Obstruction to venous return
  - Pericardial tamponade, $\uparrow$intrathoracic pressure (tension pneumothorax, $\uparrow P_{aw}$, $\uparrow$PEEP)
  - IVC obstruction ($\uparrow$intra-abdominal pressure), prone positioning, tumours, thrombus, pregnancy
- Obstruction to cardiac ejection (LV or RV)
  - Massive PE (blood, tumour, air, amniotic)
  - Dynamic RV or LV obstruction (HOCM, tetralogy of Fallot physiology)

Spinal shock
- Anatomical or anaesthetic (spinal/epidural anaesthesia)
  - Vasodilatation below the cord lesion
  - Cardiac depression (lesions above T4)

Miscellaneous causes
- Metabolic: thyroid storm, severe myxoedema, phaeochromocytoma, poisons (CO, CN)

Mixed
- Combination of above

CPB = cardiopulmonary bypass; PEEP = positive end-expiratory pressure; HOCM = hypertrophic obstructive cardiomyopathy; AS = aortic stenosis; PHT = pulmonary hypertension, HPV = hypoxic pulmonary vasoconstriction; PE = pulmonary embolus; P_{aw} = airway pressure; IVC = inferior vena cava; ARDS = adult respiratory distress syndrome; SAM = systolic anterior motion of the mitral valve; SIRS = systemic inflammatory response syndrome; CO = carbon monoxide; CN = cyanide; IABP = intra-aortic balloon pump.

patients; the primary findings seen on echocardiography are summarised in Table 1.3. However, it is crucial to note that the diagnosis of postoperative tamponade remains a clinical diagnosis, and a negative TOE may at times be misleading.

Postcardiotomy cardiogenic shock

Transient myocardial depression following cardiotomy is frequently observed due to post cardiopulmonary bypass stunning, often multifactorial, and is confounded by

Table 1.2 Haemodynamic monitoring in the presence of tricuspid regurgitation

Central venous pressure
Mixed venous saturation (Svo_2)
Doppler
- TOE, conventional TTE, handheld TTE
- Transoesophageal Doppler (CardiacQ)
Fick method
- Oxygen:
  - Estimate O_2 consumption
  - Indirect calorimetry
- Carbon dioxide:
  - Partial CO_2 rebreathing (NICO)
Dilution
Lithium chloride (LiDCO)
Pulse contour analysis
Bioimpedance

TOE = transoesophageal echocardiography; TTE = transthoracic echocardiography.

Table 1.3 Summary of echocardiographic findings in hypotension

Category	EF	EDA
Hypovolaemic shock	↑	↓
Myocardial ischaemia/infarct	↓	n or
Obstructive shock		
Tamponade	n or	↓
Distributive shock (e.g. sepsis)		
Classic high-output septic shock	n or	n or ↓
'Cold' sepsis	↓	n or
Neurogenic shock		
High (above T4)	n or ↓	n or ↓
Low (below T4)	n or	↓

EF = ejection fraction; EDA = end-diastolic area; n = normal.

hypothermia, metabolic derangements, hypovolaemia and/or end-organ failure (see Table 1.1).[14] Management involves making a prompt, early diagnosis, and treating the underlying cause/causes. Other options will include manipulating inotropic and vasopressor agents, fluid and transfusion therapy, optimising the rate, conduction, rhythm and method of pacing (single ventricle vs biventricular), correcting metabolic abnormalities and the use of mechanical assist technologies. Although much has been written about the benefits and disadvantages of the various inotropic agents, the physiological approach in most patients involves increasing myocardial cAMP levels by stimulation of the beta-receptor complex and by inhibiting phosphodiesterase

III. This can be achieved with many different combinations of agents. These physiological manipulations, however, increase myocardial oxygen consumption and may potentially lead to ischaemia. Levosimendan, a calcium-sensitising agent and inodilator, represents a new class of agents that improve left ventricular systolic function while decreasing myocardial oxygen extraction, thus improving myocardial efficiency.[15] However, no large-scale trial has been conducted in postsurgical cardiac patients. In fact, no outcome studies suggest one combination of inotropic drugs being superior to another. Despite the considerable progress in the areas of surgical and anaesthetic techniques, cardiopulmonary bypass and myocardial protection, about 2–6% of postcardiotomy patients require aggressive therapy for severe low cardiac output syndromes.[16] New treatment modalities exist to manage challenging clinical scenarios, such as left ventricular diastolic dysfunction, right heart failure and pulmonary hypertension.

Left ventricular diastolic dysfunction

The diagnosis of diastolic dysfunction is made on the basis of a normal ejection fraction and evidence of abnormal left ventricular relaxation, filling, diastolic distensibility or diastolic stiffness.[17] Patients with ischaemia or left ventricular hypertrophy secondary to valvular or hypertensive disease are particularly at risk.[18] The diagnosis is made by having a low cardiac output state in the face of a normal ejection fraction, absence of pericardial, valvular or conduction problems and a TOE that demonstrates abnormal ventricular relaxation and restrictive filling patterns.[19] The data derived from a pulmonary artery catheter can be very misleading.[20] The development of atrial fibrillation (AF) is particularly detrimental, as these patients are very dependent on the atrial component of ventricular filling; atrial fibrillation may result in acute pulmonary oedema, hypotension and cardiogenic shock. The treatment strategies for diastolic dysfunction include maintaining sinus rhythm, rate control and/or cardioversion of rapid AF. Occasionally, the epicardial pacing can be optimised to achieve (1) mechanical atrial and ventricular synchrony and (2) optimal diastolic filling, which may involve pacing with a short PR interval, as this allows adequate time for passive filling, followed by an atrial contraction. Lusitropy can be enhanced by administration of drugs such as phosphodiesterase III inhibitors. There are now some emerging data that natriuretic peptides may have positive lusitropic actions, but their role in postcardiotomy diastolic dysfunction is not well established. Pre-existing systemic hypotension requires the careful titration of volume resuscitation and alpha-agonistic drugs to counteract a potential further decrease in systemic vascular resistance.

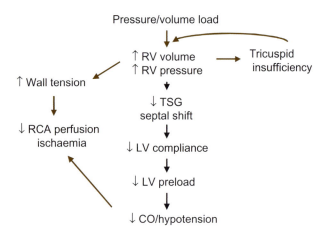

Figure 1.1
Ventricular interdependence. Adapted from Reference 17.

Right ventricular failure

Failure of the right ventricle is either the result of ischaemic failure (right coronary artery (RCA) ischaemia, poor preservation), failure secondary to increased pulmonary artery (PA) pressures or a combination of the two causes. The physiology of right ventricle (RV) failure is complex, and is summarised in Figure 1.1.[21]

The management of RV failure should follow the principles demonstrated in Table 1.4. It is crucial to note that many of the inotropic agents that are deemed favourable for RV contractility and pulmonary vascular resistance (PVR), may have their beneficial effects offset by systemic vasodilation. As the RCA blood flow is very dependent on systemic aortic pressure, this can lead to RV ischemia (Figure 1.1). Therefore, systemic vasopressors such as phenylephrine or norepinephrine are often used in combination with dobutamine or a phosphodiesterase inhibitor to offset the effect on RCA blood flow. However, they may in fact increase the PVR, and therefore the net effect on RV output may be limited. These problems have been largely overcome by the experience with vasopressin and the use of selective PA vasodilators. Vasopressin has been shown in animal models to cause little or no pulmonary artery vasoconstriction, and in fact may cause a slight decrease in PVR. It may therefore be a more prudent choice of vasopressor to sustain systemic vascular tone in the presence of RV dysfunction.

The selective inhaled PA vasodilators commonly used nowadays include inhaled prostaglandins (prostacyclin by continuous nebulisation or intermittently as inhaled iloprost). These agents have been shown to be as effective as inhaled NO, and do not have the toxicity and prohibitive cost associated with inhaled NO. Even though NO is a generic compound that has been used for years, the inhalational use of this agent has become prohibitively expensive.[22]

Table 1.4 Principles of managing RV dysfunction

Optimise rate/ and rhythm
- Maintain ↑ HR (↓ TR), SR, AV pacing, optimise AV interval

Optimise RV preload
- High CVP is detrimental (↑ TR)
- Low CVP is also deleterious

↑ RV contractility
- 'RV' inotropes (those that ↓ PVR)
- Maintain RCA blood flow

↓ RV afterload
- Ventilation strategies
  - High $F_{I}O_{2}$ (↓ hypoxic pulmonary vasoconstriction)
  - Treatment of acidosis, hypercarbia
  - Minimise peak inspiratory pressure
- ↓ Alveolar oedema
  - Recruitment manoeuvres, optimal PEEP, diuretics, appropriate fluid management
- Optimise LV functioning (and thereby ↓ PA pressures)
- Inotropes, IABP, diuretics
- ↓ PA vasoconstrictor agents
- Blood products, protamine, α-agonists
- Selective PA vasodilators

Mechanical assist devices

Patients with refractory low cardiac output syndromes, persistent cardiogenic shock and acute mitral regurgitation should be identified early by the multidisciplinary care team and earmarked for implementation of cardiovascular support in the form of mechanical assist devices. Although, a persistent cardiac index of <2.0 L/min/m² typically is regarded as the lower cut-off limit, the practitioner should be guided specifically by clinical symptoms and signs of decreased tissue perfusion.

Intra-aortic balloon pump (IABP) counterpulsation increases myocardial function by improving coronary perfusion and by decreasing left ventricular afterload. Preoperative insertion of an IABP in selected high-risk patients seems to be beneficial,[23,24] although it is debatable whether a modest rise in cardiac output by maximally 20% will translate into decreased postoperative short- and long-term mortality. As the IABP also increases right coronary perfusion, and thus right ventricular function, it is speculated that it may also be useful in right ventricular failure and help to balance the complex ventricular interactions.[25,26] However, this clinical benefit remains largely unproven, as afterload-reducing effects are diminished by the increased myocardial oxygen demand of ongoing inotropic support.

In contrast to IAPB, a ventricular assist device (VAD) provides complete unloading of the ventricle with a decrease in inotropic support and myocardial oxygen consumption while improving end-organ recovery, including reversal of a stunned myocardium. It can serve as destination therapy or bridge to heart transplant. It is crucial to identify early the cases of severe, refractory postcardiotomy cardiac dysfunction, so that earlier use of a VAD can prevent the cycle of low perfusion and multiple organ system dysfunction. A detailed discussion of VAD is beyond the scope of this chapter.

Postcardiotomy vasodilatory shock

Approximately 10% of patients experience severe vasodilation after cardiopulmonary bypass (CPB), which usually responds to traditional vasopressor agents. However, many patients, especially those on vasodilators (including angiotensin-converting enzyme inhibitors and angiotensin receptor blockers, phosphodiesterase inhibitors and others), those with other causes of severe vasodilation (Table 1.1), or after heart transplantation and VAD insertion, can remain refractory to high doses of norepinephrine.

Role of vasopressin

Arginine vasopressin is an endogenous peptide hormone with antidiuretic, haemostatic and vasoconstrictive effects via V_1 and V_2 receptors. It was first shown that vasopressin levels are inappropriately low in patients with septic shock,[27] and that the administration of VP reduced catecholamine vasopressor requirements. There appears to be a relative vasopressin deficiency in these patients. Similarly, there is now ample evidence that vasopressin is a very effective pressor after CPB, and that the response is independent of plasma levels in those patients with postcardiotomy systemic inflammatory response syndrome shock.[28,29] Vasopressin causes arterial smooth muscle cell contraction through a non-catecholamine receptor pathway, reduces catecholamine requirements, results in a lower heart rate than when catecholamine infusions are used alone and causes less vasoconstriction of the pulmonary vascular bed. This makes it a potentially useful agent in vasodilated patients who have increased pulmonary vascular resistance and right heart dysfunction. Low-dose (<0.04 U/min) vasopressin is now commonly used in the treatment of vasodilatory shock, although no randomised clinical trials support vasopressin as a first-line agent.[30] However, the future role and safety of vasopressin has to be clarified, as it can have a deleterious effect on the thrombocyte count and splanchnic perfusion.[31] Its role needs to be defined in a prospective, randomised trial of patients with refractory vasodilatory states, ideally addressing vasodilatory postcardiotomy shock, shock from systemic inflammatory response syndrome and hyperdynamic vasodilatory septic shock as distinct entities.[32]

The benefit of vasopressin in cardiac arrest is controversial. There has been some suggestion that the rates of successful resuscitation in out-of-hospital cardiac arrest are better with vasopressin than with epinephrine, and the American Heart Association and the European Resuscitation Council have recommended that vasopressin could be used as an alternative to epinephrine for the treatment of adult cardiac arrest. However, a recent systemic review and meta-analysis shows no clear benefit of vasopressin over epinephrine .[33]

Postoperative arrhythmias

Atrial arrhythmias remain a common problem, with an incidence of atrial fibrillation of between 10% and 65%, usually on the second or third postoperative day.[34] Risk factors identified by univariant and multivariant logistic regression analysis are summarised in Table 1.5,[35–41] but are mainly obtained from CABG patients as opposed to cardiac valvular patients.

Postoperative AF is associated with increased hospital length of stay (LOS), incidence of infection, stroke, cognitive and renal dysfunction, ventricular arrhythmias and indication for permanent pacemaker insertion, with even higher rates following recurrent AF as opposed to a single episode.[37]

There are currently no consensus guidelines for the primary prevention of AF that are *specific* to cardiac surgery patients. Digoxin, despite widespread use, and procainamide and verapamil have not been proven to reduce the incidence of postoperative AF[42] and may even be proarrhythmic.[43] Recently, a risk prediction model was validated in a large multicentre cohort of over 4000 patients.[37] With a multitude of risk factors, no specific single strategy has proven to be superior, and prevention of postoperative AF most probably involves a multidimensional approach with expert opinion favouring preoperative beta-blockade, which should be recommended as soon as the patient is haemodynamically stable in the postoperative period. Although prophylactic preoperative use of amiodarone[44,45] has led to a reduction in postoperative AF,[46,47] the *routine* use of postoperative *intravenous* amiodarone is not justified because of high cost and associated toxicities, including its proarrhythmic effects and potential for acute pulmonary and hepatic toxicity;[48] it should be reserved for patients with contraindications to beta-blockade. Prophylactic single-chamber and biatrial overdrive atrial pacing to prevent postoperative AF requires further investigation. With regards to the treatment of postoperative AF, the Consensus Practice Guidelines from the American College

Table 1.5 Risk factors for the development of postoperative atrial fibrillation[31–36]

Preoperative risk factors
Advanced age*
Caucasian
History of congestive heart failure
History of paroxysmal AF
History of chronic obstructive pulmonary disease
History of cardiac surgery
History of cerebrovascular accident
History of smoking
Mitral stenosis*
Angina
Chronic renal failure
Hypertension
Myocardial infarction
Pericarditis
Peripheral vascular disease
Proximal aortic arteriosclerosis
Preoperative use of digoxin
No preoperative beta-blockers
Withdrawal of ACE inhibitor
Withdrawal of beta-blocker therapy
Preoperative use of inotropes
Presence of supraventricular tachycardia
P-wave duration >110 ms
Increased P-wave dispersion
>300 supraventricular beats on preoperative 24 h ECG
Left atrial enlargement*
Left ventricular hypertrophy
Decreased LVEF
Increased LVEDP
Increased BNP

Surgical factors
Bicaval venous cannulation
Use of systemic hypothermia
Use of a warm blood cardioplegic solution and normothermia
Prolonged aortic cross-clamp time
Valve surgery
Increased cardiopulmonary bypass time
Left ventricular apical venting
Pulmonary venting

Postoperative factors
Postoperative administration of inotropic agents
Postoperative prolonged assisted ventilation
Postoperative acidosis
Postoperative atrial or atrioventricular pacing
Postoperative electrolyte imbalance
Postoperative low cardiac output

ACE = angiotensin-converting enzyme; AF = atrial fibrillation; ECG = electrocardiogram; LVEDP = left ventricular end-diastolic pressure; LVEF = left ventricular ejection fraction; BNP = brain natriuretic peptide.
Adapted and modified from Reference 37.

of Cardiology, the American Heart Association and the European Society of Cardiology again recommend the use of beta-blockers.[49] Intravenous amiodarone is favoured in haemodynamic compromise, when even the use of ultra-short-acting beta-blockers such as esmolol is undesirable.

Most recent evidence supports the concept of *heart rate* control in AF, rather than *rhythm* control.[50,51] Immediate electrical cardioversion is still indicated whenever haemodynamic instability is present (Figure 1.2). All patients with atrial fibrillation persisting for more than 24–48 hours are at increased risk for embolic events, and should receive anticoagulation, unless contraindicated.

Left atrial (LA) appendage thrombus should be excluded with TOE before *elective* cardioversion is used. However, anticoagulation is recommended for 3–4 weeks before and after cardioversion for patients with AF of unknown duration or with AF for more than 48 hours.[52] There is no solid clinical evidence that cardioversion followed by prolonged maintenance of sinus rhythm effectively reduces thromboembolism in AF patients. It is thus unclear at present whether efforts to restore and maintain sinus rhythm are justified for the specific purpose of preventing stroke. Recovery of mechanical function may be delayed for several weeks. This could explain why some patients with no demonstrable LA thrombus on TOE before cardioversion subsequently experience thromboembolic events. Presumably, thrombus forms during the period of stunning and is expelled after the return of mechanical function.[52]

Cardiac valvular surgical patients are at higher risk of developing significant bradyarrhythmias that may require temporary pacing. Sustained ventricular tachycardia and ventricular fibrillation are rare in patients after cardiac surgery and are associated with increased mortality.[53] Prophylactic suppression of non-sustained ventricular arrhythmias after cardiac surgery with lidocaine does not improve outcome. A detailed discussion of ventricular arrhythmias is beyond the scope of this section.

Sepsis

The true incidence of severe sepsis in the cardiothoracic intensive care unit (ICU) is unknown, but is probably less than the reported 10 ± 4% in general ITU.[54] It is an important cause of death in ITU patients, and the management remains a major challenge to the healthcare provider. Expeditious and goal-directed care improves the outcomes in treatment of these patients.[55,56]

Antibiotics and source control

Gram-positive bacteria and fungal organisms are now recognised as increasingly common causes of sepsis.[57]

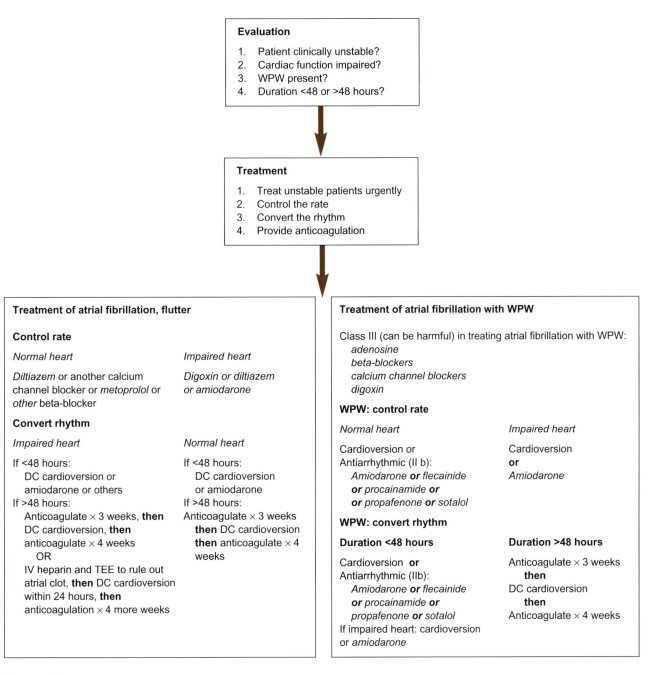

Figure 1.2
Treatment of atrial fibrillation and atrial fibrillation with Wolff–Parkinson–White (WPW) syndrome. Modified from ACLS.

Obvious sources of infection, such as vascular access catheters, should be drained or removed as soon as possible. Two or more blood cultures should be obtained peripherally, preferably before appropriate antibiotic administration,[58] complemented by cultures from other body fluids based on the clinical scenario. The benefits of imaging studies to search for a source of the infection should be weighed against the risk of transporting an unstable patient, exposure to potential nephrotoxic con-trast medium and interruption of other therapies. Delays in diagnosis and in instituting suitable, broad-spectrum antimicrobial coverage increases mortality,[59] whereas appropriate choice and dose of broad-spectrum antibi-otics, including loading doses where appropriate, can reduce the hospital mortality by 50%.[60] A quality assurance process should be in place to track antibiotic administra-tion in sepsis, and 100% of antibiotic doses should be administered within 60 minutes of the diagnosis of sepsis.[56]

The actual choice of antibiotics will be dictated by the clinical scenario, as well as unit- and/or hospital-specific antibiograms. Vancomycin has been demonstrated to improve survival in patients with severe sepsis or septic shock and an unidentified organism.[61] Combination antimicrobial therapy for *Pseudomonas* remains controversial.[62,63] Neutropenic patients should receive broad-spectrum antibiotics for the entire course of their neutropenia. Immune-compromised patients are at risk for atypical infections, including viral, fungal, mycobacterial and parasitic infections. In these patients, a careful search for these microorganisms must be conducted, and early, broad-spectrum therapy may have to be started while awaiting the results of specialised cultures, polymerase chain reaction (PCR) and serology.

The duration of antibiotic coverage remains controversial, but should be directed by clinical data and microbiology. The general aim is to narrow the coverage[57] as soon as possible so as to limit to the appearance of drug-resistant organisms and other antibiotic-associated complications (fungal superinfections[64] and *Clostridium difficile* colitis). In patients with ventilator-associated pneumonia (the commonest ITU infection), 8 days of therapy was as effective as 15 days of antibiotic treatment (with the possible exception of non-fermenting, Gram-negative bacillus infections),[65] and this resulted in a reduction of multi-resistant pathogens.

Early goal-directed therapy

The early, good, resuscitation of septic patients (so called 'goal-directed therapy in sepsis') improves 28-day mortality, and includes optimum fluid therapy, blood transfusion when required and use of invasive monitoring.[66] Invasive therapy includes central venous pressure (CVP) monitoring, monitoring superior vena cava saturation with an oximetric CVP catheter (instead of mixed venous saturation monitoring, which would have required a PA catheter) and manipulating fluids, inotropes and transfusion therapy to keep the superior vena cava saturation >70%.

Use of vasopressors and inotropic drugs

Initiation of vasopressor therapy is indicated for refractory hypotension despite an acceptable fluid challenge or for life-threatening hypotension, even when hypovolaemia has not yet been fully corrected. Although norepinephrine or dopamine have been advocated as first-line choice, replacement dose of vasopressin (0.01–0.04 U/min) or terlipressin can restore vascular tone, as vasopressin defiance con-tributes to refractory shock associated with sepsis (and refractory cardiogenic shock).[30,67–70] Although vasopressin consistently results in a higher mean arterial pressure and a reduction in other vasopressor use in sepsis, its effect on mortality is not known, and it should not be used as a first-line agent at this stage. This is particularly concerning as some patients with sepsis have a reduced cardiac output (cold sepsis), and vasopressin would be deleterious in these situations, as inotropic therapy would be required. Vaso-pressin should therefore not be used in septic patients without cardiac output monitoring. Cardiac output should be normalised (as evidenced by lack of acidosis and normal venous oxygen tension), and not increased to some prede-fined, elevated level, as two large prospective trials failed to demonstrate benefit from increasing oxygen delivery to supranormal levels.[71,72] There are no outcome studies comparing different inotropes in sepsis. The largest experience in treating sepsis has been with the use of dobutamine, although the use of phosphodiesterase inhibitors has also been described.[56] Epinephrine has been postulated to increase the lactic acidosis associated with sepsis, and to possibly reduce tissue perfusion.

Activated protein C

The current understanding of the pathophysiology of sepsis encompasses a triad of inflammation, coagulopathy and reduced fibrinolysis, leading to microvascular thrombosis and end-organ dysfunction[73] with activation of protein C playing a key modulatory role (Figure 1.3).[74] In contrast to two other anticoagulants (antithrombin III and tissue factor-pathway inhibitor), which failed as treatments of sepsis in large, well-designed studies,[75,76] administration of recombinant human activated protein C (APC) in patients with severe sepsis resulted in a 19.4% reduction in the relative risk of death and an absolute risk reduction of 6.1%.[77] Currently, the use of APC is restricted in many hospitals to patients who meet the criteria for severe sepsis specified by the Acute Physiology and Chronic Health Evaluation scoring system (APACHE II Score >25): i.e. those who have severe organ dysfunction and the highest likelihood of death. In contrast, a Food and Drug Administration (FDA) required phase 3B study addressing the issue of the role of APC in less severe sepsis was discontinued after enrolling only 25% of the 11 000 patients based on ineffectiveness. A major risk is haemorrhage:[77–79] 3.5% of patients had serious bleeding (intracranial haemorrhage, a life-threatening bleeding episode or a requirement for 3 or more units of blood), as compared with 2% of patients who received placebo ($p < 0.06$). With open-label use of APC after the trial, 2.5% had intracranial haemorrhage. Caution is advised when using APC in patients with an international normalised ratio (INR) >3.0 or a platelet count of less than

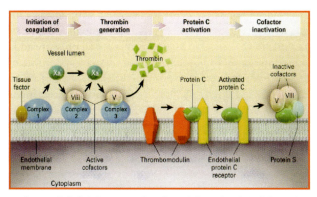

Sepsis → endothelial damage → thrombomodulin and endothelial protein C receptor becomes soluble → protein C cannot be activated

Properties of activated protein C
Inactivates factors Va and VIIIa
Prevents the generation of thrombin
Decreases inflammation by inhibiting platelet activation, neutrophil recruitment and mast-cell degranulation
Direct anti-inflammatory properties, including blocking of the production of cytokines by monocytes and blocking cell adhesion
Modulates the abnormal fibrinolytic response during severe sepsis

Figure 1.3
Activation of protein C and its normal function. Modified, with permission, from Reference 74.

30 000/mm³. The actual role of APC in severe sepsis remains an area of debate in the sepsis community, with many valid criticisms having been raised about the design and conduct (and early termination) of the trial that led to the approval of the agent.

Corticosteroids

In contrast to worsening outcome with the administration of high doses of corticosteroids in the late 1990s, a decrease of mortality in patients with septic shock with relative adrenal insuffiency is noted with the administration of low doses.[80] This group is identified by a cortisol response of 9 μg/dl or less to a 250 μg corticotrophin (ACTH) stimulation test. In these 'non-responders' with relative adrenal insufficiency, low-dose hydrocortisone (100 mg IV 6-hourly) together with enteral fludrocortisone (50 μg/day) for 7 days, led to an absolute risk reduction in mortality of 10% in septic shock.[81] However, there has been valid design and methodological criticism of this study, and validation of the results is needed. In addition, this and all earlier studies of cortisol levels in sepsis measured total cortisol level. Although total serum glucocorticoid response is low in critically ill patients with hypoproteinaemic states, concentration of the bioactive, 'free' cortisol may be normal.[82] In 35% of ITU patients, total cortisol is low, but free corti-

sol is normal. It is therefore conceivable that the results of many of the studies that have relied on total cortisol levels are invalid. Free cortisol levels are currently not routinely available. Thus, until free cortisol concentrations become available and are validated in critically ill patients, care should be taken not to overdiagnose relative adrenal insufficiency in ITU and not to prescribe glucocorticoid therapy, especially for those patients with hypoproteinaemia.

Respiratory failure

Lung protective ventilation strategies

Lung protective ventilatory strategies for adult respiratory distress syndrome (ARDS) reduce morbidity and mortality by utilising lower tidal volumes, lower airway pressures, permissive hypercarbia and optimising positive end-expiratory pressure (PEEP). Although results were inconsistent in several outcome studies,[83–85] a large multicentre, randomised trial by the ARDS Network on reduced tidal volumes in ARDS, demonstrated a 9% decrease in all-cause mortality.[86] A reduction in tidal volumes over 1 to 2 hours to a low tidal volume (6 ml/kg lean body weight) should be implemented (as opposed to 12 ml/kg) while aiming to maintain end-inspiratory plateau pressures at <30 cmH₂O.[87] It is crucial to use lean body mass, and not total body mass, when calculating tidal volume. These volume–pressure goals may need to be modified, based on patients' thoracoabdominal compliance. However, of note is that a recent Cochrane review concluded that there is no significant difference in outcome between small and conventional tidal volume ventilation if plateau pressure is ≤31 cmH₂O.[88]

To allow for lower tidal volumes and pressures, permissive hypercarbia can be used. It is generally well-tolerated in patients with acute lung injury (ALI)/ARDS.[89–91] Although no upper limit for $P_a\mathrm{CO_2}$ has been established, authorities recommend to maintain a pH at >7.20–7.25, which can be achieved by a slow infusion of sodium bicarbonate. Pre-existing metabolic acidosis limits the use of permissive hypercarbia. Raised intracranial pressure and severe pulmonary hypertension are contraindications to its use.[92]

Minimum goals of oxygen therapy include maintaining a $P_a\mathrm{O_2}$ of >58–60 mmHg or an oxygen saturation of 90. Higher PEEP level improves oxygenation, which in turn allows recruitment of lung units. It is prudent to try to minimise potentially toxic levels of oxygen ($F_i\mathrm{O_2}$ <0.60), although the deleterious effect of prolonged, increased inhaled oxygen concentration on adult lungs is not well-established.

The level of PEEP does not affect outcome in ARDS patients. In a large multicentre trial in patients with ALI/ARDS, if low tidal volumes were used and the plateau pressure was limited to 30 cmH$_2$O, the level of PEEP did not affect outcome.[93] An acceptable approach is therefore to set a minimum amount of PEEP based on severity of oxygenation deficit and to prevent atelectasis.

Prone ventilation

The role of the prone position in treating refractory hypoxaemia remains controversial. Although it temporarily improves gas exchange,[94] reduction in mortality is not clear, and may occur only in the most severe cases of hypoxaemia.[95–97] Prone positioning requires considerable expertise and equipment and may have potential life-threatening consequences such as obstruction of the endotracheal tube, main stem intubation, dislodgement of the central venous catheters, haemodynamic instability and pressure necrosis of the skin. The risks and benefits of prone ventilation in patients requiring potentially injurious levels of F_iO_2 or plateau pressures should be carefully balanced, particularly in light of other 'salvage' methods to improve refractory hypoxaemia, e.g. selective pulmonary artery vasodilators (see below).

High-frequency oscillatory ventilation

Some studies have suggested that high-frequency oscillatory ventilation (HFOV) may improve oxygenation[98] when used as rescue therapy after proven lung protective strategies have failed, especially when combined with inhaled nitric oxide.[99] However, it does not improve mortality rates.[100] HFOV does, however, appear to be safe in adults with ARDS/ALI who have failed conventional methods of mechanical ventilation.

Extracorporeal membrane oxygenation

Several case reports describe successful outcomes in patients where extracorporeal membrane oxygenation (ECMO) was used as salvage therapy.[101] It is only likely to be successful in those patients where the underlying pulmonary injury is acutely reversible, e.g. in some reperfusion injuries after lung transplantation and in some inflammatory conditions that may acutely respond to immune therapy. Improved mortality rates have been reported with ECMO since the introduction of heparin-coated circuits, the use of centrifugal as opposed to roller pumps and a better understanding of anticoagulation management (including monitoring for heparin levels and activity, regular measurements of anti-Xa and antithrombin III levels). However, there has been no published randomised clinical trial comparing current ventilatory strategies of ARDS with that of ECMO.

Early versus late tracheostomy

The optimum timing to perform tracheostomy in ITU is controversial, and remains largely institution-specific. However, there is increasing evidence that early tracheostomy may reduce the time on mechanical ventilation and ITU resource utilisation.[102,103] Early tracheostomy may also reduce the risks associated with failed extubation, which has been shown to be associated with adverse outcome.[104] The complication rates of percutaneous versus open tracheostomy, and operating room (OR)- or ITU-based procedures, are comparable, although overall resource use is less with ITU-based procedures. The choice of type and location of the tracheostomy should therefore depend on factors such as operator preference, neck anatomy and institutional logistics. It is uncertain, however, whether tracheostomy increases the risk of deep sternal wound infection, mediastinitis and mortality in open heart surgical patients[105] as several epidemiological studies of mediastinitis have failed to demonstrate an association between mediastinitis and tracheostomy.[106–109]

Non-invasive mechanical ventilation

Non-invasive mechanical ventilation has been enthusiastically received in the last decade, and has been increasingly used in acute respiratory failure. The exact role of non-invasive ventilation is continuing to evolve. It has been shown to reduce the need for intubation in some patient populations. However, its use is not without danger. In a recent multicentre study, 221 patients were randomly assigned to either non-invasive ventilation or standard medical therapy after failed extubation. The trial was stopped early after an interim analysis showed that there was no difference between the non-invasive ventilation group and the standard therapy group in the need for reintubation, but that the mortality was higher in the non-invasive group (25% vs 14%, relative risk = 1.78; 95% CI 1.03–3.20; $p = 0.048$).[110] In another recent observational study, delayed intubation after a period of non-invasive ventilation was also associated with an increased mortality

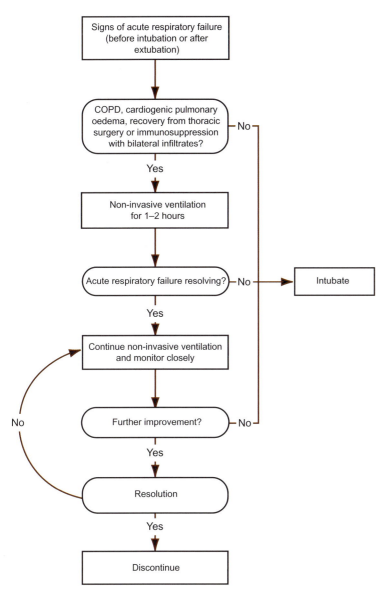

Figure 1.4
Suggested use of non-invasive ventilation in ITU. Modified, with permission, from Reference 162.

Role of selective pulmonary arterial vasodilators

The role of selective pulmonary artery vasodilators in hypoxaemic respiratory failure is limited. Inhaled nitric oxide (iNO) temporarily improves oxygenation in patients with ALI/ARDS,[112–116] but does not alter mortality or other clinically relevant end-points (ventilator-free days, ICU stay). Because of its temporary effect on oxygenation, its associated toxicities and prohibitive cost, iNO has little or no role. There are significant problems associated with suppression of endogenous NO production, leading to potentially serious rebound effects if acutely stopped.

There are other selective, inhaled pulmonary artery vasodilators that are as effective as iNO, much cheaper and are devoid of toxicity issues and monitoring. These include inhaled sodium nitroprusside, glyceryl trinitrate, phosphodiesterase V inhibitors, milrinone, prostaglandin E1 (PGE$_1$, alprostadil), prostaglandin I$_2$ (PGI$_2$, prostacyclin) and iloprost (the stable analogue of PGI$_2$).[117] The most experience is with inhaled prostacyclin. In addition to being effective as a treatment of pulmonary hypertension and RV dysfunction, inhaled PGI$_2$ is an effective rescue therapy in the treatment of refractory hypoxaemia.[22,118–120] It improves oxygenation, does not have any systemic vasodilating effects and has no appreciable tolerance after 4–6 hours of administration. Despite a theoretical concern about the potential antiplatelet effects of iPGI$_2$, several studies have now attested to its safety, with no increased risk of bleeding.[22,121] Compared to iNO, it is less expensive, easier to administer (although it needs to be suspended in a glycine diluent and requires a continuous nebulisation), relatively free of side effects and requires no special toxicity monitoring.[22] Inhaled iloprost, a synthetic analogue of prostacyclin which is stable at normal pH and can be given by intermittent nebulisation, is therefore likely to replace the use of inhaled prostacyclin. Although rebound after acute withdrawal of inhaled prostaglandin was thought not to occur, it has been recently described.

rate.[111] The mechanisms of increased mortality are speculative, and include cardiac ischaemia, increased respiratory muscle fatigue, respiratory arrest, aspiration, complications of emergency intubation and factors related to less-effective respiratory parameter monitoring while on non-invasive ventilation. A high level of expertise and vigilance is required when using non-invasive ventilation; nursing a patient with hypoxaemic respiratory failure with non-invasive ventilation usually requires one nurse to one patient. Intubation should be performed expeditiously in those patients who do not respond. A proposed scheme for using non-invasive ventilation is shown in Figure 1.4.

Fluid therapy in the intensive therapy unit

Crystalloid versus colloid controversy

A Cochrane Injuries Group meta-analysis in 1998 noted an overall increase in mortality in patients treated with albumin as opposed to crystalloids, with 1 additional death for every 17 critically ill patients treated. However, a second, larger meta-analysis could not confirm these findings, even suggesting a reduced mortality when assessing only trials of higher methodological quality.[122] In an effort to address this ongoing controversy, a large Australian/New Zealand trial was conducted: the Saline vs Albumin Fluid Evaluation (SAFE) study comparing 4% human albumin solution with 0.9% sodium chloride (saline) in over 7000 critically ill patients showed identical mortality rate, number of organ failures, and ICU LOS in patients receiving albumin or saline.[123] Subgroup analysis revealed that albumin demonstrated a trend towards benefit in patients with severe sepsis and a trend towards harm in trauma patients. Although it was thought that approximately three times more volume of crystalloid is required than colloid, the SAFE study revealed the actual ratio for comparable haemodynamic end-point to be 1.4 to 1.

Adverse effects of fluid therapy

Fluids with a high chloride concentration cause hyperchloraemic, non-anion gap metabolic acidosis, which may impair cellular mechanisms, decrease renal blood flow, gastric motility and perfusion and increase PA pressure[124] and, most importantly, may be confused by the clinician with anion gap acidosis and respiratory acidosis. Impaired ability for compensatory hyperventilation with ensuing severe acidaemia may be observed in patients with compromised respiratory function and in those receiving narcotics, both common situations after cardiac valve surgery.

Crystalloid solutions have been associated with hypercoagulability, whereas non-protein colloids are associated with impaired haemostasis, platelet dysfunction and excessive bleeding.[125–130] Hydroxyethyl starches have been linked to increased bleeding complications and ICU LOS in cardiac surgery.[131] In contrast, albumin has minimal effects on coagulation. Furthermore, 6% hydroxyethyl starch (200 kDa, 0.60–0.66 substitution) administration was associated with higher frequencies of acute renal failure, oliguria and higher serum creatinine concentrations than gelatin administration in patients with severe sepsis or septic shock.[132] Differences are also noted in septic, hypovolaemic patients, with gelatin administration increasing gastric intramucosal pH and hydroxyethyl starches decreasing gastric intramucosal pH.[133]

Fluid administration also affects immunological function: isotonic crystalloids cause immune activation[134] and dextran and Hespan (hydroxyethyl starch) cause neutrophil activation and cellular injury.[135,136] Activation of the immune system has not been demonstrated with fresh frozen plasma and albumin.

The volume of fluids used in ICU patients has also come under increasing scrutiny. Clearly, inadequate fluid therapy is deleterious, but similarly, high volumes of crystalloids may be deleterious. Large amounts of crystalloid impair tissue oxygenation and wound healing,[137] and have been associated with increased death rates from respiratory failure and cardiovascular events.[137,138] In a recent trial of patients undergoing abdominal surgery, a restrictive fluid strategy was associated with significantly less complications and had a trend towards fewer deaths.[139]

Blood transfusion strategies in the intensive care unit

The optimum transfusion trigger in ITU patients remains uncertain, especially in patients with cardiovascular disease and tissue hypoperfusion. Two retrospective studies, one in the perioperative period and one in critically ill patients, showed that severe anaemia was associated with increased mortality in patients with cardiac disease.[140,141] However, the multicentre Canadian Transfusion Requirements in Critical Care (TRICC) trial demonstrated that a restrictive transfusion (transfuse if haemoglobin concentration <7 g/dl) was associated with an improved outcome compared with a liberal transfusion strategy (transfusion trigger <10 g/dl).[142] In the less severely ill patients and in those younger than 55 years old, the restrictive group was half as likely to die within 30 days. A subsequent analysis of TRICC patients with cardiovascular disease concluded that a restrictive strategy is safe in most critically ill patients with cardiovascular disease, with the possible exception of patients with acute coronary syndromes (ACS).[143] In support of this position, in elderly patients with ACS, anaemia was associated with worse outcomes, and transfusion appeared to reduce the mortality.[144] Similarly, several recent studies have shown that patients with congestive cardiac failure and chronic renal failure may benefit from higher haemoglobin levels and possibly from blood transfusions.[145,146] However, this thesis has recently again been challenged by a posthoc analysis of clinical trials of patients with ACS. This report demonstrated that blood transfusion in the setting of ACS may increase mortality.[147] Many clinicians believe that a state of clinical equipoise exists regarding the transfusion threshold in patients with cardiac disease, and that a randomised trial is needed. How these results are to be applied to postoperative cardiac surgery ITU patients is also uncertain. Despite these concerns, many experts endorse the findings of the TRICC trial. However, what is concerning is that, despite the TRICC data, transfusion practice has changed little over the past decade, with the mean pretransfusion haemoglobin concentration still being 8.5 ± 1.5 g/dl.[148] Only 30% of patients had a transfusion trigger of <8 g/dl, and in only 7.5% was the trigger <7 g/dl. Until further evidence is forthcoming, expert opinion suggests a more liberal transfusion in some ITU patients (Table 1.6).

Table 1.6 Conditions that may require a higher haemoglobin level (adapted from Zimmerman[140])

Acute cardiovascular instability?
Cardiovascular disease
- Severe coronary artery disease
- Acute coronary syndromes
- Low cardiac output
Pulmonary disease?
- Severe arterial hypoxaemia
Organ or tissue ischaemia
- Severe mixed venous desaturation
- Elevated lactate level

Why is liberal transfusion not associated with improved outcomes? Either anaemia has beneficial effects and/or transfusion has adverse effects. The adverse effects of transfusion include infections (including known and yet undiscovered agents), haemolytic reactions, contamination, allergic reactions, anaphylaxis, transfusion-related ALI, fluid-overload pulmonary oedema and immune modulation. It is thought that transfused allogeneic leucocytes trigger an immune response, leading to an increased risk of infection, earlier recurrence of malignancy and increased mortality. A significant association between the number of red blood cells (RBCs) transfused and the risk of nosocomial infections has been reported.[149] A recent study showed that the adoption of a leucoreduction pathway potentially decreases mortality, fever episodes and antibiotic use.[150]

Sedation and paralysis

Inappropriate use of sedation and oversedation of ITU patients is common. Intubation and mechanical ventilation does not always require continuous sedative infusion. Each patient's needs have to be individualised, with the treatment spectrum encompassing no psychoactive medications, a nocturnal sleep aide, intermittent patient-requested analgesia or anxiolysis, medication for delirium, to that of continuous sedation and analgesic infusions. Inappropriate use of sedation and paralysis significantly increases morbidity such as critical illness polyneuropathy.[151] Practice guidelines have now been established for the use of sedation and neuromuscular blockade (NMB).[152–154] The sedation guidelines published by the Society of Critical Care Medicine are shown in Figure 1.5. Good ITU practice requires that sedation be minimised and interrupted daily if continuous infusion is required and that neuromuscular blockers be avoided wherever pos-

sible. Sedation and paralysis should be monitored with validated means, such as sedation scales and with the use of train-of-four monitoring.[155–157] Propofol is being increasingly utilised in ITU, and is generally a safe drug when used appropriately. However, the propofol infusion syndrome has been described and consists of cardiac failure, rhabdomyolysis, severe metabolic acidosis and renal failure. It is often fatal, and occurs when high doses (>5 mg/kg/h) are used in critically ill patients for prolonged periods (>48 hours).[158] Sepsis and the use of catecholamine infusions and steroids, may act as a trigger.

The exact role of the highly selective alpha$_2$-adrenoreceptor agonist dexmedetomidine, in ITU sedation has to be established.[159,160] It has novel properties such as anxiolysis, reduced narcotic requirements and minimal effect of the respiratory drive. However, it currently only has approval for use for 24 hours in ITU, limiting its usefulness in many patients.

Glucose control

Insulin therapy in critically ill patients has a beneficial effect on short-term[161] as well as long-term mortality. Aggressive glucose control in mechanically ventilated patients with a target blood glucose level of between 80 and 110 mg/dl (4.4–6.1 mmol/L) resulted in a 3.4% absolute risk reduction in 1-year mortality irrespective of a history of diabetes, with the greatest benefit seen in patients with a 5 day or ICU LOS or multi-organ failure secondary to sepsis. Significant relative risk reduction in the range of 34–50% was seen in in-hospital mortality, bloodstream infections, acute renal failure, critical illness polyneuropathy, prolonged ventilation and ICU LOS. Future studies are needed:

- to determine whether less tight control of blood glucose – e.g. a blood glucose level of 120–160 mg/dl (6.7–8.9 mmol/L) – provides similar benefits
- to define the role of insulin protocols in the prevention of hypoglycaemic events.

Intensivist-led multidisciplinary intensive care unit team

A growing body of evidence supports the intensivist-led, multidisciplinary critical care model:[162,163] high-intensity ICU physician staffing (i.e. mandatory intensivist consultation, or closed ICU – all care directed by intensivist) is associated with reduced ICU and hospital mortality and ICU and hospital LOS compared with a model of

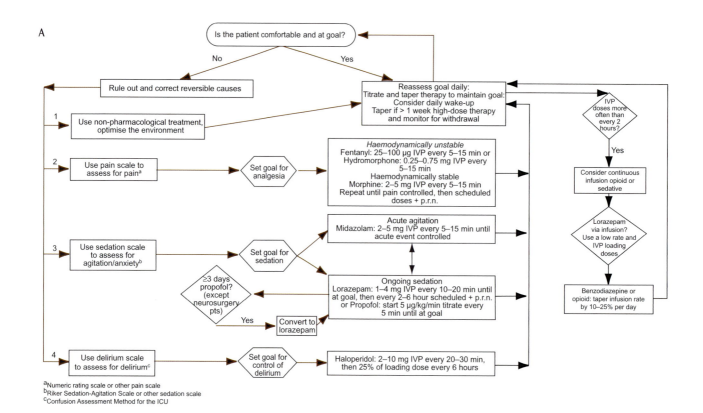

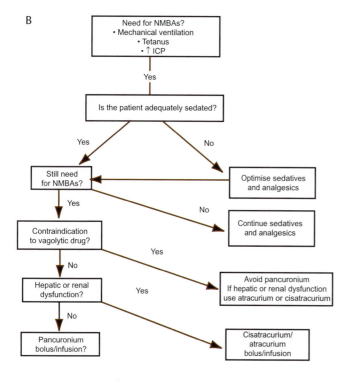

low-intensity ICU physician service (i.e. no intensivist, or elective intensivist consultation only). The implementation of this critical care model, which is widely accepted in Europe, Australia and New Zealand, is estimated to save 162 000 lives annually in the United States. Even under conservative assumptions, a financial analysis demonstrated cost saving for US hospitals. From 2001 to 2003, surveys report a doubling in the number of US hospital ICU staffed by intensivists,[164] as recommended by the Leapfrog Group, a coalition of large US healthcare purchasers, in their publication on the *Intensive Care Unit Physician Staffing standard*.[165]

Summary

Many of the recent advances in the management of critically ill patients apply to current clinical practice. However, simple cost-effective general measures such as maximal sterile barriers during procedures, hand disinfections, early goal-directed resuscitation with appropriate fluids, inotropes and antibiotics and surgical source control of infected foci should still form the basis of clinical practice. High quality of care in the ICU (see Tables 1.7 and 1.8) is a result of a multi-team approach and should be safe, efficient, effective, patient-centred, timely and equitable. Even

Figure 1.5

(A) Sedation and (B) use of neuromuscular blockers practice guidelines of the Society of Critical Care Medicine. Reproduced with permission from References 146 and 147.

Table 1.7 Summary of interventions that reduce mortality in critical care patients. Adapted from Pronovost[162]

Intervention	Mortality without intervention	Absolute risk reduction
Early goal-directed therapy in severe sepsis and septic shock[62]	46.5	16
Low-dose corticosteroids in septic shock and relative adrenal insuffiency[77]	63	10
Low tidal volume ventilation in ARDS[82]	39.8	8.8
Activated protein C in severe sepsis[73]	30.8	6.1
High-intensity vs low-intensity ICU physician staffing[157]	12	4
Intensive insulin therapy to maintain glucose at 80–110 mg/dl[164]	8	3.4
Adequate antimicrobial treatment for infections[57]*	52.1	39.9

* = Denotes observational trial.

Table 1.8 Intensive care unit quality measures

	Outcome measure	RRR	ARR	NNT
Daily interruption of sedation for at least 12 hours or until patient follows commands[151]	Reduction of duration of mechanical ventilation by 2.4 days and ICU LOS by 3.5 days			
Appropriate use of blood transfusions[137]	Reduced 30 day mortality Reduced 60 day mortality	20% 14%	4.6% 3.8%	21 26
Appropriate peptic ulcer prophylaxis[165]	Reduced upper GI haemorrhage	25%	2.1%	47
Head of bed elevation >30º[166]	Reduction in ventilator-associated pneumonia	78%	18%	5.5

RRR = relative risk reduction; ARR = absolute risk reduction; NNT = numbers needed to treat.

with successful translation of evidence-based intensive care practice into daily praxis, challenges such as improvement in global long-term outcome in ICU survivors as measured by health-related quality of life remain ahead.[166]

References

1. Lee TW, Jacobsohn E. Pro: tracheal extubation should occur routinely in the operating room after cardiac surgery. J Cardiothorac Vasc Anesth 2000; 14(5):603–10.
2. Myles PS, Daly DJ, Djaiani G, Lee A, Cheng DC. A systematic review of the safety and effectiveness of fast-track cardiac anesthesia. Anesthesiology 2003; 99(4):982–7.
3. Edwards FH, Peterson ED, Coombs LP, et al. Prediction of operative mortality after valve replacement surgery. J Am Coll Cardiol 2001; 37(3):885–92.
4. Higham H, Sear JW, Sear YM, et al. Peri-operative troponin I concentration as a marker of long-term postoperative adverse cardiac outcomes – a study in high-risk surgical patients. Anaesthesia 2004; 59(4):318–23.
5. Sandham JD, Hull RD, Brant RF, et al. A randomized, controlled trial of the use of pulmonary-artery catheters in high-risk surgical patients. N Engl J Med 2003; 348(1):5–14.
6. Richard C, Warszawski J, Anguel N, et al; French Pulmonary Artery Catheter Study Group. Early use of the pulmonary artery catheter and outcomes in patients with shock and acute respiratory distress syndrome: a randomized controlled trial. JAMA 2003; 290(20):2713–20.
7. Yu DT, Platt R, Lanken PN, et al. Relationship of pulmonary artery catheter use to mortality and resource utilization in patients with severe sepsis. Crit Care Med 2003; 31(12):2734–41.
8. Gnaegi A, Feihl F, Perret C. Intensive care physicians' insufficient knowledge of right-heart catheterization at the bedside: time to act? Crit Care Med 1997; 25(2):213–20.
9. Jacka MJ, Cohen MM, To T, Devitt JH, Byrick R. Pulmonary artery occlusion pressure estimation: how confident are anesthesiologists? Crit Care Med 2002; 30(6):1197–203.

10. Iberti TJ, Fischer EP, Leibowitz AB, et al. A multicenter study of physicians' knowledge of the pulmonary artery catheter. Pulmonary Artery Catheter Study Group. JAMA 1990; 264(22):2928–32.

11. Balik M, Pachl J, Hendl J. Effect of the degree of tricuspid regurgitation on cardiac output measurements by thermodilution. Intensive Care Med 2002; 28(8):1117–21.

12. Heerdt PM, Blessios GA, Beach ML, Hogue CW. Flow dependency of error in thermodilution measurement of cardiac output during acute tricuspid regurgitation. J Cardiothorac Vasc Anesth 2001; 15(2):183–7.

13. Berton C, Cholley B. Equipment review: new techniques for cardiac output measurement – oesophageal Doppler, Fick principle using carbon dioxide, and pulse contour analysis. Crit Care 2002; 6(3):216–21.

14. Goldstein DJ, Oz MC. Mechanical support for postcardiotomy cardiogenic shock. Semin Thorac Cardiovasc Surg 2000; 12(3):220–8.

15. Michaels AD, McKeown B, Kostal M, et al. Effects of intravenous levosimendan on human coronary vasomotor regulation, left ventricular wall stress, and myocardial oxygen uptake. Circulation 2005; 111(12):1504–9.

16. Vigilance DW, Oz MC. Strategies for management of postcardiotomy cardiogenic shock following valvular heart surgery. Adv Cardiol 2004; 41:140–9.

17. Aurigemma GP, Gaasch WH. Clinical practice. Diastolic heart failure. N Engl J Med 2004; 351(11):1097–105.

18. Yamada H, Goh PP, Sun JP, et al. Prevalence of left ventricular diastolic dysfunction by Doppler echocardiography: clinical application of the Canadian consensus guidelines. J Am Soc Echocardiogr 2002; 15(10 Pt 2):1238–44.

19. Garcia MJ, Thomas JD, Klein AL. New Doppler echocardiographic applications for the study of diastolic function. J Am Coll Cardiol 1998; 32(4):865–75.

20. Vinch CS, Aurigemma GP, Hill JC, et al. Usefulness of clinical variables, echocardiography, and levels of brain natriuretic peptide and norepinephrine to distinguish systolic and diastolic causes of acute heart failure. Am J Cardiol 2003; 91(9):1140–3.

21. Wiedemann HP, Matthay RA. Acute right heart failure. Crit Care Clin 1985; 1(3):631–61.

22. De Wet CJ, Affleck DG, Jacobsohn E, et al. Inhaled prostacyclin is safe, effective, and affordable in patients with pulmonary hypertension, right heart dysfunction, and refractory hypoxemia after cardiothoracic surgery. J Thorac Cardiovasc Surg 2004; 127(4):1058–67.

23. Suzuki T, Okabe M, Handa M, Yasuda F, Miyake Y. Usefulness of preoperative intraaortic balloon pump therapy during off-pump coronary artery bypass grafting in high-risk patients. Ann Thorac Surg 2004; 77(6):2056–9; discussion 2059–60.

24. Kang N, Edwards M, Larbalestier R. Preoperative intraaortic balloon pumps in high-risk patients undergoing open heart surgery. Ann Thorac Surg 2001; 72(1):54–7.

25. Nordhaug D, Steensrud T, Muller S, Husnes KV, Myrmel T. Intraaortic balloon pumping improves hemodynamics and right ventricular efficiency in acute ischemic right ventricular failure. Ann Thorac Surg 2004; 78(4):1426–32.

26. Arafa OE, Geiran OR, Andersen K, et al. Intraaortic balloon pumping for predominantly right ventricular failure after heart transplantation. Ann Thorac Surg 2000; 70(5):1587–93.

27. Landry DW, Levin HR, Gallant EM, et al. Vasopressin deficiency contributes to the vasodilation of septic shock. Circulation 1997; 95(5):1122–5.

28. Dunser MW, Hasibeder WR, Wenzel V, et al. Endocrinologic response to vasopressin infusion in advanced vasodilatory shock. Crit Care Med 2004; 32(6):1266–71.

29. Argenziano M, Choudhri AF, Oz MC, et al. A prospective randomized trial of arginine vasopressin in the treatment of vasodilatory shock after left ventricular assist device placement. Circulation 1997; 96(9 Suppl):II-286–90.

30. Dunser MW, Mayr AJ, Ulmer H, et al. Arginine vasopressin in advanced vasodilatory shock: a prospective, randomized, controlled study. Circulation 2003; 107(18):2313–19.

31. Martikainen TJ, Uusaro A, Tenhunen JJ, Ruokonen E. Dobutamine compensates deleterious hemodynamic and metabolic effects of vasopressin in the splanchnic region in endotoxin shock. Acta Anaesthesiol Scand 2004; 48(8):935–43.

32. Westphal M, Bone HG. Are vasodilatory shock states due to sepsis and cardiovascular surgery like two peas in a pod? Crit Care Med 2004; 32(6):1411–12.

33. Aung K, Htay T. Vasopressin for cardiac arrest: a systematic review and meta-analysis. Arch Intern Med 2005; 165(1):17–24.

34. Maisel WH, Rawn JD, Stevenson WG. Atrial fibrillation after cardiac surgery. Ann Intern Med 2001; 135(12):1061–73.

35. Asher CR, Miller DP, Grimm RA, Cosgrove DM 3rd, Chung MK. Analysis of risk factors for development of atrial fibrillation early after cardiac valvular surgery. Am J Cardiol 1998; 82(7):892–5.

36. Amar D, Shi W, Hogue CW Jr, et al. Clinical prediction rule for atrial fibrillation after coronary artery bypass grafting. J Am Coll Cardiol 2004; 44(6):1248–53.

37. Mathew JP, Fontes ML, Tudor IC, et al; Investigators of the Ischemic Research and Education Foundation; Multicenter Study of Perioperative Ischemia Research Group. A multicenter risk index for atrial fibrillation after cardiac surgery. JAMA 2004; 291(14):1720–9.

38. Orlowska-Baranowska E, Baranowski R, Michalek P, et al. Prediction of paroxysmal atrial fibrillation after aortic valve replacement in patients with aortic stenosis: identification of potential risk factors. J Heart Valve Dis 2003; 12(2):136–41.

39. Ducceschi V, D'Andrea A, Galderisi M, et al. Risk predictors of paroxysmal atrial fibrillation following aortic valve replacement. Ital Heart J 2001; 2(7):507–12.

40. Wazni OM, Martin DO, Marrouche NF, et al. Plasma B-type natriuretic peptide levels predict postoperative atrial fibrillation in patients undergoing cardiac surgery. Circulation 2004; 110(2):124–7.

41. DiDomenico RJ, Massad MG. Pharmacologic strategies for prevention of atrial fibrillation after open heart surgery. Ann Thorac Surg 2005; 79(2):728–40.

42. Amar D, Roistacher N, Burt ME, et al. Effects of diltiazem versus digoxin on dysrhythmias and cardiac function after pneumonectomy. Ann Thorac Surg 1997; 63(5):1374–81; discussion 1381–12.

43. Rose MR, Glassman E, Spencer FC. Arrhythmias following cardiac surgery: relation to serum digoxin levels. Am Heart J 1975; 89(3):288–94.

44. Mooss AN, Wurdeman RL, Sugimoto JT, et al. Amiodarone versus sotalol for the treatment of atrial fibrillation after open heart surgery: the Reduction in Postoperative Cardiovascular Arrhythmic Events (REDUCE) trial. Am Heart J 2004; 148(4):641–8.

45. Kerstein J, Soodan A, Qamar M, et al. Giving IV and oral amiodarone perioperatively for the prevention of postoperative atrial fibrillation in patients undergoing coronary artery bypass surgery: the GAP study. Chest 2004; 126(3):716–24.

46. White CM, Giri S, Tsikouris JP, et al. A comparison of two individual amiodarone regimens to placebo in open heart surgery patients. Ann Thorac Surg 2002; 74(1):69–74.

47. Cochrane AD, Siddins M, Rosenfeldt FL, et al. A comparison of amiodarone and digoxin for treatment of supraventricular arrhythmias after cardiac surgery. Eur J Cardiothorac Surg 1994; 8(4):194–8.

48. Camus P, Martin WJ 2nd, Rosenow EC 3rd. Amiodarone pulmonary toxicity. Clin Chest Med 2004; 25(1):65–75.

49. Fuster V, Ryden LE, Asinger RW, et al. ACC/AHA/ESC guidelines for the management of patients with atrial fibrillation. A report of the American College of Cardiology/American Heart Association Task Force on Practice Guidelines and the European Society of Cardiology Committee for Practice Guidelines and Policy Conferences

(Committee to Develop Guidelines for the Management of Patients with Atrial Fibrillation) developed in collaboration with the North American Society of Pacing and Electrophysiology. Eur Heart J 2001; 22(20):1852–923.

50. Wyse DG, Waldo AL, DiMarco JP, et al. A comparison of rate control and rhythm control in patients with atrial fibrillation. N Engl J Med 2002; 347(23):1825–33.

51. Van Gelder IC, Hagens VE, Bosker HA, et al. A comparison of rate control and rhythm control in patients with recurrent persistent atrial fibrillation. N Engl J Med 2002; 347(23):1834–40.

52. Fuster V, Ryden LE, Asinger RW, et al. ACC/AHA/ESC guidelines for the management of patients with atrial fibrillation: executive summary. A Report of the American College of Cardiology/ American Heart Association Task Force on Practice Guidelines and the European Society of Cardiology Committee for Practice Guidelines and Policy Conferences (Committee to Develop Guidelines for the Management of Patients With Atrial Fibrillation): developed in collaboration with the North American Society of Pacing and Electrophysiology. J Am Coll Cardiol 2001; 38(4):1231–66.

53. Yeung-Lai-Wah JA, Qi A, McNeill E, et al. New-onset sustained ventricular tachycardia and fibrillation early after cardiac operations. Ann Thorac Surg 2004; 77(6):2083–8.

54. Linde-Zwirble WT, Angus DC. Severe sepsis epidemiology: sampling, selection, and society. Crit Care 2004; 8(4):222–6.

55. Padkin A, Goldfrad C, Brady AR, et al. Epidemiology of severe sepsis occurring in the first 24 hrs in intensive care units in England, Wales, and Northern Ireland. Crit Care Med 2003; 31(9):2332–8.

56. Dellinger RP, Carlet JM, Masur H, et al. Surviving Sepsis Campaign guidelines for management of severe sepsis and septic shock. Crit Care Med 2004; 32(3):858–73.

57. Martin GS, Mannino DM, Eaton S, Moss M. The epidemiology of sepsis in the United States from 1979 through 2000. N Engl J Med 2003; 348(16):1546–54.

58. O'Grady NP, Barie PS, Bartlett J, Bleck T, Garvey G, Jacobi J, et al. Practice parameters for evaluating new fever in critically ill adult patients. Task Force of the American College of Critical Care Medicine of the Society of Critical Care Medicine in collaboration with the Infectious Disease Society of America. Crit Care Med 1998; 26(2):392–408.

59. Yu DT, Black E, Sands KE, et al. Severe sepsis: variation in resource and therapeutic modality use among academic centers. Crit Care 2003; 7(3):R24–34.

60. Jimenez MF, Marshall JC. Source control in the management of sepsis. Intensive Care Med 2001; 27 (Suppl 1):S49–62.

61. Kollef MH, Sherman G, Ward S, Fraser VJ. Inadequate antimicrobial treatment of infections: a risk factor for hospital mortality among critically ill patients. Chest 1999; 115(2):462–74.

62. Safdar N, Handelsman J, Maki DG. Does combination antimicrobial therapy reduce mortality in Gram-negative bacteraemia? A meta-analysis. Lancet Infect Dis 2004; 4(8):519–27.

63. Paul M, Benuri-Silbiger I, Soares-Weiser K, Leibovici L. Beta lactam monotherapy versus beta lactam-aminoglycoside combination therapy for sepsis in immunocompetent patients: systematic review and meta-analysis of randomised trials. BMJ 2004; 328(7441):668.

64. Michalopoulos AS, Geroulanos S, Mentzelopoulos SD. Determinants of candidemia and candidemia-related death in cardiothoracic ICU patients. Chest 2003; 124(6):2244–55.

65. Chastre J, Wolff M, Fagon JY, et al. Comparison of 8 vs 15 days of antibiotic therapy for ventilator-associated pneumonia in adults: a randomized trial. JAMA 2003; 290(19):2588–98.

66. Rivers E, Nguyen B, Havstad S, et al. Early goal-directed therapy in the treatment of severe sepsis and septic shock. N Engl J Med 2001; 345(19):1368–77.

67. Kam PC, Williams S, Yoong FF. Vasopressin and terlipressin: pharmacology and its clinical relevance. Anaesthesia 2004; 59(10): 993–1001.

68. Dunser MW, Mayr AJ, Ulmer H, et al. The effects of vasopressin on systemic hemodynamics in catecholamine-resistant septic and post-cardiotomy shock: a retrospective analysis. Anesth Analg 2001; 93(1):7–13.

69. Argenziano M, Chen JM, Choudhri AF, et al. Management of vasodilatory shock after cardiac surgery: identification of predisposing factors and use of a novel pressor agent. J Thorac Cardiovasc Surg 1998; 116(6):973–80.

70. Dunser MW, Mayr AJ, Stallinger A, et al. Cardiac performance during vasopressin infusion in postcardiotomy shock. Intensive Care Med 2002; 28(6):746–51.

71. Gattinoni L, Brazzi L, Pelosi P, et al. A trial of goal-oriented hemodynamic therapy in critically ill patients. SvO$_2$ Collaborative Group. N Engl J Med 1995; 333(16):1025–32.

72. Hayes MA, Timmins AC, Yau EH, et al. Elevation of systemic oxygen delivery in the treatment of critically ill patients. N Engl J Med 1994; 330(24):1717–22.

73. Hotchkiss RS, Karl IE. The pathophysiology and treatment of sepsis. N Engl J Med 2003; 348(2):138–50.

74. Faust SN, Levin M, Harrison OB, et al. Dysfunction of endothelial protein C activation in severe meningococcal sepsis. N Engl J Med 2001; 345(6):408–16.

75. Warren BL, Eid A, Singer P, et al. Caring for the critically ill patient. High-dose antithrombin III in severe sepsis: a randomized controlled trial. JAMA 2001; 286(15):1869–78.

76. Abraham E, Reinhart K, Opal S, et al. Efficacy and safety of tifacogin (recombinant tissue factor pathway inhibitor) in severe sepsis: a randomized controlled trial. JAMA 2003; 290(2):238–47.

77. Bernard GR, Vincent JL, Laterre PF, et al. Efficacy and safety of recombinant human activated protein C for severe sepsis. N Engl J Med 2001; 344(10):699–709.

78. Dhainaut JF, Laterre PF, Janes JM, et al. Drotrecogin alfa (activated) in the treatment of severe sepsis patients with multiple-organ dysfunction: data from the PROWESS trial. Intensive Care Med 2003; 29(6):894–903.

79. Dhainaut JF, Laterre PF, LaRosa SP, et al. The clinical evaluation committee in a large multicenter phase 3 trial of drotrecogin alfa (activated) in patients with severe sepsis (PROWESS): role, methodology, and results. Crit Care Med 2003; 31(9):2291–301.

80. Annane D, Bellissant E, Bollaert PE, et al. Corticosteroids for severe sepsis and septic shock: a systematic review and meta-analysis. BMJ 2004; 329(7464):480.

81. Annane D, Sebille V, Charpentier C, et al. Effect of treatment with low doses of hydrocortisone and fludrocortisone on mortality in patients with septic shock. JAMA 2002; 288(7):862–71.

82. Hamrahian AH, Oseni TS, Arafah BM. Measurements of serum free cortisol in critically ill patients. N Engl J Med 2004; 350(16): 1629–38.

83. Stewart TE, Meade MO, Cook DJ, et al. Evaluation of a ventilation strategy to prevent barotrauma in patients at high risk for acute respiratory distress syndrome. Pressure- and Volume-Limited Ventilation Strategy Group. N Engl J Med 1998; 338(6):355–61.

84. Brochard L, Roudot-Thoraval F, Roupie E, et al. Tidal volume reduction for prevention of ventilator-induced lung injury in acute respiratory distress syndrome. The Multicenter Trail Group on Tidal Volume reduction in ARDS. Am J Respir Crit Care Med 1998; 158(6):1831–8.

85. Brower RG, Shanholtz CB, Fessler HE, et al. Prospective, randomized, controlled clinical trial comparing traditional versus reduced tidal volume ventilation in acute respiratory distress syndrome patients. Crit Care Med 1999; 27(8):1492–8.

86. The Acute Respiratory Distress Syndrome Network. Ventilation with lower tidal volumes as compared with traditional tidal volumes for acute lung injury and the acute respiratory distress syndrome. N Engl J Med 2000; 342(18):1301–8.

87. Eichacker PQ, Gerstenberger EP, Banks SM, Cui X, Natanson C.

Meta-analysis of acute lung injury and acute respiratory distress syndrome trials testing low tidal volumes. Am J Respir Crit Care Med 2002; 166(11):1510–14.

88. Petrucci N, Iacovelli W. Ventilation with lower tidal volumes versus traditional tidal volumes in adults for acute lung injury and acute respiratory distress syndrome. Cochrane Database Syst Rev 2004(2):CD003844.

89. Hickling KG, Walsh J, Henderson S, Jackson R. Low mortality rate in adult respiratory distress syndrome using low-volume, pressure-limited ventilation with permissive hypercapnia: a prospective study. Crit Care Med 1994; 22(10):1568–78.

90. Bidani A, Tzouanakis AE, Cardenas VJ Jr, Zwischenberger JB. Permissive hypercapnia in acute respiratory failure. JAMA 1994; 272(12):957–62.

91. Laffey JG, Tanaka M, Engelberts D, et al. Therapeutic hypercapnia reduces pulmonary and systemic injury following in vivo lung reperfusion. Am J Respir Crit Care Med 2000; 162(6):2287–94.

92. Tasker RC, Peters MJ. Combined lung injury, meningitis and cerebral edema: how permissive can hypercapnia be? Intensive Care Med 1998; 24(6):616–19.

93. Brower RG, Lanken PN, MacIntyre N, et al. Higher versus lower positive end-expiratory pressures in patients with the acute respiratory distress syndrome. N Engl J Med 2004; 351(4):327–36.

94. Jolliet P, Bulpa P, Chevrolet JC. Effects of the prone position on gas exchange and hemodynamics in severe acute respiratory distress syndrome. Crit Care Med 1998; 26(12):1977–85.

95. Gattinoni L, Tognoni G, Pesenti A, et al. Effect of prone positioning on the survival of patients with acute respiratory failure. N Engl J Med 2001; 345(8):568–73.

96. Mancebo J, Fernandez R, Gordo F. Prone vs supine position in ARDS patients: results of a randomized multicenter trial. Am J Respir Crit Care Med 2003; 167:A180.

97. Guerin C, Gaillard S, Lemasson S, et al. Effects of systematic prone positioning in hypoxemic acute respiratory failure: a randomized controlled trial. JAMA 2004; 292(19):2379–87.

98. Fort P, Farmer C, Westerman J, et al. High-frequency oscillatory ventilation for adult respiratory distress syndrome – a pilot study. Crit Care Med 1997; 25(6):937–47.

99. Mehta S, MacDonald R, Hallett DC, et al. Acute oxygenation response to inhaled nitric oxide when combined with high-frequency oscillatory ventilation in adults with acute respiratory distress syndrome. Crit Care Med 2003; 31(2):383–9.

100. Derdak S, Mehta S, Stewart TE, et al. High-frequency oscillatory ventilation for acute respiratory distress syndrome in adults: a randomized, controlled trial. Am J Respir Crit Care Med 2002; 166(6):801–8.

101. Lewandowski K. Extracorporeal membrane oxygenation for severe acute respiratory failure. Crit Care 2000; 4(3):156–68.

102. Hsu CL, Chen KY, Chang CH, et al. Timing of tracheostomy as a determinant of weaning success in critically ill patients: a retrospective study. Crit Care 2005; 9(1):R46–52.

103. Arabi Y, Haddad S, Shirawi N, Al Shimemeri A. Early tracheostomy in intensive care trauma patients improves resource utilization: a cohort study and literature review. Crit Care 2004; 8(5):R347–52.

104. Rothaar RC, Epstein SK. Extubation failure: magnitude of the problem, impact on outcomes, and prevention. Curr Opin Crit Care 2003; 9(1):59–66.

105. Curtis JJ, Clark NC, McKenney CA, et al. Tracheostomy: a risk factor for mediastinitis after cardiac operation. Ann Thorac Surg 2001; 72(3):731–4.

106. Abboud CS, Wey SB, Baltar VT. Risk factors for mediastinitis after cardiac surgery. Ann Thorac Surg 2004; 77(2):676–83.

107. Crabtree TD, Codd JE, Fraser VJ, et al. Multivariate analysis of risk factors for deep and superficial sternal infection after coronary artery bypass grafting at a tertiary care medical center. Semin Thorac Cardiovasc Surg 2004; 16(1):53–61.

108. Sakamoto H, Fukuda I, Oosaka M, Nakata H. Risk factors and treatment of deep sternal wound infection after cardiac operation. Ann Thorac Cardiovasc Surg 2003; 9(4):226–32.

109. Swenne CL, Lindholm C, Borowiec J, Carlsson M. Surgical-site infections within 60 days of coronary artery by-pass graft surgery. J Hosp Infect 2004; 57(1):14–24.

110. Esteban A, Frutos-Vivar F, Ferguson ND, et al. Noninvasive positive-pressure ventilation for respiratory failure after extubation. N Engl J Med 2004; 350(24):2452–60.

111. Esteban A, Anzueto A, Frutos F, et al. Characteristics and outcomes in adult patients receiving mechanical ventilation: a 28–day international study. JAMA 2002; 287(3):345–55.

112. Rossaint R, Falke KJ, Lopez F, et al. Inhaled nitric oxide for the adult respiratory distress syndrome. N Engl J Med 1993; 328(6):399–405.

113. Fiser SM, Cope JT, Kron IL, et al. Aerosolized prostacyclin (epoprostenol) as an alternative to inhaled nitric oxide for patients with reperfusion injury after lung transplantation. J Thorac Cardiovasc Surg 2001; 121:981–2.

114. Weinberger B, Laskin DL, Heck DE, Laskin JD. The toxicology of inhaled nitric oxide. Toxicol Sci 2001; 59(1):5–16.

115. Kaisers U, Busch T, Deja M, Donaubauer B, Falke KJ. Selective pulmonary vasodilation in acute respiratory distress syndrome. Crit Care Med 2003; 31(4 Suppl):S337–42.

116. Sokol J, Jacobs SE, Bohn D. Inhaled nitric oxide for acute hypoxemic respiratory failure in children and adults. Cochrane Database Syst Rev 2003(1):CD002787.

117. Lowson SM. Inhaled alternatives to nitric oxide. Anesthesiology 2002; 96(6):1504–13.

118. Walmrath D, Schneider T, Schermuly R, et al. Direct comparison of inhaled nitric oxide and aerosolized prostacyclin in acute respiratory distress syndrome. Am J Respir Crit Care Med 1996; 153(3):991–6.

119. Zwissler B, Kemming G, Habler O, et al. Inhaled prostacyclin (PGI$_2$) versus inhaled nitric oxide in adult respiratory distress syndrome. Am J Respir Crit Care Med 1996; 154(6 Pt 1):1671–7.

120. van Heerden PV, Barden A, Michalopoulos N, Bulsara MK, Roberts BL. Dose-response to inhaled aerosolized prostacyclin for hypoxemia due to ARDS. Chest 2000; 117(3):819–27.

121. Haraldsson A, Kieler-Jensen N, Wadenvik H, Ricksten SE. Inhaled prostacyclin and platelet function after cardiac surgery and cardiopulmonary bypass. Intensive Care Med 2000; 26(2):188–94.

122. Wilkes MM, Navickis RJ. Patient survival after human albumin administration. A meta-analysis of randomized, controlled trials. Ann Intern Med 2001; 135(3):149–64.

123. Finfer S, Bellomo R, Boyce N, et al. A comparison of albumin and saline for fluid resuscitation in the intensive care unit. N Engl J Med 2004; 350(22):2247–56.

124. Wilkes NJ, Woolf R, Mutch M, et al. The effects of balanced versus saline-based hetastarch and crystalloid solutions on acid-base and electrolyte status and gastric mucosal perfusion in elderly surgical patients. Anesth Analg 2001; 93(4):811–16.

125. Knutson JE, Deering JA, Hall FW, et al. Does intraoperative hetastarch administration increase blood loss and transfusion requirements after cardiac surgery? Anesth Analg 2000; 90(4):801–17.

126. Cope JT, Banks D, Mauney MC, et al. Intraoperative hetastarch infusion impairs hemostasis after cardiac operations. Ann Thorac Surg 1997; 63(1):78–82; discussion 82–3.

127. Boldt J. Fluid choice for resuscitation of the trauma patient: a review of the physiological, pharmacological, and clinical evidence. Can J Anaesth 2004; 51(5):500–13.

128. Boldt J, Haisch G, Suttner S, Kumle B, Schellhase F. Are lactated Ringer's solution and normal saline solution equal with regard to coagulation? Anesth Analg 2002; 94(2):378–84.

129. Ng KF, Lam CC, Chan LC. In vivo effect of haemodilution with saline on coagulation: a randomized controlled trial. Br J Anaesth 2002; 88(4):475–80.

130. Entholzner EK, Mielke LL, Calatzis AN, et al. Coagulation effects of

a recently developed hydroxyethyl starch (HES 130/0.4) compared to hydroxyethyl starches with higher molecular weight. Acta Anaesthesiol Scand 2000; 44(9):1116–21.

131. Wilkes MM, Navickis RJ, Sibbald WJ. Albumin versus hydroxyethyl starch in cardiopulmonary bypass surgery: a meta-analysis of postoperative bleeding. Ann Thorac Surg 2001; 72(2):527–33; discussion 534.

132. Schortgen F, Lacherade JC, Bruneel F, et al. Effects of hydroxyethylstarch and gelatin on renal function in severe sepsis: a multicentre randomised study. Lancet 2001; 357(9260):911–16.

133. Asfar P, Kerkeni N, Labadie F, et al. Assessment of hemodynamic and gastric mucosal acidosis with modified fluid versus 6% hydroxyethyl starch: a prospective, randomized study. Intensive Care Med 2000; 26(9):1282–7.

134. Rhee P, Koustova E, Alam HB. Searching for the optimal resuscitation method: recommendations for the initial fluid resuscitation of combat casualties. J Trauma 2003; 54(5 Suppl):S52–62.

135. Deb S, Martin B, Sun L, et al. Resuscitation with lactated Ringer's solution in rats with hemorrhagic shock induces immediate apoptosis. J Trauma 1999; 46(4):582–8; discussion 588–9.

136. Deb S, Sun L, Martin B, et al. Lactated Ringer's solution and hetastarch but not plasma resuscitation after rat hemorrhagic shock is associated with immediate lung apoptosis by the up-regulation of the Bax protein. J Trauma 2000; 49(1):47–53; discussion 53–5.

137. Lang K, Boldt J, Suttner S, Haisch G. Colloids versus crystalloids and tissue oxygen tension in patients undergoing major abdominal surgery. Anesth Analg 2001; 93(2):405–9.

138. Arieff AI. Fatal postoperative pulmonary edema: pathogenesis and literature review. Chest 1999; 115(5):1371–7.

139. Brandstrup B, Tonnesen H, Beier-Holgersen R, et al. Effects of intravenous fluid restriction on postoperative complications: comparison of two perioperative fluid regimens: a randomized assessor-blinded multicenter trial. Ann Surg 2003; 238(5):641–8.

140. Carson JL, Duff A, Poses RM, et al. Effect of anaemia and cardiovascular disease on surgical mortality and morbidity. Lancet 1996; 348(9034):1055–60.

141. Hebert PC, Wells G, Tweeddale M, et al. Does transfusion practice affect mortality in critically ill patients? Transfusion Requirements in Critical Care (TRICC) Investigators and the Canadian Critical Care Trials Group. Am J Respir Crit Care Med 1997; 155(5): 1618–23.

142. Hebert PC, Wells G, Blajchman MA, et al. A multicenter, randomized, controlled clinical trial of transfusion requirements in critical care. Transfusion Requirements in Critical Care Investigators, Canadian Critical Care Trials Group. N Engl J Med 1999; 340(6):409–17.

143. Hebert PC, Yetisir E, Martin C, et al. Is a low transfusion threshold safe in critically ill patients with cardiovascular diseases? Crit Care Med 2001; 29(2):227–34.

144. Wu WC, Rathore SS, Wang Y, Radford MJ, Krumholz HM. Blood transfusion in elderly patients with acute myocardial infarction. N Engl J Med 2001; 345(17):1230–6.

145. McClellan WM, Flanders WD, Langston RD, Jurkovitz C, Presley R. Anemia and renal insufficiency are independent risk factors for death among patients with congestive heart failure admitted to community hospitals: a population-based study. J Am Soc Nephrol 2002; 13(7):1928–36.

146. Jurkovitz CT, Abramson JL, Vaccarino LV, Weintraub WS, McClellan WM. Association of high serum creatinine and anemia increases the risk of coronary events: results from the prospective community-based atherosclerosis risk in communities (ARIC) study. J Am Soc Nephrol 2003; 14(11):2919–25.

147. Rao SV, Jollis JG, Harrington RA, et al. Relationship of blood transfusion and clinical outcomes in patients with acute coronary syndromes. JAMA 2004; 292(13):1555–62.

148. Corwin HL, Gettinger A, Pearl RG, et al. The CRIT Study: anemia and blood transfusion in the critically ill – current clinical practice in the United States. Crit Care Med 2004; 32(1):39–52.

149. Taylor RW, Manganaro L, O'Brien J, et al. Impact of allogenic packed red blood cell transfusion on nosocomial infection rates in the critically ill patient. Crit Care Med 2002; 30(10):2249–54.

150. Hebert PC, Fergusson D, Blajchman MA, et al. Clinical outcomes following institution of the Canadian universal leukoreduction program for red blood cell transfusions. JAMA 2003; 289(15):1941–9.

151. Herridge MS, Cheung AM, Tansey CM, et al. One-year outcomes in survivors of the acute respiratory distress syndrome. N Engl J Med 2003; 348(8):683–93.

152. Jacobi J, Fraser GL, Coursin DB, et al. Clinical practice guidelines for the sustained use of sedatives and analgesics in the critically ill adult. Crit Care Med 2002; 30(1):119–41.

153. Murray MJ, Cowen J, DeBlock H, et al. Clinical practice guidelines for sustained neuromuscular blockade in the adult critically ill patient. Crit Care Med 2002; 30(1):142–56.

154. Nasraway SA Jr, Jacobi J, Murray MJ, Lumb PD. Sedation, analgesia, and neuromuscular blockade of the critically ill adult: revised clinical practice guidelines for 2002. Crit Care Med 2002; 30(1):117–18.

155. Schweickert WD, Gehlbach BK, Pohlman AS, Hall JB, Kress JP. Daily interruption of sedative infusions and complications of critical illness in mechanically ventilated patients. Crit Care Med 2004; 32(6):1272–6.

156. Kress JP, Pohlman AS, O'Connor MF, Hall JB. Daily interruption of sedative infusions in critically ill patients undergoing mechanical ventilation. N Engl J Med 2000; 342(20):1471–7.

157. Mascia MF, Koch M, Medicis JJ. Pharmacoeconomic impact of rational use guidelines on the provision of analgesia, sedation, and neuromuscular blockade in critical care. Crit Care Med 2000; 28(7):2300–6.

158. Vasile B, Rasulo F, Candiani A, Latronico N. The pathophysiology of propofol infusion syndrome: a simple name for a complex syndrome. Intensive Care Med 2003; 29(9):1417–25.

159. Maze M, Angst MS. Dexmedetomidine and opioid interactions: defining the role of dexmedetomidine for intensive care unit sedation. Anesthesiology 2004; 101(5):1059–61.

160. Herr DL, Sum-Ping ST, England M. ICU sedation after coronary artery bypass graft surgery: dexmedetomidine-based versus propofol-based sedation regimens. J Cardiothorac Vasc Anesth 2003; 17(5):576–84.

161. Pittas AG, Siegel RD, Lau J. Insulin therapy for critically ill hospitalized patients: a meta-analysis of randomized controlled trials. Arch Intern Med 2004; 164(18):2005–11.

162. Pronovost PJ, Angus DC, Dorman T, et al. Physician staffing patterns and clinical outcomes in critically ill patients: a systematic review. JAMA 2002; 288(17):2151–62.

163. Higgins TL, McGee WT, Steingrub JS, et al. Early indicators of prolonged intensive care unit stay: impact of illness severity, physician staffing, and pre-intensive care unit length of stay. Crit Care Med 2003; 31(1):45–51.

164. Altman DE, Clancy C, Blendon RJ. Improving patient safety – five years after the IOM report. N Engl J Med 2004; 351(20):2041–3.

165. Galvin R, Milstein A. Large employers' new strategies in health care. N Engl J Med 2002; 347(12):939–42.

166. Wu A, Gao F. Long-term outcomes in survivors from critical illness. Anaesthesia 2004; 59(11):1049–52.

2

Rehabilitation

Christa Gohlke-Bärwolf and Hans H Björnstad

Introduction

Successes in surgery, improvements in perioperative management and economical constraints have led to a marked abbreviation of in-hospital care of patients after valve surgery within recent years. Yet, on the other hand, more elderly and multimorbid patients are undergoing valve surgery, increasing the requirements for intensive medical management during the first weeks after heart valve surgery. Therefore, the postoperative management of these patients has become an integral part of cardiac rehabilitation in some European countries, such as in Switzerland, Austria, Hungary, Poland, France and Germany, where it is mostly practised as institutional rehabilitation. In Germany, this was instituted by law, and the cost of rehabilitating these patients is borne by the retirement funds of those still working and the sickness funds of those who have retired, with 80% of patients participating in rehabilitation after surgery. In Scandinavian countries, rehabilitation has mostly been performed on an outpatient basis. In other European countries, there are wide variations in the resources currently available for and the present provision of rehabilitation facilities.[1]

There is abundant literature on the positive effects of rehabilitation after myocardial infarction and bypass surgery as well as on chronic coronary artery disease,[2–10] and recommendations are available concerning the type and structure of rehabilitation programmes.[11–14]

In contrast, rehabilitation after valve surgery has received less attention and there is no official recommendation available as to the type and structure of the optimal rehabilitation programme after valve surgery.

But in a recent study it was shown that patients after valve surgery had the same improvement after physical training (relative increase in peak Vo_2 of 25.9%) as patients with coronary artery disease (Figure 2.1).[15]

The major core components of cardiac rehabilitation/ secondary prevention programmes defined for cardiovascular and pulmonary rehabilitation in general can also be applied to patients after valve surgery. These components need to be broadened by the specific valve-related

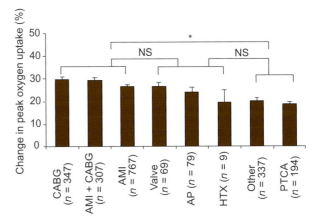

Figure 2.1
Comparison of training effects for peak Vo_2 ($F = 7.76$; $p < 0.001$) in patients with various cardiac pathologies, expressed as relative change. The Tukey test was used for post-hoc comparisons, $p < 0.05$. Data are presented as mean ±SEM. CABG, coronary artery bypass grafting; AMI, myocardial infarction; Valve, artificial valve implantation; AP, angina pectoris; HTX, heart transplantation; PTCA, percutaneous transluminal coronary angioplasty. *Significantly different; NS, not significantly different. Reproduced with permission from Reference 15.

issues. This underlines the need for guidelines concerning the content and requirements for rehabilitation after valve surgery in support of the recommendation that a multidisciplinary rehabilitation programme should be available for all patients undergoing cardiac procedures and acute coronary syndromes.[4]

Definition of rehabilitation by the World Health Organisation

Rehabilitation includes all measures that are required to achieve for a cardiac patient the best possible physical, psychological and social conditions that enable him/her to obtain out of his own strength and as normal as possible place in society and to lead an active and productive life.[16]

This definition, initially developed for patients with coronary artery disease, also applies to patients with valvular heart disease, particularly after valve replacement, since implantation of a replacement valve is a palliative procedure. As a result of the complexity and multiplicity of problems associated with valve surgery and the current abbreviated hospital stay, these patients are particularly well suited for comprehensive cardiac rehabilitation. A number of patients either remain in or develop heart failure late after valve replacement and thus represent a special group requiring prolonged professional care and intensive rehabilitative measures.

Purposes and aims of cardiac rehabilitation

Cardiac rehabilitation after valve surgery encompasses an even wider spectrum of goals than for patients with coronary disease for several reasons:

1. up to 50% of patients with valve diseases may also suffer from coronary disease, thus requiring the multifactorial comprehensive programmes directed at patients with coronary artery disease
2. these patients present with medical problems unique to them, such as bacterial endocarditis, requiring special attention and oral anticoagulation
3. several of the well-known atherosclerotic risk factors such as smoking and hypercholesterolaemia are also important thromboembolic and stroke risk factors that need to be controlled.

The various goals of rehabilitation include optimisation and adjustment of medical treatment and early recognition of complications (Table 2.1). Early ambulation and physical training, assessment and improvement in symptomatic status and of functional performance are important aspects as well as risk stratification for future cardiovascular events and medical treatment of complications.

A major part of rehabilitation of these patients consists of education on valve-specific and valve-related topics, including anticoagulation, bacterial endocarditis prophylaxis, recognition and management of patients with heart failure, the correct use of fluid restriction, weight control and use of diuretics. Furthermore, education and counselling of the patients and family about a health-conscious lifestyle and risk factor reduction, psychological support in

Table 2.1 Purposes and aims of cardiac rehabilitation

Optimisation and adjustment of medical treatment
Early recognition of complications
Early ambulation and physical training
Assessment and improvement of symptoms and functional performance
Risk stratification for future cardiovascular events (thromboembolic and valve thrombosis)
Education about valve-specific topics
Education about health-conscious lifestyle
Psychological support in adjustment to chronic disease
Vocational counselling

adjusting to chronic disease and vocational counselling are included in rehabilitation. There are other special features to rehabilitation after valve surgery in that a rapidly increasing number of elderly, multimorbid patients, particularly female, present for rehabilitative measures. Their medical, physical and psychosocial problems are very complex and divergent, and require intensive individualised management, education and counselling.

Optimisation and adjustment of medical treatment and early recognition of complications

Clinical evaluation

Careful history and daily physical examinations of these patients are mandatory during the early postoperative period. Thorough auscultation of the heart allows the identification of the normal sounds and murmurs of the artificial heart valve, together with deviations from the normal auscultatory findings, and is one of the most important and cost-effective examinations during the early and long-term follow-up of these patients. The initial auscultatory findings are of particular importance and should serve as the patient's own control in the follow-up assessment. Pericardial rubs are frequently heard in the early postoperative period and may occasionally make the interpretation of the auscultatory findings difficult.

The opening and closing sound of the artificial heart valves – the clicks, their intensity, character and associated murmurs – depend on the type and location of the prosthesis, the heart rate and rhythm and the underlying haemodynamic status. Also, lung auscultation and percussion is important to detect pleural effusion, pleural rubs and/or atelectasis.

Echocardiography should be performed prior to the initiation of cardiac rehabilitation to determine valve function, left ventricular size and function, presence of pulmonary hypertension and pericardial effusion.

The need for diuretics, digitalis, angiotensin-converting enzyme (ACE) inhibitors, beta-blockers and antiarrhythmic drugs should be assessed. Intensity of anticoagulation should be optimised according to valve type, position and risk factors.

Optimal control of blood pressure should be achieved (<140/80 mmHg; in diabetics <125/80 mmHg) and glycated haemoglobin of diabetes (HbA1c <6.5%).

Discontinuation of smoking is also an important goal for valve patients for thromboembolic prevention.

A health-orientated, low-fat diet, rich in vegetables and fruits, should be taught.

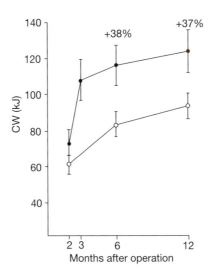

Figure 2.2
Physical training and improvement in cumulative work capacity (CW) after aortic valve replacement. ●, trained patients; ○, untrained patients. Modified from Reference 25.

Exercise training

A coordinated multidisciplinary cardiac exercise programme is essential to overcome the physical and psychosocial problems associated with cardiac surgery.

The known positive effects of training on cardiovasculatory fitness are an improvement in general circulatory response to exercise with reduced heart rate and blood pressure and greater exercise tolerance.[17] Attenuated progression of coronary artery disease makes a physical training programme for patients after valve replacement specifically advisable, since there are still patients who present for valve surgery after years of severe restriction of physical activity. This applies particularly to elderly patients. Also patients with heart failure can profit from regular exercise.[17–20]

Cardiorespiratory fitness is further impaired by surgical trauma and postoperative bedrest, so patients recovering from successful cardiac surgery can be in a markedly reduced state of cardiorespiratory fitness, especially those with rheumatic heart disease and impairment of cardiac performance.

The most recent developments in valve surgery, with excellent results in reconstructive surgical techniques, have led to recommendations to operate at an earlier state of the disease, even in the asymptomatic state.[21] This applies particularly to younger patients who are in generally good condition, who wish to exercise and return to work early after surgery.

The effect of exercise training on patients after valve replacement has been examined in only a few studies,[22–25] and has demonstrated an increase in exercise tolerance without serious risks (Figure 2.2): 6 and 12 months after prosthetic aortic valve replacement, the training group had a 38% and 37% higher physical work capacity compared with the untrained group.[25]

In a small study of women after prosthetic mitral valve replacement, slight haemolysis occurred, without serious valve dysfunction. Patients undergoing an 8-week exercise training programme improved their metabolic equivalent capacity by 19% and their physical working capacity by 25%, whereas control patients did not improve.[26] A total of 49 patients after aortic and/or mitral valve replacement/reconstruction underwent a 3-month exercise rehabilitation programme of moderate intensity, commencing 9 weeks postoperatively. The V_{O_2} at the maximum stage of exercise tolerance testing increased significantly ($p < 0.05$) by 25% for the training group (4.89 ± 5.0 ml/kg/min) and control (5.11 ± 4.48 ml/kg/min), without significant differences between the groups. This was because more than half of the control group also exercised on their own.[27]

Improvement in quality of life was also demonstrated by exercise training[28] (Figure 2.3).

Patients after valve surgery can improve to the same extent with exercise as for patients with other conditions, such as with coronary disease or after percutaneous transluminal coronary angioplasty (PTCA) or bypass surgery.[15]

Exercise haemodynamics

Haemodynamics improve significantly at rest and during exercise after surgery in patients with aortic stenosis and impaired left ventricular function preoperatively. In contrast, patients after mitral valve replacement not only have a markedly lower exercise tolerance but also only 40–60% of patients have normal haemodynamics at rest and only

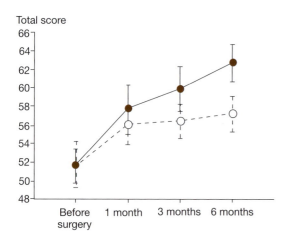

Figure 2.3
Improvement in quality of life with exercise training after valve replacement in patients with aortic and mitral insufficiency. Reproduced with permission from Reference 28.

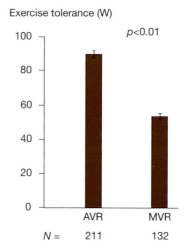

Figure 2.4
Exercise tolerance in 211 patients after aortic valve replacement (AVR) and 132 patients after mitral valve replacement (MVR) under the age of 56 years. Reproduced with permission from Reference 23.

25% during exercise.[23] Abnormal rest and exercise haemodynamics may persist for 6–12 months after surgery.[23,24,29,30]

In patients with mitral stenosis, pulmonary capillary wedge pressure falls significantly after surgery as does pulmonary hypertension. The degree of pulmonary hypertension preoperatively and the speed of postoperative regression are of importance for further management.[23,24]

To determine the type of rehabilitative measures, several other factors need to be taken into account, including the postoperative course of regression of left ventricular hypertrophy and improvement in left ventricular function following correction of the various valve lesions.

Evaluation for exercise training

General aspects

Patients with mitral valve disease have a markedly lower exercise tolerance postoperatively than those with aortic valve disease, and thus are candidates for a different, low-level training programme (Figure 2.4). Patients who can be expected to be candidates for exercise training postoperatively are those with pure aortic stenosis and normal ventricular function, those with aortic insufficiency and preserved left ventricular function pre- and postoperatively and an uncomplicated postoperative course. Patients with isolated mitral valve insufficiency preoperatively on the basis of mitral valve prolapse, especially if they have undergone mitral valve reconstruction, with an uncomplicated postoperative course, can be included in an exercise programme (Figures 2.5 and 2.6).

Patients with mitral stenosis and combined mitral valve lesion usually have a low exercise tolerance postoperatively.

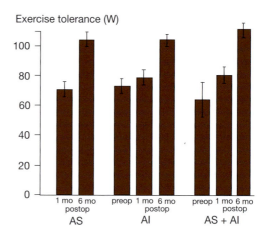

Figure 2.5
Exercise tolerance after aortic valve replacement pre-, 1 and 6 months postoperatively, in patients with aortic stenosis (AS), aortic insufficiency (AI), and mixed aortic lesion (AS + AI) (*n* = 307). Reproduced with permission from Reference 23.

In addition, the residual gradient across the valve and the marked increase in gradient with rising heart rate make an exercise programme for these patients particularly challenging. Before conditioning begins, the heart rate needs to be controlled by medication, both at rest and during exercise. This is particularly important for patients with atrial fibrillation. A decision should be made if atrial fibrillation

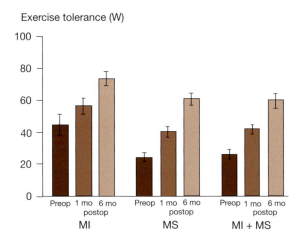

Figure 2.6
Exercise tolerance after mitral valve replacement pre-, 1 and 6 months postoperatively, in patients with mitral stenosis (MS), mitral insufficiency (MI) and mixed mitral lesion ($n = 258$). Reproduced with permission from Reference 23.

can be converted to sinus rhythm. A programme specifically designed for these patients, including walking, callisthenics, gymnastics and a low-level bicycle ergometry with special consideration of the heart rate achieved, appears to be of particular benefit. These patients could follow the training groups for heart failure patients.

Recommendations concerning exercise and recreational activity in patients after valve replacement should take into account the factors outlined in Table 2.2. Furthermore, psychological problems influencing exercise tolerance should be acknowledged and treated appropriately.[31]

Baseline information to be obtained during exercise test

Information comprises assessment of heart rate and rhythm, symptoms, ST-segment changes, and exercise capacity. Occasionally, non-invasive exercise haemodynamics using Doppler echocardiography to determine valve gradients and pulmonary pressures may be helpful.

As a simple guide to determine the optimal training level, the results of the exercise test and, in some cases, the exercise haemodynamics, are very useful. That level of activity or exercise that is still associated with normal haemodynamics can be taken as a guide for leisure-time activities. If haemodynamics are not available, a rating of perceived exertion such as the Borg scale[32] or the 'talk test' are valuable measurements of the intensity of exertion. The talk test refers to that level of exertion at which the patient can still lead a conversation.

Table 2.2 Factors influencing exercise recommendations after valve replacement*

Age of patient
Weight
Previous level of training
Type of cardiac disease and valve replaced
Postoperative functional status, determined by:
- clinical assessment
- echocardiographic determination of left ventricular function and size
- exercise testing with and without spiroergometry
- measurement of haemodynamics
- Holter monitoring for evaluation of arrhythmias

Type of exercise

Dynamic, aerobic types of exercise such as walking, jogging and cycling are preferable to isometric exercise. However, in elderly patients who present with problems of muscle weakness, a high-intensity strength training to improve muscle strength and coordination has been shown to be of benefit.[20,33–35] Swimming is associated with an energy requirement equivalent to 100–150 W, as far as the response of heart rate, norepinephrine and lactate levels are concerned.[36] Patients should be informed about the amount of energy expenditure associated with different types of exercise and advised about the activities suited to them.

A submaximal exercise test can be performed after completion of early mobilisation and climbing two flights of stairs without symptoms. This is usually the case 2 weeks after surgery; a symptom-limited maximal exercise test can be performed 3–4 weeks after surgery.

Table 2.3 Exercise prescription

For aerobic exercise
Intensity (50–80% of exercise capacity), heart rate guided: <130 beats/min
Duration 20–60 minutes
Frequency 3–5 times/week
Modality: walking, cycling, treadmill, stair climbing, arm ergometry, etc.

For resistance exercise
Intensity: 5 repetitions for strength training, 8–15 repetitions for endurance training
Duration: 1–3 sets of 6–10 different upper- and lower-body exercises (20–30 minutes)
Frequency 2–3 times/week
Modality: elastic bands, cuff weights, free weights, weight machines

Recommendations

Exercise prescription should include advice for aerobic and resistance training and should specify intensity, duration, frequency and modality (Table 2.3).

Training can be started at low intensity by 2 weeks for patients with aortic valve replacement and normal left ventricular function and also for patients after mitral valve repair with normal left ventricular function. In patients with mitral valve replacement and those with impaired left ventricular function, the start of training may need to be delayed to the third week, increasing slowly thereafter.

Swimming can be commenced when the sternal wound is completely healed (usually after 3 weeks) and the sternum is fixed (usually after 2 months). Breast stroke swimming may still cause sternal pain for 2 months; it corresponds to at least 75 W of energy expenditure. Swimming can also lead to rhythm disturbances.

Expected outcomes

Exercise leads to improvement of functional capacity, enhanced muscular endurance, strength and flexibility and contributes to overall lowering of cardiovascular risk. Physical conditioning and individually tailored exercise training are advisable for most patients after valve replacement, taking into account left ventricular function, the type of valve replaced, pulmonary hypertension and heart rate. The general circulatory responses to exercise – such as decreased heart rate and blood pressure at a given exercise load and increased exercise tolerance – are of benefit to most of these patients and could enable them to participate

better in social activities and live a more active and productive life. However, further studies are needed to determine the type, structure, effects and risks of exercise programmes in the various valve lesions.

Education

Education of patients with valvular heart disease and after valve surgery is of utmost importance during rehabilitation. In addition to the educational aspects applied in coronary patients, with regard to risk factor reduction and lifestyle changes, extensive information and education is required in valve-related specific topics. The patient needs to become an expert on his/her own disease (Table 2.4).

Vocational rehabilitation and return to work after valve replacement

Controversial results have been published concerning the influence of valve replacement on the return to work rate; it has been reported to be between 24% and 80%.[23,24,34,37–39]

The return to work rate after valve replacement is determined by a complex interplay of several medical and non-medical factors; in multivariate analysis, preoperative employment status, gender and functional status after surgery are the most important determinants of postoperative employment. Patients with aortic valve replacement, particularly for aortic stenosis, have a higher return to work rate than those with mitral valve replacement for rheumatic valve disease.[23,24]

Functional evaluation and improvement should have a high priority in comprehensive cardiac rehabilitation and vocational assessment of patients after valve replacement.

Exercise tolerance and the ability to return to work and to participate in recreational activities such as sports are important parameters which determine quality of life.

Early rehabilitation is one important means of improving the degree to which these activities can be performed after surgery. Rehabilitation can also enable the patient to cope with the palliative aspects of valve surgery.

Table 2.4 Educational aspects

The type of valve prosthesis and possible complications
The implications of symptoms and other problems
Medical therapy
Oral anticoagulation, dosing, control and complications
Possibility of patient-regulated anticoagulation and self-assessment of anticoagulation intensity, determined by international normalised ratio (INR)
Bacterial endocarditis and endocarditis prophylaxis
Meticulous dental hygiene
In case of persistent heart failure after operation, information on salt and fluid restriction, daily weight control, use of diuretics, etc.
Risk factor control – avoiding smoking, hypertension and obesity, to reduce the risk of thromboembolism and the need for reoperation in case of structural valve failure or for newly occurring coronary artery disease
Health-orientated lifestyle

Summary

Successful valve replacement leads to an overall improvement in symptoms, functional performance, quality of life and longevity. The degree of subjective and objective improvement depends on multiple preoperative factors, such as NYHA status, left ventricular function, valve lesion and type of valve replaced, as well as peri- and postoperative factors such as the occurrence of perioperative myocardial infarction, the degree of intraoperative myocardial damage, the type of valve replacement and the speed and degree of postoperative regression of left ventricular hypertrophy and dilatation, regression of pulmonary hypertension and improvement of left ventricular function.

Exercise tolerance and the ability to return to work and to participate in recreational activities such as sports are important parameters which determine quality of life. Early rehabilitation is one important means of improving the degree to which these activities can be performed after surgery. Rehabilitation can also enable the patient to cope with the palliative aspects of valve surgery. Therefore cardiac rehabilitation, as a multifactorial intervention programme including physical therapy, exercise training and optimisation of medical therapy, should be an integral part of the early cardiological management after valve surgery.

References

1. Vanhees L, McGee HM, Dugmore LD, Schepers D, van Daele P; Carinex Working Group: CArdiac Rehabilitation INformation EXchange. A representative study of cardiac rehabilitation activities in European Union Member States: the Carinex survey. J Cardiopulm Rehabil 2002; 22:264–72.

2. Fox KF, Nuttall M, Wood DA, et al. A cardiac prevention and rehabilitation programme for all patients at first presentation with coronary artery disease. Heart 2001; 85:533–8.

3. Wright DK, Williams SG, Riley R, Marshall P, Tan LB. Is early, low level, short term exercise cardiac rehabilitation following coronary bypass surgery beneficial? A randomised controlled trial. Heart 2002; 88:83–4.

4. Giannuzzi P, Saner H, Björnstad H, et al. Secondary prevention through cardiac rehabilitation: position paper of the Working Group on Cardiac Rehabilitation and Exercise Physiology of the European Society of Cardiology. Eur Heart J 2003; 24:1273–8.

5. Saner H, Saner B, Staubli R. Initial results with a comprehensive ambulatory rehabilitation program for heart patients. Schweiz Med Wochenschr 1994; 124:2075–82.

6. Belardinelli R, Georgiou D, Cianci G, et al. Randomized, controlled trial of long-term moderate exercise training in chronic heart failure: effects on functional capacity, quality of life, and clinical outcome. Circulation 1999; 99:1173–82.

7. Dubach P, Myers J, Dziekan G, et al. The effect of high intensity exercise training on central haemodynamic response to exercise in men with reduced left ventricular function. J Am Coll Cardiol 1997; 29:1591–98.

8. Gohlke H, Gohlke-Bärwolf C. Cardiac rehabilitation: Where are we going? Eur Heart J 1998; 19 (Suppl O):O5–12.

9. Gohlke H. Gohlke-Bärwolf C. Cardiac rehabilitation. Eur Heart J 1998; 19(7):1004–10.

10. Cottin Y, Cambou JP, Casillas JM, et al. Specific profile and referral bias of rehabilitated patients after an acute coronary syndrome. J Cardiopulm Rehabil 2004; 24(1):38–44.

11. Fletcher GF, Balady GJ, Amsterdam EA, et al. Exercise standards for testing and training: a statement for healthcare professionals from the American Heart Association. Circulation 2001; 104:1694–740.

12. Balady GJ, Ades PA, Comoss P, et al. Core components of cardiac rehabilitation/secondary prevention programmes: a statement for healthcare professionals from the American Heart Association and the American Association of Cardiovascular and Pulmonary Rehabilitation Writing Group. Circulation 2000; 102:1069–73.

13. McGee HM, Hevey D, Horgan JH. Cardiac rehabilitation service provision in Ireland: the Irish Association of Cardiac Rehabilitation survey. Ir J Med Sci 2001; 170:159–62.

14. Task force of the Working Group on Cardiac Rehabilitation of the European Society of Cardiology 1992. Long-term comprehensive care of cardiac patients – recommendations by the Working Group on Rehabilitation of the ESC. Cardiac rehabilitation: definition and goals. Eur Heart J 1992; 13(Suppl C):1–2.

15. Vanhees L, Stevens AN, Schepers D, et al. Determinants of the effects of physical training and of the complications requiring resuscitation during exercise in patients with cardiovascular disease. Eur J Cardiovasc Prev Rehabil 2004; 11:304–12.

16. Report of the WHO expert Committee on Disability Prevention and Rehabilitation. Disability, prevention and rehabilitation. WHO Tech Series No. 668. Geneva: World Health Organisation, 1981.

17. Hambrecht R, Gielen S, Linke A, et al. Effects of exercise training on left ventricular function and peripheral resistance in patients with chronic heart failure: a randomized trial. JAMA 2000; 283:3095–101.

18. Hambrecht R, Fiehn E, Weigl C, et al. Regular physical exercise corrects endothelial dysfunction and improves exercise capacity in patients with chronic heart failure. Circulation 1998; 98(24):2709–15.

19. Pina IL, Apstein CS, Bulady GJ, et al. Exercise and heart failure: a statement from the American Heart Association Committee on exercise, rehabilitation, and prevention. Circulation 2003; 107:1210–25.

20. Hare DL, Ryan TM, Selig SE, et al. Resistance exercise training increases muscle strength, endurance and blood flow in patients with chronic heart failure. Am J Cardiol 1999; 83:1674–7.

21. Iung B, Gohlke-Bärwolf C, Tornos P, et al. Recommendations on the management of the asymptomatic patient with valvular heart disease. Eur Heart J 2002; 23:1253–66.

22. Newell JP, Kappagoda CT, Stoker JB, et al. Physical training after heart valve replacement. Br Heart J 1980; 44:638–49.

23. Gohlke-Bärwolf C, Gohlke H, Samek L, et al. Exercise tolerance and working capacity after valve replacement. J Heart Valve Dis 1992; 1:189–95.

24. Gohlke-Bärwolf C, Roskamm H. Ergebnisse des Herzklappenersatzes. Prognose – Arbeits- und Leistungsfähigkeit – Berufliche Wiedereingliederung. Versicherungsmedizin 1992; 44:163–8.

25. Sire S. Physical training and occupational rehabilitation after aortic valve replacement. Eur Heart J 1987; 8:1215–20

26. Habel-Verge C, Landry F, Desaulnier D, et al. L'entrainement physique apres un remplacement valvulaire mitral. Can Med Ass J 1987; 136:142–7.

27. Jairath N, Salerno T, Chapman J, Dorman J, Weisel R. The effect of moderate exercise training on oxygen uptake post-aortic/mitral valve surgery. J Cardiopulm Rehabil 1995; 15:424–30.

28. Ueshima K, Kamata J, Kobayashi N, et al. Effects of exercise training after open heart surgery on quality of life and exercise tolerance in patients with mitral regurgitation or aortic regurgitation. Jpn Heart J 2004; 45(5):789–97.

29. Carstens V, Behrenbeck DW, Hilger HH. Exercise capacity before and after cardiac valve surgery. Cardiology 1983; 70:41–9.

30. Nakamura M, Chiba M, Ueshima K, et al. Effects of mitral and/or aortic valve replacement or repair on endothelium-dependent peripheral vasorelaxation and its relation to improvement in exercise capacity. Am J Cardiol 1996; 77:98–102.

31. Bettinardi O, Bertolotti G, Baiardi P, et al. [Can anxiety and depression influence the six-minute walking test performance in post-surgical heart valve patients? A pilot study]. Monaldi Arch Chest Dis 2004; 62(3):154–61 [in Italian].

32. Borg GA. Psychophysical basis of perceived exertion. Med Sci Sports 1982; 14:377–81.

33. Fiatarone MA, Marks EC, Ryan ND, et al. High-intensity strength training in nonagenarians. Effects on skeletal muscle. JAMA 1990; 263:3029–34.

34. Lunel C, Laurent M, Corbineau H, et al. [Return to work after cardiac valvular surgery. Retrospective study in a series of 105 patients]. Arch Mal Coeur Vaiss 2003; 96:15–22 [in French].

35. Pollock ML, Franklin BA, Balady GJ, et al. AHA Science Advisory. Resistance exercise in individuals with and without cardiovascular disease: benefits, rationale, safety, and prescription: an advisory from the Committee on Exercise, Rehabilitation, and Prevention, Council on Clinical Cardiology, American Heart Association; Position paper endorsed by the American College of Sports Medicine. Circulation 2000; 101(7):828–33.

36. Samek L, Lehmann M, Keul J, Roskamm H. Rückwirkungen leichter Schwimmbelastungen bei KHK- Patienten und gesunden Kontrollpersonen and Kreislaufgrössen, Katecholamine und Laktatspiegel. In: Rieckert H, ed. Sportmedizin-Kursbestimmung. Heidelberg: Springer-Verlag, 1987: 912–15.

37. Führer U, Both G, Fischer K, et al. Sozialanamnestische und hämodynamische Untersuchungen 4 bis 6 Jahre nach prothetischem Klappenersatz. Z KardioI 1977; 66:251–6.

38. Walter TPJ, Ibe B, Gottwik M. Return to work after heart valve replacement. In: Walter TPJ, ed. Return to work after coronary artery bypass surgery. Heidelberg: Springer-Verlag, 1985: 125–33.

39. Mattem H, Wisshirchen KJ, Fricke G, Bernard A. Belastbarkeit und berufliche Wiedereingliederung nach prothetischem Klappenersatz in Abhängigkeit von der postoperativen Hämodynamik. Z Kardiol 1979; 68:36–40.

3

Follow-up after valve surgery

Bertrand Cormier, Bernard Iung and Alec Vahanian

Follow-up after valve surgery

Although significant changes in valve design, prosthetic materials and surgical techniques have improved postoperative results after heart valve surgery, the haemodynamic performance of prosthetic valves remains inferior to that of native valves and life expectancy after valve replacement is reduced in comparison to age-matched controls,[1-4] although patient-related factors have a major influence. Patients with prosthetic heart valves are prone to complications, which vary according to the type of prosthetic valve used. The design of biological valves can be divided into true biological valves, represented by the homograft and the autograft, and heterograft valves constructed of biological material rendered immunologically inactive by treatment with glutaraldehyde. Whatever the type of biological valve considered, the main complication of these substitutes is late primary valve failure, especially in patients aged <70 years old. Mechanical valves include caged-ball valves, tilting disc valves and bileaflet valves. All require life-long anticoagulation to prevent valve thrombosis and thromboembolism. Thus, patients who have undergone valve replacement are not cured and should be followed with the same care as patients with native valve disease.

Despite this necessity, there is very little consensus as regards the required frequency of routine follow-up.[5,6] Follow-up should therefore be tailored according to the individual patient, the type of prosthesis used and available outcome data, which establish certain fundamentals:

1. There is a very low rate of structural deterioration with mechanical valves, whatever the design of prosthesis used.
2. When adequate anticoagulation is used with a mechanical prosthesis, the risk of thromboembolism does not exceed that of a bioprosthesis, in particular in the subgroup of low-risk patients (aortic position, sinus rhythm, etc.; see Chapter 8).
3. The incidence of bleeding depends mainly on the intensity of anticoagulation, co-morbidities and age.

4. Structural valve deterioration of bioprostheses occurs more rapidly in younger patients and in the mitral position.

It is generally accepted that the first postoperative visit should take place within 3 months of operation; however, no consensus has been reached on the frequency of routine late follow-up. In one recent study routine outpatient examination of asymptomatic patients with mechanical valve prosthesis had limited therapeutic impact due to the low rate of structural deterioration.[7] However, ACC/AHA guidelines recommend yearly visits in asymptomatic patients. Shorter time intervals have been suggested for patients with bioprostheses that have been implanted for more than 5 years or those showing new structural abnormalities upon echocardiography. One important argument for regular routine follow-up of asymptomatic patients by a cardiologist is the fact that many alterations in valve function and clinical status of the patient may begin with subtle changes that are not recognised by the patient himself (in the form of symptoms) or by a non-specialist not trained in cardiology. These include pathological valve sounds associated with insidious subacute valve thrombosis, new murmurs, new asymptomatic atrial fibrillation and incipient heart failure. In addition to these routine evaluations, a cardiologist should always be consulted when new symptoms or changes in the clinical status of the patient occur.

During each follow-up visit to a cardiologist, the quality of anticoagulation should be reviewed and important patient educational aspects re-emphasised (e.g. anticoagulation control and endocarditis prophylaxis – see Chapters 8 and 12).

Modalities of follow-up depend on the type of surgery (valve repair versus valve replacement), the type of prosthesis (mechanical versus biological), aetiology of valve disease (degenerative, dystrophic, rheumatic), stage of disease (functional class, left ventricular (LV) dysfunction, atrial fibrillation), associated lesions (coronary artery disease, aortic disease, other valve pathology) and patient characteristics (age, co-morbidities).

Clinical evaluation should be the cornerstone of follow-up, as changes in symptoms or physical findings are usually the first indication of any complication such as prosthetic valve dysfunction, LV dysfunction or associated valvular or coronary disease. The clinical findings will determine the further investigations required (see also Figure 10.3).

Early follow-up

During the first evaluation after operation, it is important to review the operative report (cross-clamping time, operative procedures, difficulties in weaning from bypass, etc.) and any in-hospital complications such as excessive bleeding, wound infection, pericardial effusion, arrhythmias or prolonged intensive therapy unit (ITU) stay. The outcome of postoperative rehabilitation and improvement in functional performance should also be reviewed to detect any problems suitable for early correction. It is important to be aware that prosthetic valves have specific auscultation characteristics. Most prosthetic valves, in particular aortic prostheses of small size, usually have some degree of obstruction compared with native valves. Thus, a mild systolic murmur is usually audible in patients with aortic or pulmonic valve prostheses. Caged-ball valves have loud opening and closing clicks. Disc valves, especially bileaflet, have no opening click but do have an audible closing click. The valve sounds of normally functioning bioprostheses are difficult to distinguish from native valves that are healthy or which have undergone successful repair. Finally, homografts in the aortic position have the best haemodynamic performance and do not even present a mild systolic murmur if functioning normally.

Late follow-up

Any deterioration in clinical status, such as changes in baseline auscultatory findings and/or unexplained appearance of clinical signs of heart failure, should prompt evaluation of prosthetic function. However, prosthetic valve dysfunction is not the only cause of late deterioration. Progression of coexistent valve disease, LV dysfunction, uncontrolled systemic hypertension, coronary artery disease, development of arrhythmias (in particular atrial fibrillation) and aortic wall complications may also be responsible for worsening or new symptoms.

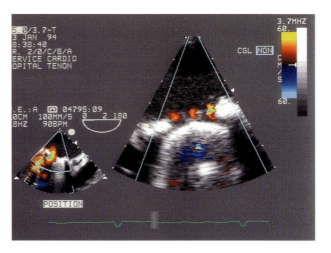

Figure 3.1
Bileaflet prosthesis in mitral position (color Doppler transoesophageal echocardiography): physiological transvalvular regurgitation.

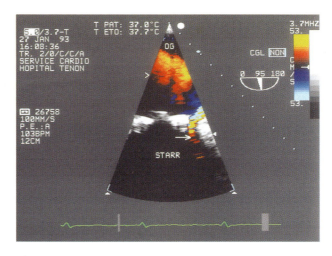

Figure 3.2
Caged-ball valve in mitral position (transoesophageal echocardiography): small paravalvular leak.

detect complications, to assess LV function and to identify other coexisting abnormalities.[8] Therefore, echocardiography combined with clinical examination is currently the method of choice for routine evaluation of prosthetic valves and detection of complications and has largely replaced cardiac catheterisation (see Chapters 4 and 5).

Echocardiography

Echocardiography has emerged as the principal method to evaluate prosthetic valve function (Figures 3.1–3.5), to

Early echocardiographic follow-up

The first post-discharge evaluation is ideally performed after 1 month, when the main parameters likely to alter

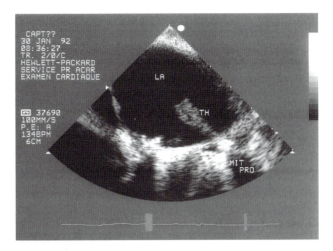

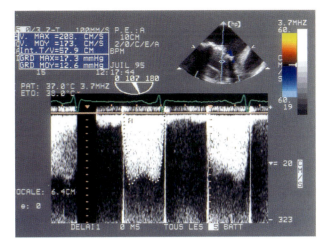

Figure 3.3
Non-obstructive thrombus on the left atrial side of a bileaflet prosthesis in mitral position (transoesophageal echocardiography).

Figure 3.5
Same patient: continuous wave (CW) Doppler recording an increase in transvalvular gradient (mean ΔP = 12.5 mmHg).

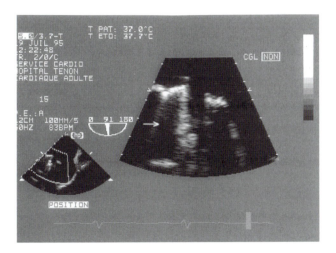

Figure 3.4
Obstructive thrombosis of a bileaflet mitral thrombosis ($\rightarrow$) (transoesophageal echocardiography).

cardiac output, such as fever, anaemia and inflammatory processes, are normalised. It should certainly be performed within 3 months of discharge. This baseline evaluation serves as the reference for future examinations with regard to prosthetic valve function, ventricular remodelling and haemodynamics.[9]

Late echocardiographic follow-up

The value of routine yearly evaluation remains debatable in patients with valve replacement or repair in whom there has been no change in clinical signs and valvular dysfunction is not suspected. During late follow-up (>5 years) the risk of primary degeneration of bioprostheses and homografts increases progressively and evaluation may detect subtle subclinical anatomical abnormalities, which would necessitate changes in the frequency of follow-up. Transthoracic evaluation is mandatory in patients with an increase in clinical signs and symptoms or in suspected prosthetic dysfunction, including endocarditis. Transoesophageal echocardiography (TOE), which provides high-resolution imaging of valvular and paravalvular structures, is necessary if endocarditis or mitral prosthetic dysfunction is suspected (see Chapters 4 and 16).

Echocardiography provides a wide variety of information on valve structure and function. Two-dimensional and M-mode echocardiography, which evaluate the structure of the prosthesis, the motion of the occluder and the stability of the valve ring, allow identification of possible causes or mechanisms of valve dysfunction. Transthoracic echocardiography (TTE) can identify calcification on a bioprosthesis, which may precede valve dysfunction. However, TTE is often limited in the evaluation of the structure of mechanical valves. Doppler echo provides haemodynamic information on valve gradients (Figure 3.5), effective valve areas and valve regurgitation (Figures 3.1 and 3.2).[10–14] In addition to information on the valve itself, echocardiography offers unique information about cardiac structures adjacent to the prosthesis as well as cardiac size and function and estimated pulmonary artery pressure.[15]

The same Doppler principles and formulae used for native valve stenosis are applied to prosthetic valves.[16] A normal prosthetic valve in the aortic position will resemble mild native aortic stenosis with maximal velocity of between 2 and 3 m/s. However, higher gradients may be seen with normally functioning smaller valves, as velocities and gradients across normal prosthetic valves are determined by valve type, valve size and flow through the valve, which explains the difficulty of differentiating malfunctioning from normal prosthetic valves in high flow states with small prostheses. In this situation it is important to compare observed values with previous serial measurements and to use supplementary methods to assess valve function, such as effective orifice areas using the continuity equation. Body size is important in assessing possible valve prosthesis–patient mismatch, considered severe when the aortic valve area is <0.6 cm^2/m^2, with potential significant deleterious effects.[17,18] In contrast to prosthetic aortic valves, mitral gradients are less dependent on the size of the prosthesis and are mainly influenced by heart rate, which should be systematically reported during the evaluation.

It has been suggested that stress or exercise echocardiography could be useful in evaluating rise in mean gradient and increase in systolic pulmonary artery pressure when compared with resting evaluation, but there is no reference threshold to define a definite diagnosis of dysfunction.

Aortic homografts are often considered as the substitutes of choice for infective endocarditis, but there are still concerns about their superiority to bioprostheses in terms of durability.[19] In the aortic position, homografts have a similar appearance to native valves.[20] Occasionally, sutures can be seen around the valve annulus. The valve slowly degenerates and this may result in calcification, with stenotic dysfunction, or in rupture, with prolapse and regurgitation. Progressive dilatation of the sinotubular junction may result in aortic regurgitation and can benefit from early detection. Follow-up of patients with aortic homografts should probably be the same as for patients with bioprostheses. Mitral homografts are not widely used and results have been disappointing.[21] For further discussion, see Chapter 6.

Given their availability, the experience of their use, and the standardisation of surgical techniques, mechanical and biological prostheses are by far the most widely used valves.[22–27] The stents on which xenograft valves are mounted are echogenic and cast acoustic shadows, making it difficult to investigate behind them. Primary degeneration of both pericardial and porcine xenografts results in calcification, which causes valvular stenosis and regurgitation or tearing of a cusp with consequent severe regurgitation. As compared with stented bioprostheses, unstented valves generally provide a larger effective orifice area in relation to the patient's body surface area and permit avoidance of mismatch in patients with a small aortic root.[28,29] Superior haemodynamics may result in quicker and more complete regression of LV hypertrophy than with stented valves. However, there are no data on long-term outcome, and durability has yet to be proven.

Valvular obstruction is usually detected by TTE, but the identification of the underlying pathology (thrombus or pannus) is better assessed by TOE.[30,31] All mechanical prosthetic valves have a degree of physiological transvalvular regurgitation that must be differentiated from pathological transvalvular regurgitation due to interference with occluder closure and from pathological paravalvular regurgitation. The ability of TTE to detect and localise regurgitation depends on the position of the valve and TOE may be required, particularly in the mitral position.[32]

Although it is more complex and difficult, the Ross procedure has the advantage in children that the valve is able to grow as the child grows (see Chapter 18). The incidence of thromboembolism is very low, as is that of infective endocarditis.[33,34] The problems which need to be detected by echocardiographic surveillance are progressive dilatation of the aortic root, with associated aortic regurgitation, and progressive stenosis of the pulmonary homograft (see Chapter 6).

Aortic complications are common in patients with connective tissue disorders, particularly Marfan's syndrome. Even though life expectancy improves after surgical repair of the aortic aneurysm, a significant number of patients still require further surgery for the aortic or the mitral valve. Thus it is important to follow these patients with regular clinical examinations to identify new symptoms or murmurs and to continue imaging the hearts of patients with Marfan's syndrome throughout their lifetime.

After aortic valve replacement for aortic insufficiency, the risk of postoperative dissection or rupture relates to the size of the ascending aorta at the time of aortic valve replacement. This phenomenon clearly indicates the importance of indexing the absolute aortic dimension to body surface area, particularly in women.[35,36] Other risk factors for aortic wall complications include the rate of aortic expansion and the underlying pathology. Bicuspid aortic valves are frequently associated with aortic root dilatation, annuloaortic ectasia and aortic dissection and the risk persists after aortic valve replacement.[37–39]

Other investigations

Routine haematology and biochemistry blood tests are usually performed at the first post-discharge evaluation, together with tests for haemolysis, particularly in patients with multiple mechanical prostheses or in patients in whom echocardiography reveals a paravalvular leak. A regular electrocardiogram (ECG) is useful during early follow-up and yearly examinations to assess the regression of LV hypertrophy, to detect any new abnormalities, to identify conduction defects, particularly after aortic valve replacement or in patients with LV dysfunction, and to identify asymptomatic atrial or ventricular arrhythmias. In the latter case, 24-hour Holter monitoring may be required.

A baseline chest X-ray is useful to detect any residual pulmonary or pleural abnormality and to assess cardiac size. The role of cinefluoroscopy has decreased since the advent of ultrasound techniques, in particular TOE, but it remains useful in detecting limitation of occluder movement, particularly in bileaflet valves, in which angles of opening and closing can be measured accurately. In this way it can play a complementary role in patients with suspected valve thrombosis or pannus ingrowth, especially in the aortic position. Catheterisation is rarely necessary in patients with prosthetic heart valves, since echocardiography, with its different modalities such as TOE and stress echo, has become the reference method in this setting.

Specific problems

Chest pain

Chest pain may have many cardiac and non-cardiac causes. If the associated symptoms and signs raise suspicion of possible endocarditis, C-reactive protein (CRP) level, blood cultures and echocardiography should be performed as soon as possible. Absence of regional wall motion abnormalities has a high negative predictive accuracy regarding the likelihood of acute ischaemia. Detection of segmental LV wall motion abnormalities is helpful when clinical history and ECG are inconclusive; however, they can also be seen in patients with transient myocardial ischaemia.

Typical angina and/or myocardial infarction can occur in young patients with no coronary risk factors and result from coronary occlusion related to an embolic event, in particular in patients with mechanical prosthesis or in endocarditis with valvular vegetations. Other causes of ischaemic symptoms are anaemia, from bleeding or haemolysis, severe aortic regurgitation, from valvular dehiscence or thrombus, and increased wall stress, whatever the cause (pannus, mismatch, thrombus).

In addition to ischaemia, the main cardiovascular sources of chest pain are pericarditis and aortic dissection. Pericardial effusion is common during the first postoperative days, but it can also occur later during the course of the first postoperative month. It commonly causes chest pain, fever, pericardial or pleural rubs and increased CRP and sedimentation rate. Aortic dissection is less common but has been described in patients with previous aortic valve replacement without concomitant replacement of an associated dilated ascending aorta. It should be specifically excluded as a cause of chest pain in young patients with previous aortic valve replacement for degenerative aortic regurgitation, including those with Marfan's syndrome. In all of these situations, echocardiography helps to make a clinical decision and select patients in whom coronary angiography or additional investigations such as magnetic resonance imaging (MRI) should be performed.

Heart failure

The management of low cardiac output in the immediate postoperative period is discussed in Chapter 1. Intractable early heart failure or new 'late' heart failure after valve replacement may result from several causes, which can be found alone or in combination:

- preoperative LV dysfunction that persists after surgery in patients operated on for aortic or mitral regurgitation
- associated coronary artery disease and/or hypertension
- perioperative myocardial damage (myocardial infarction or suboptimal myocardial protection)
- prosthetic heart valve complications (obstruction or paravalvular leak)
- progression of valve disease at another site
- arrhythmia with very rapid heart rate.

Preoperative heart failure in patients undergoing surgery for aortic or mitral regurgitation usually persists early after operation. In contrast, heart failure in association with aortic stenosis improves rapidly after relief of the stenosis.[6]

Two-dimensional and Doppler echocardiography should be performed to assess prosthetic function, determine the degree of LV impairment and exclude pericardial effusion or constriction. If the latter diagnosis is suspected, cardiac MRI may be useful. In patients with intraoperative myocardial infarction or unexplained deterioration in LV function postoperatively, coronary angiography should be considered to exclude a new coronary lesion or a preoperative stenosis which was not bypassed and which may be amenable to percutaneous intervention. Late tricuspid regurgitation is particularly difficult to manage;[40] prevention by appropriate tricuspid annuloplasty at the time of the original operation is preferable to the necessity for late reoperation, which carries a high mortality. This issue is discussed further in Chapter 7.

Medical management for both early postoperative heart failure and later developing heart failure involves therapy with digitalis, diuretics (including aldosterone antagonists) and angiotensin-converting enzyme (ACE) inhibitors. In stable patients with persistent systolic LV dysfunction, beta-blockers are also of benefit. Nitrates are very useful in patients with residual pulmonary hypertension to lower pulmonary artery pressure and relieve right heart failure. Reoperation must be considered in patients with documented prosthetic dysfunction or with other significant valve disease (see also Chapters 10 and 13).

Arrhythmias

Atrial fibrillation is the most common arrhythmia in the early postoperative period. It is associated with increased stroke risk and low cardiac output, in particular when there is a very fast or very slow heart rate. Sinus bradycardia and slow atrioventricular (AV) junctional rhythms may favour low cardiac output in the early postoperative period. AV block can occur more often after aortic valve replacement, in particular in patients with extensive calcification, and requires a permanent pacemaker in less than 10% of cases. The treatment of atrial fibrillation is considered in more detail in Chapter 1.

Asymptomatic paravalvular leaks

Paravalvular leaks may be observed in the early postoperative period, particularly in cases with heavy annular calcification, acute infective endocarditis or connective tissue disease. During the late postoperative period they are often related to infective endocarditis and can result in variable degrees of regurgitation and haemolysis. Doppler echocardiography and TOE help to assess the severity of the regurgitation, the origin of the jet inside or outside the prosthetic annulus and haemodynamic tolerance. Echocardiographic follow-up and laboratory evaluations – lactate dehydrogenase (LDH) and haemoglobin – will guide therapeutic decisions (see also Chapter 11).

Conclusions

Valve replacement, the second most common cardiac operation after coronary surgery, usually results in functional improvement and better quality of life. However, despite continuing progress in prosthetic valve technology, complications can occur throughout the patient's life, underlining the need for careful medical follow-up. Ultrasound techniques, mainly represented by TTE, are the main diagnostic modality for serial evaluation of prosthetic valve function as well as left ventricular function and dimensions. For future comparison, a baseline Doppler echocardiographic study performed early after operation is essential. Follow-up should also involve adequate patient education, which will hopefully decrease the incidence of complications.

References

1. Rahimtoola SH. Choice of prosthetic heart valve for adult patients. J Am Coll Cardiol 2003; 41:893–904.
2. Thourani VH, Weintraub WS, Craver JM, et al. Ten-year trends in heart valve replacement operations. Ann Thorac Surg 2000; 70:448–55.
3. Rao V, Christakis GT, Weisel RD, et al. Changing pattern of valve surgery. Circulation 1996; 94 (Suppl 9):II113–20.
4. Bach DS. Choice of prosthetic heart valves: update for the next generation. J Am Coll Cardiol 2003; 42:1717–19.
5. Guidelines for the management of patients with valvular heart disease. Circulation 1998; 98:1949–82.
6. Gohlke-Bärwolf C, Gohlke H, Roskamm H. Follow-up and rehabilitation. In: Acar J, Bodnar E, eds. Textbook of acquired heart valve disease. London: ICR Publishers, 1995: 1002–28.
7. Mahy IR, Dougall H, Buckley A, et al. Routine hospital based follow up for patients with mechanical valve prostheses: is it worthwhile? Heart 1999; 82:520–2.
8. ACC–AHA Guidelines for the clinical application of echocardiography. Circulation 1997; 95:1686–744.
9. Wiseth R, Hegrenaes L, Rossvoll O, Skjaerpe T, Hatle L. Validity of an early postoperative baseline Doppler recording after aortic valve replacement. Am J Cardiol 1991; 67:869–72.
10. Burston DJ, Nishimura RA, Bailey KR, et al. Continuous wave Doppler echocardiographic measurements of prosthetic valve gradients. A simultaneous Doppler–catheter correlative study. Circulation 1989; 80:504–14.
11. Dumesnil JG, Honos GN, Lemieux M, Beauchemin J. Validation and application of mitral prosthetic areas calculated by Doppler echocardiography. Am J Cardiol 1990; 65:1443–8.
12. Chambers J, Deverall P. Limitations and pitfalls in the assessment of prosthetic valves with Doppler ultrasonography. J Thorac Cardiovasc Surg 1992; 104:495–501.
13. Chambers J, Monaghan M, Jackson G. Colour flow Doppler mapping in the assessment of prosthetic valve regurgitation. Br Heart J 1989; 62:1–8.
14. Nanda NC, Cooper JW, Mahan III AF, Fan P. Echocardiographic assessment of prosthetic valves. Circulation 1991; 84(Suppl 1):228–39.
15. De Paulis R, Sommavira L, Colagrande L, et al. Regression of left ventricular hypertrophy after aortic valve replacement for aortic stenosis with different valve substitutes. J Thorac Cardiovasc Surg 1998; 116:590–8.
16. Hatle L, Angelsen B, Tromsdal A. Noninvasive assessment of atrioventricular pressure half time by Doppler ultrasound. Circulation 1979; 60:1096–104.
17. Rahimtoola SH. Valve prosthesis–patient mismatch: an update. J Heart Valve Dis 1998; 7:207–10.
18. Pibarot P, Dumesnil JG. Hemodynamic and clinical impact of prosthesis–patient mismatch in the aortic valve position and its prevention. J Am Coll Cardiol 2000; 36:1131–41.
19. O'Brien MF, Hancock S, Stafford EG. The homograft aortic valve: a 29-year, 99.3 % follow-up of 1,022 valve replacements. J Heart Valve Dis 2001; 10:334–44.
20. Jaffe WM, Coverdale A, Roche A, et al. Doppler echocardiography in the assessment of the homograft aortic valve. Am J Cardiol 1989; 63:1466–70.
21. Acar C, Tolan M, Berrebi A, et al. Homograft replacement of the mitral valve. Graft selection, technique of implantation, and results in forty-three patients. J Thorac Cardiovas Surg 1996; 111:367–78.
22. Butchart EG, Li HH, Payne N, Buchan K, Grunkemeier GL. Twenty years' experience with the Medtronic Hall valve. J Thorac Cardiovasc Surg 2001; 121:1090–100.
23. Peterseim DS, Chen Y-Y, Cheruvu S. Long-term outcome after biological versus mechanical aortic valve replacement in 841 patients. J Thorac Cardiovasc Surg 1999; 117:890–7.
24. Grunkemeier GL, Li HH, Naftel DC, Starr A, Rahimtoola SH. Long-term performance of heart valve prosthesis. Curr Probl Cardiol 2000; 25:73–154.
25. Orszulak TA, Schaff HV, Puga FJ, et al. Event status of the Starr-Edwards aortic valve to 20 years: a benchmark for comparison. Ann Thorac Surg 1997; 63:620–6.

26. Murday A, Hochstitzky A, Mansfield J, et al. A prospective randomized trial of St Jude versus Starr-Edwards aortic and mitral valve prostheses. Ann Thorac Surg 2003; 76:66–74.

27. Saour JN, Sieck JO, Mamo LAR, Gallus AS. Trial of different intensities of anticoagulation in patients with prosthetic heart valves. N Engl J Med 1990; 322:428–32.

28. Walther T, Falk V, Langebartels G, et al. Prospectively randomized evaluation of stentless versus conventional biological aortic valves: impact on early regression of left ventricular hypertrophy. Circulation 1999; 100(Suppl II):II6–II10.

29. Gelsomino S, Morocutti G, Frassani R, et al. Usefulness of the Cryolife O'Brien stentless supraannular aortic valve to prevent prosthesis–patient mismatch in the small aortic root. J Am Coll Cardiol 2002; 39:1845–51.

30. Dürrleman N, Pellerin M, Bouchard D, et al. Prosthetic valve thrombosis: twenty-year experience at the Montreal Heart Institute. J Thorac Cardiovasc Surg 2004; 127:1388–92.

31. Laplace G, Lafitte S, Labeque JN, et al. Clinical significance of early thrombosis after prosthetic mitral valve replacement: a postoperative monocentric study of 680 patients. J Am Coll Cardiol 2004; 43:1283–90.

32. Ionescu A, Fraser AG, Butchart EG. Prevalence and clinical significance of incidental paraprosthetic valvar regurgitation: a prospective study using transesophageal echocardiography. Heart 2003; 89:1316–21.

33. Böhm Jo, Botha CA, Hemmer W, et al. The Ross operation in 225 patients: a five-year experience in aortic root replacement. J Heart Valve Dis 2001; 10:742–9.

34. Elkins RC, Knott-Craig CJ, Ward KE. Pulmonary autograft in children: realized growth potential. Ann Thorac Surg 1994; 57:1387–92.

35. Roman MJ, Devereux RB, Kramer-Fox R, O'Loughlin J. Two-dimensional echocardiographic aortic root dimensions in normal children and adults. Am J Cardiol 1989; 64:507–12.

36. McDonald ML, Smedira NG, Blackstone EH, et al. Reduced survival in women after valve surgery for aortic regurgitation: effect of aortic enlargement and late aortic rupture. J Thorac Cardiovasc Surg 2000; 119:1205–15.

37. Prenger K, Pieters FA, Cheriex E, et al. Aortic dissection after aortic valve replacement: incidence and consequences for strategy. J Card Surg 1994; 9:495–9.

38. Pieters FA, Widdershoven JW, Gerardy AC, et al. Risk of aortic dissection after aortic valve replacement. Am J Cardiol 1993; 72:1043–7.

39. Russo CF, Mazzetti S, Garatti A, et al. Aortic complications after bicuspid aortic valve replacement: long-term results. Ann Thorac Surg 2002; 74:S1773–6.

40. Porter A, Shapira Y, Wurzel M, et al. Tricuspid regurgitation late after mitral valve replacement: clinical and echocardiographic evaluation. J Heart Valve Dis 1999; 8:57–62.

4

Echocardiographic follow-up

Pathmaja Paramsothy and Catherine M Otto

In the patient with a prosthetic heart valve, echocardiography is essential for evaluation of valve haemodynamics, ventricular function, pulmonary pressures and detection of prosthetic valve dysfunction. The echocardiographic evaluation of prosthetic valves is similar to that of native valves with a few key differences. First, normal fluid dynamics and flow velocities differ, depending on valve design and size.[1] Secondly, technical aspects, such as acoustic shadowing, make interpretation of data challenging.

Timing of examinations

There are two basic types of prosthetic valves: mechanical valves and tissue valves (see Chapter 5). Although mechanical valves are durable, they are susceptible to thrombotic complications, ranging from valve thrombosis to systemic thromboembolism. Tissue valves have fewer thrombotic complications, but have limited durability, being prone to degeneration and calcification, which results in stenosis or regurgitation.

A baseline echocardiographic evaluation of the patient with a prosthetic valve is recommended early (within the first 3 months) after surgery to document the normal appearance and haemodynamics of the prosthesis in that patient for comparison to future studies if valve dysfunction is subsequently suspected. It is helpful to review the surgical approaches used at your institution and to view an example of each type of valve prosthesis implanted at your institution for correlation with the echocardiographic image. The baseline examination may also reveal unexpected postoperative results, such as a mild paravalvular leak, and provides a postoperative baseline for left ventricular (LV) function and pulmonary artery pressures (Table 4.1).

The timing of subsequent examinations is based on:

1. the expected natural history for the type of prosthetic valve
2. any abnormalities on the baseline postoperative examination

Table 4.1 Indications for echocardiography in patients with prosthetic valves

Transthoracic echocardiogram
Baseline examination: within 3 months of valve replacement
Surveillance examinations:
- Mechanical valves: every 2–4 years
- Tissue valves: every 2–4 years for the first 10 years, then annually

Increased frequency of examination:
Persistent abnormalities of other structures post-valve replacement:
- LV hypertrophy or dilation
- LV systolic and/or diastolic dysfunction
- Pulmonary hypertension
- Other valve lesions

Any symptoms or physical findings consistent with prosthetic valve dysfunction:
- New heart failure symptoms
- Syncope or dizziness
- New or increasing murmur
- Dyspnea

Transoesophageal echocardiogram
Whenever transthoracic imaging is inadequate
Clinical signs or symptoms of prosthetic mitral valve dysfunction
Positive blood cultures or any other sign of prosthetic valve infection
Evaluation for paravalvular abscess or pseudoaneurym

3. any change in clinical symptoms or physical examination findings.

In general, examinations every 2–4 years are appropriate, with an increased frequency of examination for tissue valves after 10 years of implantation. However, many patients with prosthetic valves need more frequent evaluation because of coexisting valve lesions, residual LV hypertrophy, systolic or diastolic dysfunction or persistent pulmonary hypertension.

Table 4.2 Transthoracic echocardiography evaluation of a patient with a prosthetic valve

Parameter	View	Limitations
Valve anatomy		
Aortic valve prosthesis	Parasternal long and short axis	Shadowing and reverberations from struts or from mechanical prosthesis
Mitral valve prosthesis	Parasternal long and short axis, apical four-chamber, and long-axis views	Shadowing and reverberations from struts or from mechanical prosthesis, making imaging from left atrium by TOE preferable, especially if abnormality on atrial side
Valve haemodynamics		
Aortic velocity	From apical and suprasternal windows CW Doppler to determine the maximum aortic velocity with calculation of mean gradient	Different normal antegrade velocities for each valve size/type. Velocity underestimated if intercept angle is not parallel
LVOT velocity	PW Doppler in apical long-axis view with sample volume just proximal to aortic valve	Inaccurate if not at same site as LVOT diameter measurement or with a non-parallel intercept angle
LVOT diameter	Parasternal long-axis view, parallel and immediately adjacent to aortic valve. Use to calculate continuity equation AVA	Avoid reverberations and shadowing from valve
Mitral valve area	From apical recording of transmitral Doppler velocity, calculate mean pressure gradient and pressure half-time	Average multiple beats if in atrial fibrillation
Valve regurgitation		
Aortic regurgitation	Colour Doppler in parasternal long-axis, short-axis, apical long-axis view	Colour alone is not enough to quantify severity. Shadowing and reverberations may limit evaluation of the outflow tract, even with TOE imaging
	CW Doppler for velocity curve and density	Parallel intercept angle is needed for accurate CW assessment
	PW Doppler in descending thoracic and abdominal aorta to determine holodiastolic reversal	
Mitral regurgitation	Colour Doppler in parasternal long-axis, short-axis, apical long-axis views	Shadowing of left atrium by prosthesis limits utility of transthoracic Doppler. Look for secondary signs of regurgitation. TOE needed if MR suspected
	CW Doppler from apex	
Left ventricle		
Systolic function	Parasternal long- and short-axis, apical two- and four-chamber and long axis Measure systolic and diastolic dimensions and wall thickness (M-mode or 2D imaging) Calculate ejection fraction Evaluate regional wall motion	Contrast agents to help define the endocardial border may be helpful
Diastolic function	Mitral inflow peak E and A IVRT Pulmonary vein a velocity duration and peak Tissue Doppler velocities	With a mitral prosthesis these parameters will reflect valve function, not LV diastolic function
Pulmonary artery pressures	Peak TR velocity from multiple windows to determine the highest velocity TR jet add estimated right atrial pressure based on IVC size and collapsibility	Underestimation of pressures if intercept angle is not parallel Persistent or recurrent pulmonary hypertension suggests prosthetic mitral valve dysfunction, TOE recommended
Right heart	Parastenal short axis and RV inflow views, apical four-chamber view for evaluation of RV size and systolic function	
Ascending aorta	Parasternal long axis, suprasternal views, apical five-chamber Measure aortic dimensions at annulus, sinuses, sinotubular junction and ascending aorta	

CW = continuous wave, PW = pulsed wave, IVC = inferior vena cava, IVRT = isovolumic relaxation time, LV = left ventricular, LVOT = left ventricular outflow tract, MR = mitral regurgitation, TOE = transoesophageal echocardiography, TR = tricuspid regurgitation, RV = right ventricular, AVA = aortic valve area.

The echocardiographic approach

The echocardiographic examination focuses on imaging the prostheses and Doppler evaluation of valve haemodynamics. Other key components of the examination include assessment of LV geometry and systolic and diastolic function; estimation of pulmonary pressures; evaluation of the right heart; imaging of adjacent chambers and vessels (e.g. left atrium and aorta); and quantitation of any other valve lesions (Table 4.2).

Valve anatomy

Tissue valves

Bioprosthetic valves include homograft valves and stented and non-stented heterograft valves. Echocardiography allows evaluation of valve position and leaflet motion, and assessment of the sewing ring and adjacent structures. Aortic valve tissue prostheses are best evaluated by transthoracic echocardiography (TTE) because of the anterior position of the valve in the chest. Transoesophageal echocardiography (TOE) is appropriate when TTE images are suboptimal or when infection is suspected.

For stented aortic valves, anatomy is well demonstrated in the parasternal long- and short-axis views (Figure 4.1). The valve usually is implanted so the three leaflets are in the normal positions of the right, left and non-coronary valve cusps and the thin leaflets can be visualised in many patients. However, in some patients the echogenicity of the three struts and sewing ring result in reverberations and shadowing, limiting visualisation of the leaflets.

Tissue valves that are implanted as an intact valve and root, including aortic homografts and some heterografts, demonstrate increased thickness diffusely in the aortic wall extending from the annulus into the ascending aorta, espe-

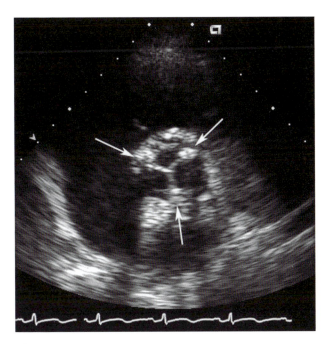

Figure 4.1
Transthoracic parasternal short-axis view of a stented tissue prosthetic valve in the aortic position. The three arrows point to the three stents.

cially at the proximal and distal suture line. Thickening of the aortic wall is most prominent early after surgery and, to some extent, regresses over time. Stentless bioprosthetic valves also may demonstrate increased echogenicity in the aortic root in the early postoperative period but often appear similar to a native aortic valve on long-term follow-up.[2]

The stents of a tissue mitral valve are seen in the parasternal long-axis view, with a typical appearance of the valve orifice directed anteriorly towards the ventricular septum (Figure 4.2). Visualisation of leaflets from the TTE approach is more difficult than for aortic valve prostheses due to the distance of the valve from the transducer and

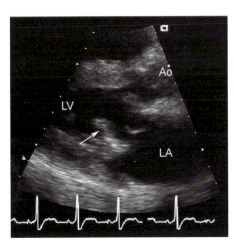
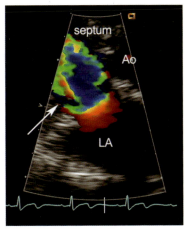

Figure 4.2
Transthoracic parasternal long-axis images of a stented tissue valve in the mitral position. Left: the arrow points to the posterior stent. Colour Doppler demonstrates that the position of the valve directs inflow anteriorly towards the septum. Right: careful evaluation of the left ventricular outflow tract is needed with these valves to ensure no evidence of obstruction. Ao = Ascending aorta, LV = left ventricle, LA = left atrium.

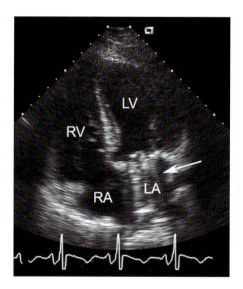

Figure 4.3
Apical four-chamber view of a bileaflet mechanical prosthesis in the mitral position. Note reverberations and shadowing from the prosthesis obscuring the left atrium from this transducer position. Shadow is marked with arrow. RA = right atrium, RV = right ventricle, LA = left atrium, LV = left ventricle.

shadowing by the valve stents, so that TOE should be considered when evaluation of the valve leaflets is needed. With a stented mitral valve prosthesis, it is also important to evaluate for LV outflow tract obstruction due to native valve remnants or excessive protrusion of the mitral valve stents into the outflow tract.[3]

Mechanical valves

Transthoracic imaging of mechanical valves in the aortic or mitral position is also performed in the standard paraster-

nal and apical views. However, image quality is limited by shadowing and reverberations. With a caged-ball valve, reverberations originate both from the metal cage and the spherical ball occluder. A tilting-disc valve results in shadowing related to the sewing ring, and reverberations due to the single circular disc opening at an angle to the annulus plane. With a bileaflet mechanical valve, imaging artefacts are due to the sewing ring and the two semicircular discs which open to form two large lateral orifices and a smaller central orifice (Figure 4.3).

On TOE imaging, an aortic prosthesis is best seen in the high oesophageal views at approximately 0° in short axis and 120° in long axis. A mitral valve prosthesis is best seen in the high oesophageal view, starting in the four-chamber image plane (approximately 0°), followed by slow rotation of the image plane to 120°, with the valve centred in the image.[4] Although shadowing and reverberations still occur, different parts of the image are obscured due to the different site of origin of the ultrasound beam (Figure 4.4). For example, the ventricular side of a mechanical mitral valve is best evaluated from a TTE apical approach, whereas the atrial side of this valve is best evaluated from a TOE approach. Thus, whenever there is clinical evidence for valve dysfunction or infection, TOE imaging is needed for mechanical valves in the mitral position.

Valve repair

Many patients now undergo mitral or tricuspid valve repair, instead of valve replacement. The first step in the echocardiographic evaluation of a repaired valve is to review the operative report to determine the exact type of surgical repair and whether an annuloplasty ring is present (Figure 4.5). The most typical mitral valve repair is quadrangular resection of the middle scallop of the posterior leaflet and placement of an annuloplasty ring. The resulting

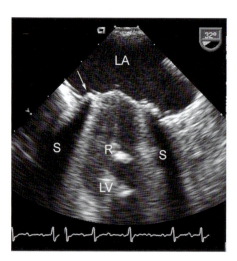
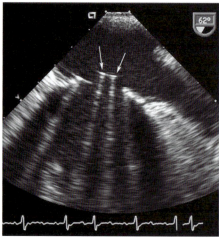

Figure 4.4
Transoesophageal four-chamber view of a bileaflet mechanical mitral prosthesis in systole (left) and diastole (right). In systole the two mechanical leaflets close at a slightly obtuse angle. The sewing ring (arrow) result in shadowing (S) and the leaflets result in reverberations (R), which obscure the left ventricle from this tranducer position. In diastole (right), the two open leaflets assume a parallel orientation (arrows) with a small central and two larger lateral orifices. LA = left atrium, LV = left ventricle.

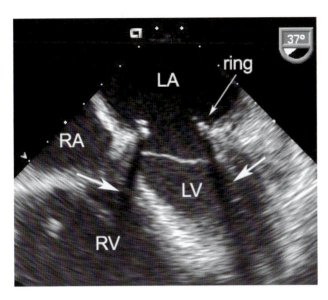

Figure 4.5
In this transesophageal 4-chamber view, a mitral annuloplasty ring is seen. As with a prosthetic valve, the annuloplasty ring causes shadowing (arrows) on echocardiographic examination.

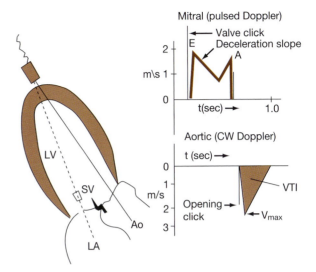

Figure 4.6
Schematic diagram of an apical view showing the correct Doppler beam alignment for accurate transaortic and transmitral flow velocity curves. The apical window usually provides an intercept parallel to flow, so that underestimation of velocities is avoided. Normal prosthetic transmitral flow (upper right) usually can be recorded using pulsed Doppler with the sample volume (SV) positioned just apical to the valve plane. The normal pattern demonstrates an early filling velocity (E), atrial contribution to flow (A) and the deceleration slope. Recording antegrade prosthetic aortic flow usually requires continuous-wave (CW) Doppler due to the higher flow velocities. Lower right: the maximum velocity (V_{max}) and velocity time integral (VTI) are used in evaluation of valve function. LV = left ventricle, LA = left atrium, Ao = aorta.

echocardiographic findings include a thickened and relatively immobile posterior mitral leaflet and an echo-dense annuloplasty ring that causes reverberations and shadowing. The annular ring also results in a slight reduction in valve area so that a modest increase in transvalvular velocity and mean gradient is typical. With a successful mitral repair, only trace to mild residual regurgitation is seen.

Echocardiographic evaluation after valve repair is performed using the same approach as for a prosthetic valve. Transthoracic imaging is performed in parasternal and apical views, along with Doppler evaluation of transmitral velocity, mean valve gradient and effective orifice area. Colour Doppler is used to evaluate for residual mitral regurgitation, although transesophageal imaging often is needed when significant regurgitation is suspected.[4a] In addition, rigid annuloplasty rings have been associated with systolic anterior motion of the anterior leaflet resulting in dynamic subaortic LV outflow obstruction.[4b]

Doppler evaluation

Doppler evaluation is a standard component of every echocardiographic examination because imaging alone has a low sensitivity and specificity for detection of valve dysfunction. Normal Doppler velocity data depend on the type, size and position of the prosthetic valve, as detailed in Chapter 5, and it is helpful to have tables of normal values for the types of prosthetic valves used at your medical centre available in the echocardiography laboratory.

As with any Doppler technique, accurate data recording requires careful attention to technical aspects of the examination (Figure 4.6). Most importantly, care is needed to ensure a parallel intercept angle between the ultrasound beam and direction of blood flow to avoid underestimation of velocities (and pressure gradients). This potential source of error is minimised by an experienced echocardiographer using multiple acoustic windows (sometimes including TOE) with careful transducer angulation to obtain the highest velocity signal.

Antegrade velocities across a mitral or tricuspid prosthesis are easily recorded from a transthoracic apical view using pulsed- or continuous-wave (CW) Doppler. Antegrade mitral velocities are sometimes recorded from a parasternal long-axis view if the valve is aimed towards the ventricular septum. In some cases, tricuspid velocity data may be recorded from a parasternal right ventricular inflow view. From the transoesophageal approach, antegrade mitral velocities are easily recorded from a high transoesophageal view in a four-chamber or long-axis image plane. Color Doppler guidance may be helpful in

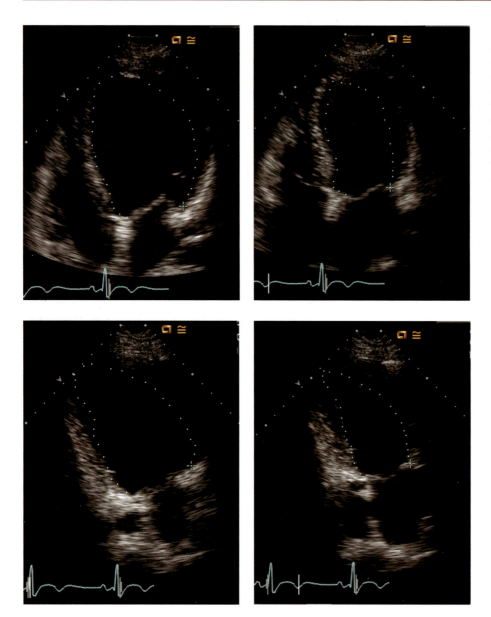

Figure 4.7
Apical images of a patient with chronic aortic regurgitation and a dilated left ventricle demonstrating the views needed for biplane ejection fraction calculations. Endocardial borders are traced in a four-chamber (top) and two-chamber (bottom) view at end-diastole (left) and end-systole (right).

alignment of the ultrasound beam in the centre of the flow stream.

Antegrade velocities across an aortic prosthesis usually are too high for measurement with pulsed Doppler so that CW Doppler is needed. A dedicated small CW Doppler probe should be used, as the smaller probe allows better angulation of the beam direction and the signal-to-noise ratio is optimal. The highest transaortic velocity may be recorded from the apex or from a suprasternal notch or high right parasternal view. All of these acoustic windows should be tried, with appropriate patient positioning to identify the highest flow velocity. On TOE examination, it is difficult to align the ultrasound beam parallel to the aortic flow stream. A signal may be obtained from a transgastric apical view, but this may underestimate velocity due to a non-parallel intercept angle.

Most prosthetic valves have a small amount of normal backflow (or regurgitation) across the valve. A combination of colour Doppler flow mapping and CW Doppler recordings are used to evaluate for prosthetic valve regurgitation. If the degree of regurgitation is greater than expected for the valve type and position, further evaluation of regurgitant severity is warranted.

The left ventricle

Patients with long-standing valve disease usually have alterations in LV size, wall thickness, diastolic, or systolic function. Chronic severe aortic regurgitation, for example, results in a dilated LV, whereas chronic severe aortic stenosis results in concentric LV hypertrophy. After valve

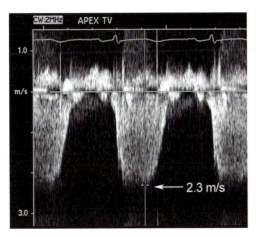 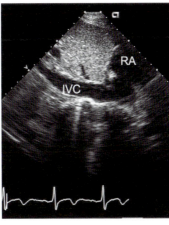

Figure 4.8
Pulmonary pressure is calculated from the continous wave (CW) Doppler recording of tricuspid regurgitation jet velocity from whatever window yields the highest velocity (left) and from the size and respiratory variation in the inferior vena cava (IVC). The peak tricuspid regurgitant jet velocity and the right atrial pressure (which is based on IVC dynamics) can be used in the simplified Bernoulli equation to estimate pulmonary artery systolic pressures. In this example, the estimated pulmonary systolic pressure is $4(2.3)^2 + 5 = 26$ mmHg (normal).

replacement these changes reverse, at least to some degree, so that periodic evaluation includes measurement of the extent of improvement in diastolic function and regression of LV hypertrophy or dilation. Evaluation of LV regional and global systolic function is based on standard views. Ideally, LV volumes and ejection fraction should be calculated based on manual tracing of endocardial borders at end-diastole and end-systole in apical four-chamber and two-chamber views, using the biplane volume formula (Figure 4.7). On TTE imaging, when endocardial border definition is suboptimal, the use of echocardiographic contrast agents that opacify the LV may be helpful.

On TOE imaging, LV function should be evaluated in standard four-chamber, two-chamber and long-axis views obtained from a high oesophageal position by rotating the image plane with the ventricular apex centred in the image. When a mitral prosthetic valve is present, reverberations and shadowing may obscure the LV; in this case, evaluation by transthoracic imaging is preferable.

In patients with a prosthetic aortic valve, LV diastolic function is assessed based on transmitral filling patterns, measurement of the isovolumic relaxation time, tissue Doppler myocardial velocities and the pulmonary vein flow pattern. However, evaluation of diastolic function is problematic in patients with a mitral prosthesis, as parameters of diastolic filling more often reflect the effects of the valve prosthesis, rather than LV diastolic function.

Pulmonary artery pressures and right heart

Long-standing valvular heart disease such as mitral stenosis often results in pulmonary hypertension. After successful valve repair or replacement, pulmonary pressures typically decrease over time and may even normalise. Thus, it is important to assess pulmonary pressures early after valve replacement for comparison with follow-up examinations. A lack of a fall in pulmonary pressures after surgery, or a rise in pulmonary pressures later in the post-operative course, should prompt consideration of mitral prosthetic valve dysfunction.

Pulmonary artery pressures (PAP) are obtained non-invasively by measuring the peak tricuspid regurgitant (TR) velocities using CW Doppler (Figure 4.8). The TR jet is examined from both parasternal and apical views with careful transducer angulation to identify the highest velocity signal. The right ventricular to right atrial systolic pressure difference is calculated using the simplified Bernoulli equation ($4V^2$) and then added to right atrial pressure (RAP):

$$PAP = 4V_{TR}^2 + RAP$$

A limitation of echocardiography is that pulmonary vascular resistance cannot be accurately measured. If this information is needed for clinical decision-making, right heart catheterisation is appropriate. Right atrial pressure is estimated from the size and respiratory variation in the inferior vena cava (IVC), visualised in the subcostal view at the junction with the right atrium.

Right ventricular (RV) size and systolic function are assessed from standard views, with evaluation of the shape, size, wall thickness and degree of wall motion. Patients with long-standing pulmonary hypertension from valvular heart disease often have RV dilation and hypertrophy. RV dilation is significant when it approaches or exceeds LV size (assuming normal LV size). RV hypertrophy is diagnosed when the right ventricular free wall thickness is >0.5 cm. Systolic function is graded qualitatively as normal, mildly, moderately or severely reduced.

Atrial enlargement

The left atrium can be evaluated in the parasternal long-axis, apical two-chamber view, apical four-chamber view and subcostal view. Left atrial dimension is commonly measured as the anterior-posterior diameter in the parasternal long-axis view, although some clinicians also measure left atrial length in an apical four-chamber view or even planimeter left atrial area in apical views. Left atrial enlargement is usually seen in patients with mitral prostheses for mitral stenosis or mitral regurgitation. Atrial enlargement typically does not regress after successful valve surgery.

Left atrial thrombi may complicate the clinical course in patients with prosthetic valves, especially in patients with atrial fibrillation. Transthoracic imaging has a very low sensitivity for detection of left atrial thombi because many are located in the atrial appendage and because the left atrium is obscured by the valve reverberations and shadowing. If evaluation for atrial thrombus is needed, TOE imaging is very accurate for this diagnosis. Occasionally, the left atrial appendage becomes inverted, simulating a left atrial mass on TOE imaging. The echocardiographer should review the operative report prior to the study, as some surgeons remove the left atrial appendage at the time of mitral valve surgery.

Aortic dilation

Aortic root dilation often is present in patients with aortic regurgitation and in some patients with aortic stenosis. In particular, a history of a bicuspid aortic valve is associated with aortic dilation and an increased risk of aortic dissection.[5] The aortic root and ascending aorta are evaluated in a high parasternal long-axis and the suprasternal notch view. The descending thoracic aorta is visualised from the suprasternal notch and from a posteriorly angulated apical two-chamber view. The proximal abdominal aorta is visualised in the subcostal view. The normal pattern of aortic antegrade flow in the descending thoracic aorta shows a peak velocity of 1 m/s and brief early diastolic flow reversal.[6] Holodiastolic flow reversal in the abdominal or descending thoracic aorta indicates significant aortic valve regurgitation, unless a patent ductus arteriosus or other aortopulmonary shunt is present.

Echocardiographic evaluation of prosthetic valve dysfunction

Prosthetic valve stenosis

If a higher than expected antegrade velocity is recorded across the valve, prosthetic valve stenosis should be considered. As with native valves, evaluation of stenosis severity is based on measurement of antegrade velocities and calcula-

tion of pressure gradients and valve area. Other clues to the pressure of prosthetic stenosis on echocardiography include persistent left ventricular hypertrophy after aortic valve replacement and persistent or recurrent pulmonary hypertension after mitral valve replacement.

Pressure gradients

Pressure gradients (ΔP) are calculated from velocities (V) using the simplified Bernoulli equation:

$$\Delta P = 4V^2$$

with the maximum velocity used to calculate the maximum pressure gradient and with averaging of the instantaneous pressure gradients in systole for calculation of the mean gradient. Clinically, mean gradients are more useful than peak gradients in evaluating prosthetic valve haemodynamics because prosthetic valves have a high peak instantaneous velocity due to a high-pressure gradient at the time of valve opening. This is evident in the more triangular shape of the antegrade velocity across a prosthetic aortic valve compared to the rounded curve seen with native aortic valve stenosis. However, mean gradients are normal because of rapid equilibration of pressures later in the cardiac cycle.[4]

Multiple studies have verified that mean and maximal gradients correspond well to simultaneous catheter data in bioprosthetic and mechanical valves in the aortic, mitral and tricuspid positions[7–12] (Table 4.3). As with any intracardiac Doppler data, velocities and pressure gradients may be underestimated if there is a non-parallel angle between the ultrasound beam and direction of blood flow. However, overestimation of gradients also can occur when the velocity proximal (or upstream) to the valve is not negligible. When the proximal velocity is >1.5 m/s, both the proximal velocity (V_1) and aortic jet velocity (V_2) should be included in the Bernoulli equation:

$$\Delta P = 4(V_2^2 - V_1^2)$$

Another cause of overestimation of prosthetic valve gradients is related to the central smaller orifice of a bileaflet mechanical valve, which results in a localised higher velocity (see Chapter 5). This high-velocity signal will be correctly recorded by CW Doppler, reflecting the localised high velocity rather than the effective mean transvalvular gradient.[10] Overestimation of gradients also may be due to pressure recovery downstream from the valve. As discussed in Chapter 5, some of the issues related to overestimation of pressure gradients with bileaflet mechanical valves are less important the greater the degree of valve stenosis.

Aortic prostheses have higher gradients than mitral prostheses because of the combination of a smaller valve

Table 4.3 Validation of Doppler echo prosthetic mean valve gradients compared with invasive data (selected series)

First author, year	Valve type/position	n	r	SEE (mmHg)	Mean difference
Sagar,[7] 1986	Hancock & B.S./mitral	19	0.93	2.5	
Sagar,[7] 1986	Hancock & B.S./aortic	11	0.94	7.4	
Wilkins,[10] 1986	Starr-Edwards, B.S./porcine/mitral	11	0.96	–	
Burstow,[8] 1989	Mixed/aortic	20	0.94	3	
	Mixed/mitral	20	0.97	1.2	
Baumgartner,[9] 1990	St. Jude	In vitro	0.98	1.9	10±3 mmHg
	Hancock	In vitro	0.98	1.4	2±1 mmHg
Stewart,[11] 1991	Bioprosthetic/aortic	in vitro	0.78–0.98		Overestimation by Doppler
Baumgartner,[12] 1992	St. Jude	In vitro	0.98	2.0	13±8 mmHg
	Medtronic–Hall	In vitro	0.99	0.5	0.8±0.6 mmHg
	Starr–Edwards	In vitro	0.97	2.0	8±4 mmHg
	Hancock	In vitro	0.99	1.5	1.9±1.6 mmHg

B.S. = Bjork–Shiley tilting-disc mechanical valve. SEE = Standard error of estimate.
Reprinted from Otto CM, Textbook of clinical echocardiography, 3rd edn. Philadelphia: WB Saunders, 2004 with permission from Elsevier.

area and higher transvalvular pressure gradient during the period of antegrade flow. Right-sided valves have lower velocities than the corresponding left-sided heart valves. For example, a maximum pressure gradient of >8 mmHg suggests stenosis[13] of a tricuspid prosthesis, but this may be a normal maximum pressure for a mitral prosthesis. Reference to normal Doppler data for various valves helps in interpretation of transvalvular gradients, especially when baseline values for that patient are not available.[13,14] In the early postoperative period, velocities and pressure gradients may be elevated due to a high output state related to sympathetic nervous system activation and anaemia. Velocities normalise to expected values by 3 months after surgery, which is the optimal time to perform the baseline echocardiogram, unless clinical signs or symptoms have necessitated earlier evaluation.

Continuity equation valve area

The use of Doppler echo has been validated in the estimation of prosthetic valve areas (Table 4.4).[7,10,15–17] As with

Table 4.4 Validation of Doppler echo prosthetic valve areas (selected series)

First author, year	Valve type/position	n	Comparison	r	SEE	Mean difference
Sagar,[7] 1986	Hancock & B.S./mitral	12	$T_{1/2}$ vs Gorlin	0.98	0.1 cm²	
Wilkins,[10] 1986	Porcine/mitral	8	$T_{1/2}$ vs Gorlin	0.65	–	–
Rothbart,[15] 1990	Bioprosthetic/aortic	22	Cont eq vs Gorlin at cath	0.93	–	–
Chafizadeh,[16] 1991	St. Jude/aortic	67	Cont eq vs. actual orifice area	0.83		Doppler effective orifice area less than actual orifice area
Baumgartner,[17] 1992	St. Jude	In vitro	Cont eq vs Gorlin	0.99	0.08	0.4–0.6 cm²
	Medtronic–Hall	In vitro		0.97	0.10	0–0.25 cm²
	Hancock aortic	In vitro		0.93	0.10	0-0.25 cm²

B.S. = Bjork–Shiley tilting-disc mechanical valve; Cont eq = continuity equation valve area with Doppler and 2D echo data; Gorlin = Gorlin formula valve area using invasive data; $T_{1/2}$ = Doppler pressure half-time method.
Reprinted from Otto CM, Textbook of clinical echocardiography, 3rd edn. Philadelphia: WB Saunders, 2004 with permission from Elsevier.

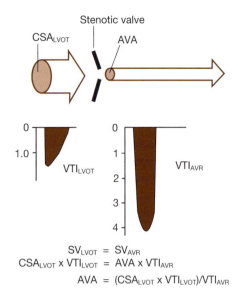

$$SV_{LVOT} = SV_{AVR}$$
$$CSA_{LVOT} \times VTI_{LVOT} = AVA \times VTI_{AVR}$$
$$AVA = (CSA_{LVOT} \times VTI_{LVOT})/VTI_{AVR}$$

Figure 4.9
The continuity equation allows calculation of stenotic valve area based on the principle that the volumes of flow proximal to and in the stenotic valve are equal. Left ventricular outflow tract (LVOT) stroke volume (SV) is represented by an arrow with the cross-sectional area (CSA) of the base of the arrow representing the LVOT-CSA and the length of the arrow representing the velocity time integral of flow (VTI). The VTI is calculated by tracing the velocity curve of flow and conceptually represents the distance the average blood cell travelled on that beat. The velocity time integral (VTI) is the product of velocity (measured in cm/s) multiplied by time (in seconds) to yield units of cm for the VTI (VTI = cm/s × s = cm). The flow through the stenotic valve is represented by the arrow with a cross-sectional area equal to the aortic valve area (AVA) and a length equal to the VTI of flow through the aortic valve replacement (AVR).

native valves, transvalvular velocities and gradients across prosthetic valves vary with volume flow rate for a given orifice area.[8] Therefore, a high velocity may be found with normal prosthetic valve function when there is an increased cardiac output such as in anaemia or a febrile illness. Conversely, a low velocity may be present despite severe stenosis if cardiac output is depressed, such as with LV dysfunction. Therefore, a flow-independent measure of prosthetic valve function is needed for assessment of valve haemodynamics. The continuity equation has been validated for central orifice tissue aortic valves with anatomy and haemodynamics similar to a native valve.[15] The continuity equation is based on the concept that the stroke volumes proximal to the valve and within the prosthetic (inherently stenotic) valve are equal (Figure 4.9). Because volume flow rate in the LV outflow tract (LVOT) and aortic valve replacement (AVR) are equal to the product of the cross-sectional area (CSA) and the velocity time integral (VTI of flow in systole):

$$CSA_{AVR} \times VTI_{AVR} = CSA_{LVOT} \times VTI_{LVOT}$$

Solving for prosthetic valve area:

$$CSA_{AVR} = (CSA_{LVOT} \times VTI_{LVOT})/VTI_{AVR}$$

LVOT diameter is measured from the septal endocardium to the anterior mitral leaflet, parallel to and immediately adjacent to the aortic valve in a parasternal long-axis view during mid-systole (Figure 4.10). The LVOT diameter should be directly measured because the implanted prosthetic valve size refers to the external diameter of the sewing ring and not the effective diameter of the subvalvular flow region. The LVOT velocity is recorded from an

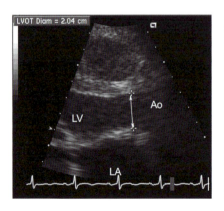
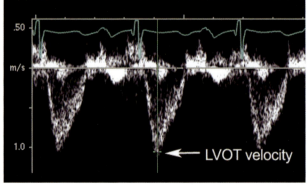

Figure 4.10
The stroke volume in the left ventricular outflow tract (LVOT) is calculated using LVOT diameter measured in a parasternal long-axis view in mid-systole from the septal endocardium to the anterior mitral leaflet, parallel to and immediately adjacent to the aortic valve (right), and the LVOT velocity is recorded from an apical approach using pulsed Doppler with the sample volume positioned immediately adjacent to the valve. Ao = ascending aorta, LV = left ventricle, LA = left atrium.

apical approach using pulsed Doppler with the sample volume positioned just proximal to the prosthetic valve, avoiding the small region of flow acceleration adjacent to the valve (Figure 4.10). The aortic jet velocity is recorded with CW Doppler from multiple windows in order to obtain the highest velocity signal (Figure 4.11). In a patient with suspected prosthetic valve stenosis, evaluation includes measurement of maximum velocity, mean gradient and continuity equation valve area (Figure 4.12).

Transvalvular velocity ratio

The continuity equation may not be as accurate with mechanical valves because of the assumption of a flat flow velocity profile within the valve orifice. Empirically, the 'velocity ratio' is a useful clinical measure; it is defined as the ratio of outflow tract maximum velocity to aortic jet maximum velocity. There are several advantages of the velocity ratio: aortic jet velocity is effectively indexed for transvalvular volume flow rate; an outflow tract diameter measurement is not needed; and the measurement is straightforward and reproducible.[16] A ratio close to 1 indicates the absence of obstruction. Because all prosthetic valves are inherently stenotic, the normal velocity ratio ranges from 0.35 to 0.50 for prosthetic valves, compared with 0.75 to 0.90 for a normal native valve. While the velocity ratio does not provide an absolute measure of valve function, it can be very useful for following serial changes in an individual patient.

Pressure half-time method

The pressure half-time ($T_{1/2}$) method has been applied to both mitral and tricuspid prosthetic valves (Figure 4.13). As with native valves, the rate of decline in diastolic pressure across the valve reflects functional valve area (Figure 4.14). With central flow tissue valves, it is reasonable to use the empiric constant of 220, derived from native mitral valve stenosis, for calculation of prosthetic mitral valve area (MVA):[18]

$$MVA = 220/T_{1/2}$$

With mechanical mitral or tricuspid valves, it is still helpful to calculate the pressure half-time (Figures 4.15 and 4.16) but, it is less clear whether it is appropriate to use the empiric constant. Our practice is to report the pressure half-time itself, and (as with the aortic velocity ratio) use the data for serial follow-up of individual patients. The pressure half-time is measured as the time interval from the peak pressure gradient to the time point corresponding to 50% of the peak gradient on the transvalvular velocity curve. The Doppler data are best recorded from an apical

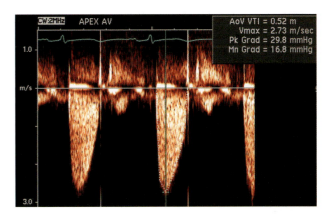

Figure 4.11
In the same patient as Figure 4.10, the maximum aortic jet is measured with continuous-wave (CW) Doppler from whichever window yields the highest velocity flow. In this patient, the highest velocity signal was obtained from the apical window. The signal has a well-defined curve, with a clear peak and opening and closing clicks.

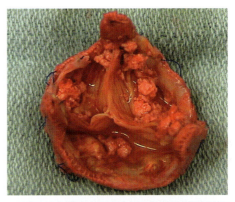

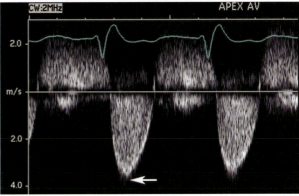

Figure 4.12
This 72-year-old woman presented 10 years after aortic valve replacement with severe exertional dyspnoea. Bottom: echocardiography showed prosthetic aortic valve stenosis, with a maximum jet velocity of 3.8 m/s and a continuity equation valve area of 0.7 cm². This was a marked change compared with her previous postoperative studies. She underwent repeat aortic valve replacement. The arrow indicates maximum jet velocity. Left: the explanted valve shows severe calcification of the prosthetic leaflets.

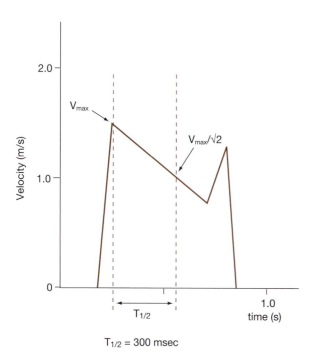

$T_{1/2} = 300 \text{ msec}$

Figure 4.13
The method for measuring pressure half-time from the mitral inflow pattern is based on the time interval from the peak pressure gradient to the point in diastole where the peak gradient falls to half of its original value. The maximum velocity (V_{max}) corresponds to the maximum pressure gradient but half the gradient is equal to the maximum velocity divided by $\sqrt{2}$, because of the quadratic relationship between velocity and the pressure gradient. When the deceleration curve is non-linear, the probe should be repositioned to obtain a better signal. If a non-linear pattern persists or if diastole is short in duration, the mid-diastolic slope is extrapolated for this measurement.

approach using pulsed or CW Doppler (depending on the velocity scale needed) on TTE and from a four-chamber or long-axis orientation on TOE imaging.

Patient–prosthesis mismatch

Patient–prosthesis mismatch (PPM), initially described in 1978 by Rahimtoola,[19] is defined as an effective orifice area (EOA) that is too small for body size. PPM results in persistent symptoms, due to inability to maintain an adequate cardiac output to meet metabolic demands, and is associated with persistent LV hypertrophy after aortic valve replacement. Patient–prosthesis mismatch is defined as an EOA <0.85 cm^2/m^2, based on studies comparing symptom status to EOA. Prospective studies have demonstrated that PPM is associated with a higher short-term and long-term

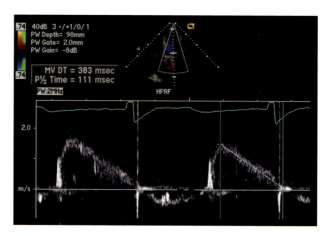

Figure 4.14
This 68-year-old patient is status post mitral valve replacement with a bioprosthetic stented mitral prosthesis for rheumatic mitral valve disease. The mitral velocity curve demonstrated a pressure half-time of 111 ms, consistent with a functional valve area of 2.0 cm^2, using the empiric constant of 220.

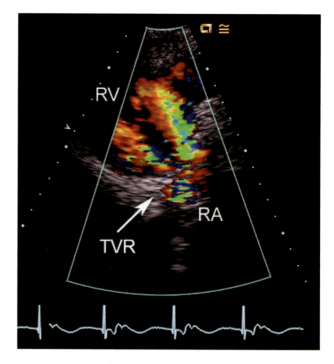

Figure 4.15
This 46-year-old man had undergone tricuspid valve replacement with a bileaflet mechanical valve several years previously. He now presents with increasing fatigue, abdominal girth and lower extremity oedema. Review of his anticoagulation records showed non-compliance, with an INR of 1.0 on admission. In the right ventricular inflow view, colour Doppler demonstrates two jets across the valve in diastole, consistent with limited valve leaflet motion and significant stenosis.

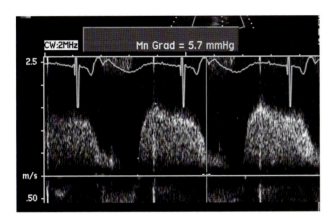

Figure 4.16
The continuous-wave (CW) Doppler recording of tricuspid inflow in the same patient as Figure 4.15 shows a prolonged pressure half-time and a mean gradient of 5.7 mmHg. At surgery, valve thrombosis was confirmed.

mortality after valve surgery, especially in patients with diminished LV systolic function.[20,21] In patients with even more severe PPM (an indexed EOA <0.65 cm^2/m^2), there is a high incidence of heart failure.

Patient–prosthesis mismatch is prevented by ensuring implantation of an adequately sized valve substitute. Before surgery, the minimal EOA needed to avoid PPM is determined by multiplying the desired postoperative-indexed EOA by the patient's BSA. A prosthesis is chosen based on published reference effective valve areas for each type and size of prosthesis.[20] The need to achieve an adequate EOA also must be balanced with other factors favouring a tissue or mechanical valve in these patients. In some cases, the surgeon may need to consider an aortic root enlarging procedure to ensure the functional valve area will be adequate for patient size. The echocardiographic evaluation of prosthetic valve haemodynamics should take into account the possibility of PPM when higher than expected transvalvular gradients are encountered.

Prosthetic valve regurgitation

Evaluation of prosthetic valve regurgitation requires integration of multiple approaches, including colour Doppler flow patterns, pulsed Doppler data and CW Doppler velocity curves. Visualisation of a flow disturbance in the left atrium in systole (for the mitral valve) or in the LVOT in diastole (for the aortic valve) is clear evidence that regurgitation is present. However, as for native valves, the size of the distal flow disturbance is a suboptimal measure of regurgitant severity.[22] Instead, the proximal flow geometry, including the proximal flow convergence region (or PISA) and vena contracta, provide more quantitative measures of

regurgitant severity.[23,24] In addition, the CW Doppler curve provides data on the volume of regurgitation based on the relative intensity of antegrade versus retrograde flow and the time course of the pressure difference between the two chambers on either side of the valve.[25] Pulsed Doppler allows detection of distal flow reversals, e.g., holodiastolic flow reversal in the descending aorta in patients with severe aortic regurgitation. Regurgitant volumes, regurgitant fraction and regurgitant orifice area can be calculated using the proximal isovelocity surface area (PISA) approach on colour flow imaging. Alternatively, regurgitant volume and orifice area can be calculated by measurement of forward stroke volume by pulsed Doppler in combination with 2D-echocardiographic measurement of total stroke volume. For example, in a patient with a mitral prosthesis, forward stroke volume is measured by Doppler across the native aortic valve and total stroke volume calculated from 2D LV volumes using the apical biplane method.

Quantifying the amount of regurgitation is challenging, in part because a small amount of regurgitation is normal for most prosthetic valves.[26,27] In addition, there is no consensus statement on the optimal approach to evaluation or quantitation of prosthetic valve regurgitation. In the absence of specific recommendations, it is reasonable to apply the criteria for regurgitation severity of native valves developed by the American Society of Echocardiography to evaluate prosthetic regurgitation (Table 4.5).

Table 4.5 Definition of regurgitant severity based on American Society of Echocardiography Guidelines*

Parameter	Mild	Severe
Aortic regurgitation		
Jet width/LVOT	<25%	>65%
Vena contracta	<0.3 cm	>0.6 cm
Pressure half-time	>500 ms	<200 ms
Regurgitant volume	>30 ml/beat	≥60 ml/beat
Regurgitant fraction	<30%	≥50%
Regurgitant orifice area	<0.10 cm^2	>0.30 cm^2
Mitral regurgitation		
Jet area	<20% LA area	>40% LA area
Vena contracta	<0.3 cm	≥0.7 cm
Regurgitant volume	<30 ml	≥60 ml
Regurgitant fraction	<30%	≥50%
Regurgitant orifice area	<0.20 cm^2	≥0.40 cm^2

LA = left atrial, LVOT = left ventricular outflow tract.
*Criteria are specifically for native valves. Formal criteria do not exist for prosthetic valves but it is probably reasonable to apply these criteria to prosthetic valves. Reprinted from Otto CM, Textbook of clinical echocardiography, 3rd edn. Philadelphia: WB Saunders, 2004 with permission from Elsevier.

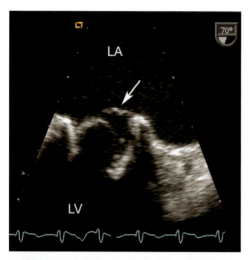

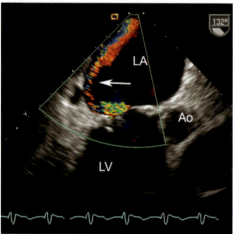

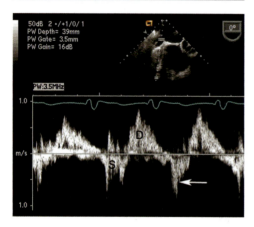

Figure 4.17

This 86-year-old patient with an 18-year-old mitral valve replacement presented with severe dyspnoea at rest, pulmonary crackles on examination and a loud holosystolic murmur. Transoesophagal images demonstrate a flail posterior mitral leaflet (arrow) during systole. Colour Doppler shows severe eccentric anteriorly directed mitral regurgitation due to the flail posterior leaflet. Pulsed Doppler examination of flow in the right upper pulmonary vein demonstrates systolic flow reversal consistent with severe mitral regurgitation. LA = left atrium, LV = left ventricle.

For aortic regurgitation, a simple approach is first to look for a regurgitant jet on transthoracic colour flow imaging. Next, the CW Doppler velocity curve is examined for signal intensity and diastolic slope. Finally, pulsed Doppler is recorded in the descending thoracic and proximal abdominal aorta to detect holodiastolic flow reversal. In the rare case where further quantitation is needed, parameters of regurgitant severity can be calculated from the difference between transmitral stroke volume (forward stroke volume) and 2D total stroke volume based on tracing endocardial LV borders.

For mitral regurgitation, the sensitivity of the transthoracic examination is limited by three key factors:

- there is a higher degree of normal regurgitation in prosthetic valves than normal valves
- the prosthetic valve has a higher antegrade velocity
- acoustic shadowing, reverberations and other artefacts make evaluation of prosthetic regurgitation more difficult.

TOE imaging is needed for evaluation of prosthetic mitral regurgitation because the left atrium is shadowed by the prosthesis on transthoracic imaging (Figure 4.17). TOE colour flow imaging is directed towards detection and measurement of the vena contracta and PISA, as well as evaluation of the size and shape of the regurgitant jet. Other helpful parameters are the CW Doppler signal and the flow pattern in the pulmonary veins, with systolic flow reversal suggesting severe regurgitation.[28–31]

Prosthetic valve endocarditis

The echocardiographic evaluation for prosthetic valve endocarditis involves interrogation of the entire valve apparatus, because infection of a mechanical valve often involves the sewing ring and annulus. Although isolated mild paravalvular regurgitation is not diagnostic of endocarditis, pathological regurgitation, especially if a new finding, is consistent with endocarditis. TTE has only a limited ability to detect vegetations because of acoustic shadowing and reverberations. TOE is highly sensitive for detecting prosthetic valve vegetations (Figure 4.18) and paravalvular abscess.[32–34] A paravalvular abscess appears as an irregularly shaped echolucent area adjacent to the valve sewing ring. The presence of valve dehiscence, pseudoaneurysms, fistulae, moderate-to-severe paravalvular regurgitation or vegetations seen in various combinations have high positive and negative predictive value.[35]

Prosthetic valve thrombosis

Prosthetic valve thrombosis may present as new regurgitation, an increased transvalvular gradient or a systemic

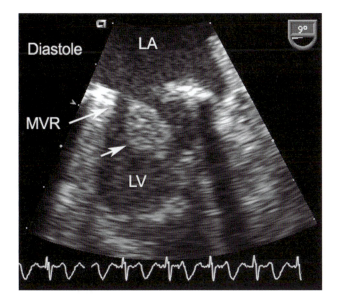

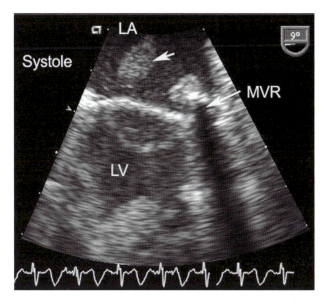

Figure 4.18
This 56-year-old woman, status post mitral valve replacement (MVR) 5 years previously for rheumatic mitral stenosis, presented with leucocytosis, hypotension and staphylococcus bacteraemia. The transoesophageal four-chamber images show the mechanical bileaflet mitral valve with two large vegetations (arrow) seen in the left ventricle (LV) in diastole (bottom), prolapsing into the left atrium (LA) in systole (top). The long arrow points to the valve sewing ring.

embolic event. Echocardiographic evaluation for thrombosis involves imaging the prosthetic valve, measuring the gradient through the valve and finding regurgitation. TOE is often needed to detect mitral prosthesis thrombosis, because thrombus most often involves the left atrial side of the valve sewing ring.[36–38] Despite use of TTE and TOE, determination of valve thrombosis can be difficult. Shadowing and other artefacts may make it difficult to see leaflets or mechanical discs. Cinefluoroscopy can be used for mechanical valves, imaging the discs to determine their motion.[39] In a patient with a prosthetic valve and a systemic embolic event, the presumed 'source of embolus' is always the prosthetic valve, even if the echocardiogram appears

normal; thrombus may be too small to be detected or may no longer be on the valve after the embolic event. The absence of visible thrombus on echocardiography should not dissuade the physician from an appropriate increase in antithrombotic therapy.

Aneurysms and pseudoaneurysms

Left ventricular pseudoaneurysm formation can complicate mitral valve replacement.[40–43] It is characterised by disruption in the integrity of the LV wall at the posterior

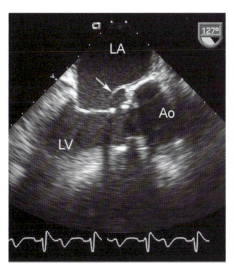

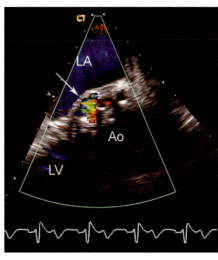

Figure 4.19
Transoesophageal image of a patient with persistent fevers after mitral valve replacement demonstrating an aneurysm of the aorta–mitral intervalvular fibrosa (arrow). Colour Doppler demonstrates flow within the aneurysm into the aneurysm from the left ventricular outflow tract. LA = left atrium, LV = left ventricle, Ao = ascending aorta.

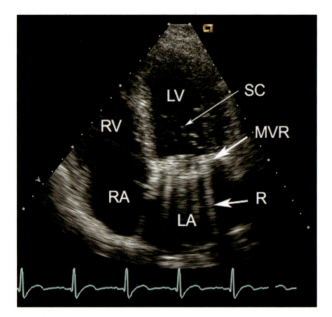

Figure 4.20
In this 36-year-old woman with mechanical mitral valve replacement for mitral valve prolapse that was not amenable to valve repair, spontaneous contrast (SC) is seen on the left ventricular (LV) side of the mitral valve replacement (MVR). Reverberations (R) from the prosthesis are also seen obscuring the left atrium (LA). RA = right atrium, RV = right ventricle.

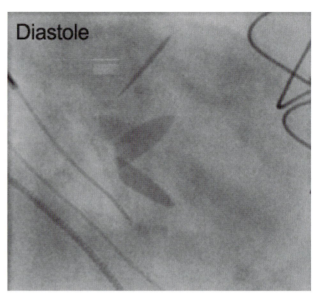

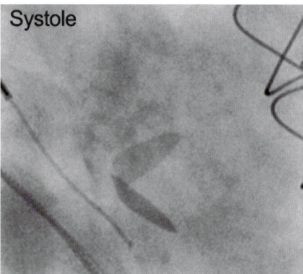

Figure 4.21
Cinefluoroscopy of a mechanical bileaflet prosthetic valve in the tricuspid position in a patient who presented with right heart failure and was non compliant with anticoagulation therapy. In diastole (top), the valve leaflets do not open fully (the leaflets should assume a near parallel orientation). Notice that the bileaflet mechanical aortic valve is closed with a normal appearance. In systole (bottom) the tricuspid valve does not close. The aortic prosthesis is not well seen as the open leaflets are parallel to the X-ray beam.

mitral valve annular suture line, allowing blood to escape into a thin-walled sac lined by pericardial adhesions. The echocardiographic features of an LV pseudoaneurysm consist of a thin-walled chamber that communicates with the LV through a narrow neck. Classically, the ratio of the aneurysm neck diameter to the total aneurysm diameter is less than 0.5. Also, an abrupt transition is seen from normal myocardium to the opening of the aneurysm. Doppler imaging may demonstrate blood flow in and out of the pseudoaneurysm.[44–46] Transthoracic images may be suboptimal due to artefact created by the prosthesis, so that TOE imaging may be needed.[47,48]

An aneurysm of the mitral–aortic intervalvular fibrosa can also occur after aortic or mitral valve surgery (Figure 4.19) and is often a sign of infection.[49] In a long-axis view, an echolucent area is seen at the base of the anterior mitral leaflet, disrupting the normal continuity of this leaflet with the posterior aortic root. Blood flow in and out of the aneurysm typically occurs from the LVOT side of the valve.

Aortic pseudoaneurysms rarely occur after aortic valve replacement. Dehiscence at the suture line between the valve and native aorta results in a collection of blood/haematoma that is contained by adhesions. Doppler evaluation may demonstrate flow into and out of the aneurysm.[50]

Spontaneous contrast

Spontaneous contrast or 'microbubbles' are high-intensity echo signals seen in up to 90% of patients with mechanical valves, often on transthoracic and more easily on TOE imaging[51] (Figure 4.20). Patients with EF <45%, larger valve sizes and a longer duration of implantation are more likely to have spontaneous contrast.[51–53] The mechanism of spontaneous contrast with prosthetic valves is thought to be microcavitation related to the velocity of prosthetic valve closure, resulting in formation of small gas bubbles.[51,54,55]

Other approaches

When echocardiography is nondiagnostic, cardiac catheterization may be helpful in evaluation of patients with suspected prosthetic valve dysfunction. Measurement of intracardiac pressures allows evaluation of transvalvular pressure gradients; although trans-septal puncture often is needed as most invasive cardiologists prefer to avoid retrograde passage of a catheter across a mechanical valve. Left ventricular or aortic angiography allows identification and semi-quantitation of prosthetic regurgitation. However, the most useful approach with mechanical valves is simple cinefluoroscopy of valve motion.[56] With use of an angle that shows disk motion, the pattern of motion can be compared to expected motion for that valve type. Failure of normal disk opening and closing (Figure 4.21) or erratic disk motion can be identified.

Conclusion

Echocardiography provides important information about prosthetic valve structure, haemodynamics and associated structures. The timing of echocardiographic evaluation is based on patient symptoms and the durability and possible complications of the valve. Technical limitations and complicated fluid dynamics limit the ease of echocardiographic evaluation. However, an organised and detailed approach with knowledge regarding limitations and pitfalls will allow the echocardiographer to obtain information that will help the clinician make informed decisions in the management of these patients.

References

1. Otto CM. Textbook of clinical echocardiography, 3rd edn. Philadelphia: WB Saunders, 2004.
2. Vongpatanasin W, Hillis LD, Lange RA. Prosthetic heart valves. N Engl J Med 1996; 335:405–16.
3. Reitman GW, van der Maaten JMAA, Douglas YL, Boonstra PW. Echocardiographic diagnosis of left ventricular outflow tract obstruction after mitral valve replacement with subvalvular preservation. Eur J Cardiothorac Surg 2002; 22:825–27.
4. Otto CM. Valvular heart disease, 2nd edn. Philadelphia: WB Saunders, 2004.
4a. Flameng W, Herijgers P, Bogaerts K. Recurrence of mitral valve regurgitation after mitral valve repair in degenerative valve disease. Circulation 2003; 107:1609–13.
4b. Maslow AD, Regan MM, Haering JM et al. Echocardiographic predictors of left ventricular outflow tract obstruction and systolic anterior motion of the mitral valve after mitral valve reconstruction for myxomatous valve disease. J Am Coll Cardiol 1999; 34:2096–104.
5. Borger MA, Preston M, David TE, et al. Should the ascending aorta be replaced more frequently in patients with bicuspid aortic valve disease? J Thorac Cardiovasc Surg 2004; 128(5):677–83.
6. Quinones MA, Otto CM, Stoddard M, et al. Recommendations for quantification of Doppler echocardiography: a report from the Doppler Quantification Task Force of the Nomenclature and Standards Committee of the American Society of Echocardiography. J Am Soc Echocardiogr 2002; 15:167–84.
7. Sagar KB, Wam LS, Paulsen WH, Romhilt DW. Doppler echocardiographic evaluation of Hancock and Bjork–Shiley prosthetic valves. J Am Coll Cardiol 1986; 7(3):681–7.
8. Burstow DJ, Nishimura RA, Bailey KR, et al. Continuous wave Doppler echocardiographic measurement of prosthetic valve gradients. A simultaneous Doppler-catheter study. Circulation 1989; 80:504–14.
9. Baumgartner H, Khan S, DeRobertis M, et al. Discrepancies between Doppler and catheter gradients in aortic prosthetic valves in vitro. A manifestation of localized gradients and pressure recovery. Circulation 1990; 82:1467–75.
10. Wilkins GT, Gillam LD, Kritzer GL, et al. Validation of continuous-wave Doppler echocardiographic measurement of mitral and tricuspid prosthetic valve gradients: a simultaneous Doppler-catheter study. Circulation 1986; 74:786–95.
11. Stewart SFC, Nast EP, Arabia FA, et al. Errors in pressure gradient measurement by continuous-wave Doppler ultrasound: type, size, and age effects in bioprosthetic aortic valves. J Am Coll Cardiol 1991; 18:769–99.
12. Baumgartner H, Khan S, DeRobertis M, Czer L, Maurer G. Effect of prosthetic aortic valve design on the Doppler-catheter gradient correlation: an in vitro study of normal St. Jude, Medtronic-Hall, Starr-Edwards and Hancock valves. J Am Coll Cardiol 1992; 19:324–32.
13. Sezai A, Shiono M, Akiyama K, et al. Doppler echocardiographic evaluation of St. Jude Medical valves in the tricuspid position: criteria for normal and abnormal valve function. J Cardiovasc Surg (Torino) 2001; 42:303–9.
14. Novaro GM, Connolly HM, Miller FA. Doppler hemodyanmics of 51 clinically and echocardiographically normal pulmonary valve prostheses. Mayo Clin Proc 2001; 76:155–60.
15. Rothbart RM, Castriz JL, Harding LV, et al. Determination of aortic valve area by two-dimensional and Doppler echocardiography in patients with normal and stenotic bioprosthetic valves. J Am Coll Cardiol 1990; 15:817–24.
16. Chafizadeh ER, Zoghbi WA. Doppler echocardiographic assessment of the St. Jude Medical prosthetic valve in the aortic position using the continuity equation. Circulation 1991; 83:213.
17. Baumgartner H, Khan SS, DeRobertis M, et al. Doppler assessment of prosthetic valve orifice area: an in vitro study. Circulation 1992; 85:2275–83.
18. Dumesnil JG, Honos GN, Lemieux M, Beauchemin J. Validation and applications of mitral prosthetic valvular areas calculated by Doppler echocardiography. J Am Coll Cardiol 1990; 65:1443.
19. Rahimtoola SH. The problem of valve prosthesis–patient mismatch. Circulation 1978; 58:20–4.
20. Rao V, Jameison WR, Ivanov J, et al. Prosthesis–patient mismatch affects survival following aortic valve replacement. Circulation 2000; 102:1115–19.
21. Blais C, Dumesnil JG, Baillot R, et al. Impact of valve prosthesis–patient mismatch on short-term mortality after aortic valve replacement. Circulation 2003; 108:983–8.

22. Yoshida K, Yosikawa J, Asaka T, et al. Value of acceleration flow signals proximal to the leaking orifice in assessing the severity of prosthetic mitral valve regurgitation. J Am Coll Cardiol 1992; 19:333–8.

23. Degertekin M, Gencbay M, Turan F, et al. Application of proximal isovelocity surface area method to determine prosthetic mitral valve area. J Am Soc Echocardiogr 1998; 11(11):1056–63.

24. Olmos L, Salazar G, Barbetseas J, Quinones MA, Zoghbi WA. Usefulness of transthoracic echocardiography in detecting significant prosthetic mitral valve regurgitation. Am J Cardiol 1999; 83(2):199–205.

25. Appleton CP, Hatle LK, Popp RL, et al. Flow velocity acceleration in the left ventricle: a useful Doppler echocardiographic sign of hemodynamically significant mitral regurgitation. J Am Soc Echocardiogr 1990; 3(1):35–45.

26. Flachskamf FA, O'Shea JP, Thomas JD, et al. Patterns of normal transvalvular regurgitation in mechanical valve prostheses. J Am Coll Cardiol 1991; 18:1493–8.

27. Baumgartner H, Khan S, Maurer G. Color Doppler regurgitant characteristics of normal mechanical mitral valve prostheses in vitro. Circulation 1992; 85:323–32.

28. Vitarelli A, Conde Y, Stellato S, et al. Assessment of severity of mechanical prosthetic mitral regurgitation by transoesophageal echocardiography. Heart 2004; 90:539–44.

29. Nellessen U, Schnittger I, Appleton CP, et al. Transesophageal two-dimensional echocardiography and color Doppler flow velocity mapping in the evaluation of cardiac valve prostheses. Circulation 1988; 78:848–55.

30. Bach DS. Transesophageal echocardiographic (TEE) evaluation of prosthetic regurgitation. Cardiol Clin 2000; 18:751–71.

31. Grayburn PA, Feshke W, Omran H, et al. Multiplane transesophageal echocardiographic assessment of mitral regurgitation by color flow mapping of the vena contracta. Am J Cardiol 1994; 74:912–17.

32. Taams MA, Gussenhoven EJ, Bos E, et al. Enhanced morphological diagnosis in infective endocarditis by transoesophageal echocardiography. Br Heart J 1990; 63:109–13.

33. Daniel WG, Mugg A, Martin RP, et al. Improvement in the diagnosis of abscesses associated with endocarditis by TEE echocardiography. N Engl J Med 1991; 324:795–800.

34. Yvorchuk KJ, Chan Kl. Application of transthoracic and transesophageal echocardiography in the diagnosis and management of infective endocarditis. J Am Soc Echocardiogr 1994; 7:1294–308.

35. Ronderos RE, Portis M, Stoermann W, Sarmiento C. Are all echocardiographic findings equally predictive for diagnosis in prosthetic endocarditis? J Am Soc Echocardiogr 2004; 17(6):664–9.

36. Habib G, Cornen A, Mesana T, et al. Diagnosis of prosthetic heart valve thrombosis: the respective values of transthoracic and transesophageal Doppler echocardiography. Eur Heart J 1993; 14:447–55.

37. Gueret P, Vignon P, Fournier P, et al. Transesophageal echocardiography for the diagnosis and management of nonobstructive thrombosis of mechanical mitral valve prosthesis. Circulation 1995; 19:979–81.

38. Dzavik V, Cohen G, Chan KL. Role of transesophageal echocardiography in the diagnosis and management of prosthetic valve thrombosis. J Am Coll Cardiol 1991; 18:1829–33.

39. Montorsi P, De Bernardi F, Muratori M, Cavoretto D, Pepi M. Role of cine-flouroscopy, transthoracic, and transesophageal echocardiography in patients with suspected prosthetic heart valve thrombosis. Am J Cardiol 2000; 85:58–64.

40. Roberts WC, Morrow AG. Causes of early postoperative death following cardiac valve replacement. Clinico-pathologic correlations in 64 patients studied at necropsy. J Thorac Cardiovasc Surg 1967; 54:422–37.

41. Roberts WC, Morrow AG. Late postoperative pathological findings after cardiac valve replacement. Circulation 1967; 35(4 Suppl): I48–62.

42. Bjork VO, Henze A, Rodriguez L. Left ventricular rupture as a complication of mitral valve replacement. J Thorac Cardiovasc Surg 1977; 73:14–22.

43. Karlson KJ, Ashraf MM, Berger RL. Rupture of left ventricle following mitral valve replacement. Ann Thorac Surg 1988; 46:590–7.

44. Catherwood E, Mintz GS, Segal BL, et al. Two-dimensional echocardiographic recognition of left ventricular pseudoaneurysm. Circulation 1980; 62:294–303.

45. Roelandt JR, Sutherland GR, Yoshikawa J. Improved diagnosis and characterization of left ventricular pseudoaneurysm by Doppler color flow imaging. J Am Coll Cardiol 1988; 12:807–11.

46. Olalla JJ, Vazques de Prada JA, Fernadez M, et al. Color Doppler diagnosis of left ventricular pseudoaneurysm. Chest 1988; 94:443–44.

47. Alam M, Glick C, Lewis JW. Transesophageal echocardiographic features of left ventricular pseudoaneurysm resulting after mitral valve replacement surgery. Am Heart J 1992; 123:226–8.

48. Esakof DD, Vannan MA, Bojar RM, et al. Visualization of left ventricular pseudoaneurysm with panoramic transesophageal echocardiography. J Am Soc Echocardiogr 1994; 31:259–65.

49. Afridi I, Apostolidou MA, Saad RM, Zoghbi WA. Pseudoaneurysms of the mitral-aortic intervalvular fibrosa: dynamic characterization using transesophageal echocardiographic and Doppler techniques. J Am Coll Cardiol 1995; 25:137–45.

50. Barbetseas J, Crawford ES, Zoghbi WA, et al. Doppler echocardiographic evaluation of pseudoaneurysms complicating composite grafts of the ascending aorta. Circulation 1992; 85:212–22.

51. Levy DJ, Child JS, Rambod E, et al. Microbubbles and mitral valve prostheses – transesophageal echocardiographic evaluation. Eur J Ultrasound 1999; 10(1):31–40.

52. Braekken SK, Russel D, Svennevig J, et al. Incidence and frequency of cerebral embolic signals in patients with a similar bileaflet mechanical heart valve. Stroke 1995; 26:1225–30.

53. Grosset DG, Cowburn P, Georgiadis D, et al. Ultrasound detection of cerebral emboli in patients with prosthetic heart valves. J Heart Valve Dis 1994; 3:128–32.

54. Deklunder G, Lecroart JL, Houdas Y, et al. Transcranial high-intensity Doppler signals in patients with mechanical heart valve prostheses: their relationship with abnormal intracavitary echoes. J Heart Valve Dis 1996; 5:662–67.

55. Georgiadis D, Mackay TG, Lees KR, et al. Differentiation between gaseous and formed embolic materials in vivo: application in prosthetic heart valve patients. Stroke 1994; 25:1559–63.

56. Castaneda-Zuniga W, Nicoloff D, Jorgensen C et al. In vivo radiographic appearance of the St. Jude valve prosthesis. Ann Thorac Surg 1980; 134:775–6.

5

Normal echocardiographic data of prosthetic valves

Raphael Rosenhek and Helmut Baumgartner

Introduction

Echocardiography plays a critical role in the evaluation of patients with heart valve prostheses, and Doppler echocardiography in particular has proven to be valuable for the assessment of prosthetic valve function. Similarly to native valve stenosis, pressure gradients, pressure half-time and effective orifice areas can be measured. However, the interpretation of these data is far more difficult in patients with prosthetic heart valves.

Even when prosthetic heart valves function normally, they are more or less obstructive.[1–89] This results in higher flow velocities and pressure gradients, as well as smaller effective orifice areas and increased pressure half-times compared with normal native valves. The difficulty is then to decide which measurement can be considered to be normal and when prosthetic valve dysfunction must be assumed.

Consideration of valve type and size

Every valve type has its own haemodynamic properties, resulting in specific normal values of gradients, pressure half-time and effective orifice area. Among bioprosthetic valves, the stentless valves are less obstructive than the stented valves; the modern mechanical valves are less obstructive than older valve types such as caged-ball valves. Finally, bileaflet valves are characterised by localised high velocities between the two leaflets, resulting in high Doppler gradients.[64] In addition, normal values also depend on valve size, with smaller valves being significantly more obstructive than larger valves.[64,89,90]

Thus, precise knowledge of valve type and size is indispensable for an appropriate interpretation of the Doppler data. Once this information is known, the measured values can be compared with published normal values. Tables 5.1 and 5.2 comprehensively summarise pooled data on normal Doppler values available in the literature for most aortic and mitral prosthetic heart valves.[91]

The data are classified according to valve position, type and size. For valves in the aortic position, peak velocities, peak gradients, mean gradients and effective orifice areas are indicated where available. For valves in the mitral position, peak velocities, peak gradients, mean gradients, pressure half-times and effective orifice areas are listed.

Flow dependence of Doppler measurements and specific flow phenomena

Even with this information at hand, data interpretation may remain difficult. A wide range of normal values may be encountered for selected valve types, particularly when dealing with smaller-sized valves. This variation in velocities and gradients is mainly caused by the flow dependence of these variables.[70,90] Therefore, the flow conditions should be considered when interpreting Doppler data. Ideally, normal values should be indicated for specific flow rates; however, such data are usually unavailable.

Some types of valves presenting with specific flow characteristics further complicate Doppler assessment of their function. Bileaflet valves, but also the nowadays rarely seen caged-ball valves, are characterised by a very inhomogeneous velocity profile.[73,92] Bileaflet valves have two larger side orifices and one smaller central orifice. The two leaflets allow for flow contraction in the central orifice and for the occurrence of a central low-pressure field corresponding to significantly higher velocities between the leaflets as compared to the side orifices. These high velocities are measured by Doppler echocardiography and therefore the estimated gradients significantly exceed the actual pressure

Table 5.1 Normal Doppler echocardiographic values for aortic valve prosthesis

Valve / Valve type	Size	n	Peak gradient (mmHg)	Mean gradient (mmHg)	Peak velocity (m/s)	Effective orifice area (cm²)	Reference
ATS Medical AP	16	6	47.7 ± 12	27 ± 7.3	3.44 ± 0.47	0.61 ± 0.09	1
ATS Medical Standard	19	9	47 ± 12.6	26.2 ± 7.9	3.41 ± 0.43	0.96 ± 0.18	1
bileaflet	21	15	25.5 ± 6.1	14.4 ± 3.5	2.4 ± 0.39	1.58 ± 0.37	1, 2
	23	8	19 ± 7	12 ± 4		1.8 ± 0.2	1
	25	12	17 ± 8	11 ± 4		2.2 ± 0.4	1
	27	10	14 ± 4	9 ± 2		2.5 ± 0.3	1
	29	5	11 ± 3	8 ± 2		3.1 ± 0.3	1
Biocor Stentless	21	45	35.97 ± 4.06	18 ± 4			3, 4
stentless bioprosthesis	23	115	29.15 ± 8.28	18.64 ± 7.14	3 ± 0.6	1.4 ± 0.5	3–5
	25	100	28.65 ± 6.6	17.72 ± 6.99	2.8 ± 0.5	1.6 ± 0.38	3–5
	27	55	25.87 ± 2.81	18 ± 2.8	2.7 ± 0.2	1.9 ± 0.46	4, 5
	≥29	16	24 ± 2				4
Biocor Extended	19–21	12	17.5 ± 5.8	9.7 ± 3.5		1.3 ± 0.4	6
Stentless	23	18	14.8 ± 5.9	8.1 ± 3.1		1.6 ± 0.3	6
stentless bioprosthesis	25	20	14.2 ± 3.5	7.7 ± 1.9		1.8 ± 0.3	6
Bioflo Pericardial	19	16	37.25 ± 8.65	24.15 ± 5.1		0.77 ± 0.11	7, 8
stented bioprosthesis	21	9	28.7 ± 6.2	18.7 ± 5.5		1.1 ± 0.1	8
	23	4	20.7 ± 4	12.5 ± 3		1.3 ± 0.09	8
Björk–Shiley Monostrut	19	37	46.0	26.67 ± 7.87	3.3 ± 0.6	0.94 ± 0.19	9–11
tilting disc	21	161	32.41 ± 9.73	18.64 ± 6.09	2.9 ± 0.4		3, 9, 11, 12
	23	153	26.52 ± 9.67	14.5 ± 6.2	2.7 ± 0.5		3, 9, 11, 12
	25	89	22.33 ± 7	13.3 ± 4.96	2.5 ± 0.4		3, 9, 11
	27	61	18.31 ± 8	10.41 ± 4.38	2.1 ± 0.4		3, 9, 11
	29	9	12 ± 8	7.67 ± 4.36	1.9 ± 0.2		3, 9, 11
Björk–Shiley Spherical	17	1			4.1		13
or not specified	19	2	27.0		3.8	1.1	13, 14
tilting disc	21	18	38.94 ± 11.93	21.8 ± 3.4	2.92 ± 0.88	1.1 ± 0.25	12–15
	23	41	33.86 ± 11	17.34 ± 6.86	2.42 ± 0.4	1.22 ± 0.23	12–17
	25	39	20.39 ± 7.07	11.5 ± 4.55	2.06 ± 0.28	1.8 ± 0.32	13–17
	27	23	19.44 ± 7.99	10.67 ± 4.31	1.77 ± 0.12	2.6	13–17
	29	5	21.1 ± 7.1		1.87 ± 0.18	2.52 ± 0.69	14, 15
	31	2			2.1 ± 0.14		13, 15
Carbomedics	17	7	33.4 ± 13.2	20.1 ± 7.1		1.02 ± 0.2	18
bileaflet	19	63	33.3 ± 11.19	11.61 ± 5.08	3.09 ± 0.38	1.25 ± 0.36	18–24
	21	111	26.31 ± 10.25	12.68 ± 4.29	2.61 ± 0.51	1.42 ± 0.36	19–24
	23	120	24.61 ± 6.93	11.33 ± 3.8	2.42 ± 0.37	1.69 ± 0.29	19, 20, 22, 23
	25	103	20.25 ± 8.69	9.34 ± 4.65	2.25 ± 0.34	2.04 ± 0.37	19, 20, 22, 23
	27	57	19.05 ± 7.04	8.41 ± 2.83	2.18 ± 0.36	2.55 ± 0.34	19, 20, 22, 23
	29	6	12.53 ± 4.69	5.8 ± 3.2	1.93 ± 0.25	2.63 ± 0.38	19, 22
Carbomedics reduced	19	10	43.4 ± 1.8	24.4 ± 1.2		1.22 ± 0.08	25
bileaflet							
Carbomedics	19	4	29.04 ± 10.1	19.5 ± 2.12	1.8	1 ± 0.18	26, 27
Supraannular Top Hat	21	30	29.61 ± 8.93	16.59 ± 5.79	2.62 ± 0.35	1.18 ± 0.33	26–28
bileaflet	23	30	24.38 ± 7.53	13.29 ± 3.73	2.36 ± 0.55	1.37 ± 0.37	26–28
	25	1	22.0	11.0	2.4		28
Carpentier–Edwards	19	56	43.48 ± 12.72	25.6 ± 8.02		0.85 ± 0.17	7, 29
stented bioprosthesis	21	73	27.73 ± 7.6	17.25 ± 6.24	2.37 ± 0.54	1.48 ± 0.3	15, 16, 19, 30–33
	23	100	28.93 ± 7.49	15.92 ± 6.43	2.76 ± 0.4	1.69 ± 0.45	15, 16, 19, 30–32, 34
	25	85	23.95 ± 7.05	12.76 ± 4.43	2.38 ± 0.47	1.94 ± 0.45	15, 16, 19, 30, 32, 34
	27	50	22.14 ± 8.24	12.33 ± 5.59	2.31 ± 0.39	2.25 ± 0.55	15, 16, 19, 30, 34
	29	24	22.0	9.92 ± 2.9	2.44 ± 0.43	2.84 ± 0.51	15, 16, 19, 30, 32
	31	4			2.41 ± 0.13		15, 30

Table 5.1 *Continued*

Valve type	Size	n	Peak gradient (mmHg)	Mean gradient (mmHg)	Peak velocity (m/s)	Effective orifice area (cm²)	Reference
Carpentier–Edwards	19	14	32.13 ± 3.35	24.19 ± 8.6	2.83 ± 0.14	1.21 ± 0.31	31, 35
pericardial	21	34	25.69 ± 9.9	20.3 ± 9.08	2.59 ± 0.42	1.47 ± 0.36	31, 33, 35
stented bioprosthesis	23	20	21.72 ± 8.57	13.01 ± 5.27	2.29 ± 0.45	1.75 ± 0.28	31, 35
	25	5	16.46 ± 5.41	9.04 ± 2.27	2.02 ± 0.31		35
	27	1	19.2 ± 0	5.6	1.6		35
	29	1	17.6 ± 0	11.6	2.1		35
Carpentier–Edwards	19	15	34.1 ± 2.7			1.1 ± 0.09	36
supra-annularAV	21	8	25 ± 8	14 ± 5		1.06 ± 0.16	33
(CE-SAV)							
stented bioprosthesis							
CryoLife–O'Brien	19	47		12 ± 4.8		1.25 ± 0.1	37
Stentless	21	163		10.33 ± 2		1.57 ± 0.6	37, 38
stentless bioprosthesis	23	40		8.5		2.2	38
	25	40		7.9		2.3	38
	27	39		7.4		2.7	38
Duromedics (Tekna)	19	1			3.6		30
bileaflet	21	3	19.08 ± 16	8.98 ± 5		1.3	33, 39
	23	12	19.87 ± 7	7 ± 2	2.64 ± 0.27		30, 39
	25	18	21 ± 9	5 ± 2	2.34 ± 0.38		30, 39
	27	15	22.5 ± 12	6 ± 3	1.88 ± 0.6		30, 39
	29	1	13.0	3.4	2.1		30, 39
Edwards PRIMA	19	7	30.9 ± 11.7	15.4 ± 7.4		1 ± 0.3	40
Stentless	21	30	31.22 ± 17.35	16.36 ± 11.36		1.25 ± 0.29	40, 41
stentless bioprosthesis	23	62	23.39 ± 10.17	11.52 ± 5.26	2.8 ± 0.4	1.49 ± 0.46	40–42
	25	97	19.74 ± 10.36	10.77 ± 9.32	2.7 ± 0.3	1.7 ± 0.55	40–42
	27	46	15.9 ± 7.3	7.1 ± 3.7		2 ± 0.6	40
	29	11	11.21 ± 8.6	5.03 ± 4.53		2.49 ± 0.52	40, 41
Hancock I	21	1			3.5		15
stented bioprosthesis	23	14	19.09 ± 4.35	12.36 ± 3.82	2.94 ± 0.24		15–17
	25	26	17.61 ± 3.13	11 ± 2.85	2.36 ± 0.37		15–17
	27	20	18.11 ± 6.92	10 ± 3.46	2.4 ± 0.36		15–17
	29	2			2.23 ± 0.04		15
	31	1			2.0		15
Hancock II	21	39	20 ± 4	14.8 ± 4.1		1.23 ± 0.27	43, 44
stented bioprosthesis	23	119	24.72 ± 5.73	16.64 ± 6.91		1.39 ± 0.23	43–45
	25	114	20 ± 2	10.7 ± 3		1.47 ± 0.19	43, 44
	27	133	14 ± 3			1.55 ± 0.18	43
	29	35	15 ± 3			1.6 ± 0.15	43
Ionescu–Shiley	17	11	42.0	21.1 ± 3.21		0.86 ± 0.1	34, 46
stented bioprosthesis	19	63	23.17 ± 6.58	20.44 ± 8.47	2.63 ± 0.32	1.15 ± 0.18	7, 34, 35, 46
	21	11	27.63 ± 8.34	15.1 ± 1.56	2.75 ± 0.25		7, 35
	23	5	18.09 ± 6.49	9.9 ± 2.85	2.1 ± 0.38		35
	25	1	18.0				7
	27	3	14.75 ± 2.17	8.97 ± 0.57	1.92 ± 0.14		35
	29	1	16.0	7.3 ± 0	2.0		35
Jyros Bileaflet	22	4	17.3	10.8		1.5	47
bileaflet	24	7	18.6	11.4		1.5	47
	26	8	14.4	8.4		1.7	47
	28	3	10.0	5.7		1.9	47
	30	1	8.0	6.0		1.6	47

continued

Table 5.1 Normal Doppler echocardiographic values for aortic valve prosthesis – *continued*

Valve Valve type	Size	n	Peak gradient (mmHg)	Mean gradient (mmHg)	Peak velocity (m/s)	Effective orifice area (cm²)	Reference
Lillehei–Kaster	14	1			2.7		30
tilting disc	16	2			3.43 ± 0.39		30
	18	2			2.85 ± 0.21		30
	20	1			1.7		30
Medtronic Freestyle	19	11		13.0			48
Stentless	21	85		7.99 ± 2.6		1.6 ± 0.32	48, 49
stentless bioprosthesis	23	141		7.24 ± 2.5		1.9 ± 0.5	48, 49
	25	164		5.35 ± 1.5		2.03 ± 0.41	48, 49
	27	105		4.72 ± 1.6		2.5 ± 0.47	48, 49
Medtronic Hall	20	24	34.37 ± 13.06	17.08 ± 5.28	2.9 ± 0.4	1.21 ± 0.45	10, 33, 50
tilting disc	21	30	26.86 ± 10.54	14.1 ± 5.93	2.42 ± 0.36	1.08 ± 0.17	33, 50, 51
	23	27	26.85 ± 8.85	13.5 ± 4.79	2.43 ± 0.59	1.36 ± 0.39	13, 16, 50, 51
	25	17	17.13 ± 7.04	9.53 ± 4.26	2.29 ± 0.5	1.9 ± 0.47	13, 16, 51
	27	8	18.66 ± 9.71	8.66 ± 5.56	2.07 ± 0.53	1.9 ± 0.16	13, 16, 51
	29	1			1.6		13
Medtronic Intact	19	16	39.43 ± 15.4	23.71 ± 9.3	2.5		52, 53
stented bioprosthesis	21	55	33.9 ± 12.69	18.74 ± 8.03	2.73 ± 0.44	1.55 ± 0.39	31, 32, 52, 53
	23	110	31.27 ± 9.62	18.88 ± 6.17	2.74 ± 0.37	1.64 ± 0.37	31, 32, 52–54
	25	41	27.34 ± 10.59	16.4 ± 6.05	2.6 ± 0.44	1.85 ± 0.25	32, 52–54
	27	16	25.27 ± 7.58	15 ± 3.94	2.51 ± 0.38	2.2 ± 0.17	32, 52, 54
	29	5	31.0	15.6 ± 2.1	2.8	2.38 ± 0.54	32, 52
Medtronic Mosaic	21	51		12.43 ± 7.3		1.6 ± 0.7	44, 55
Porcine	23	121		12.47 ± 7.4		2.1 ± 0.8	44, 55
stented bioprosthesis	25	71		10.08 ± 5.1		2.1 ± 1.6	44, 55
	27	30		9.0			55
	29	6		9.0			55
Mitroflow	19	4	18.7 ± 5.1	10.3 ± 3		1.13 ± 0.17	7
stented bioprosthesis	21	7	20.2	15.4	2.3		35
	23	5	14.04 ± 4.91	7.56 ± 3.38	1.85 ± 0.34		35
	25	2	17 ± 11.31	10.8 ± 6.51	2 ± 0.71		35
	27	3	13 ± 3	6.57 ± 1.7	1.8 ± 0.2		35
O'Brien–Angell Stentless	23			14.5 ± 7.77		1.15 ± 0.07	56
(annular position)	25	50		19 ± 12.72		1.12 ± 0.25	56
stentless bioprosthesis	27			18 ± 12.72		1.55 ± 0.21	56
	29			12 ± 7.07		2.05 ± 1.2	56
O'Brien–Angell Stentless	23			9 ± 1.4		1.58 ± 0.58	56
(supraannular position)	25	50		7.5 ± 0.7		2.37 ± 0.18	56
stentless bioprosthesis	27			8.5 ± 0.7		2.85 ± 0.87	56
	29			7 ± 1.4		2.7 ± 0.42	56
Omnicarbon	21	71	36.79 ± 12.59	19.41 ± 5.46	2.93 ± 0.47	1.25 ± 0.43	5, 57–59
tilting disc	23	83	29.33 ± 9.67	17.98 ± 6.06	2.66 ± 0.44	1.49 ± 0.34	5, 57–59
	25	81	24.29 ± 7.71	13.51 ± 3.85	2.32 ± 0.38	1.94 ± 0.52	5, 57–59
	27	40	19.63 ± 4.34	12.06 ± 2.98	2.08 ± 0.35	2.11 ± 0.46	5, 57–59
	29	5	17.12 ± 1.53	10 ± 1.53	1.9 ± 0.06	2.27 ± 0.23	57–59
Omniscience	19	2	47.5 ± 3.5	28 ± 1.4		0.81 ± 0.01	50
tilting disc	21	5	50.8 ± 2.8	28.2 ± 2.17		0.87 ± 0.13	50
	23	8	39.8 ± 8.7	20.1 ± 5.1		0.98 ± 0.07	50
On-X	19	6	21.3 ± 10.8	11.8 ± 3.4		1.5 ± 0.2	60
bileaflet	21	11	16.4 ± 5.9	9.9 ± 3.6		1.7 ± 0.4	60
	23	23	15.9 ± 6.4	8.5 ± 3.3		2 ± 0.6	60

Table 5.1 *Continued*

Valve Valve type	Size	n	Peak gradient (mmHg)	Mean gradient (mmHg)	Peak velocity (m/s)	Effective orifice area (cm²)	Reference
	25	12	16.5 ± 10.2	9 ± 5.3		2.4 ± 0.8	60
	27–29	8	11.4 ± 4.6	5.6 ± 2.7		3.2 ± 0.6	60
Sorin Allcarbon tilting disc	19	7	44 ± 7	29 ± 8	3.3 ± 0.3	0.9 ± 0.1	61
	21	25	36.52 ± 9.61	21.07 ± 6.72	2.93 ± 0.2	1.08 ± 0.19	51, 61
	23	37	34.97 ± 10.97	18.72 ± 6.49	2.9 ± 0.41	1.31 ± 0.2	51, 61
	25	23	22 ± 4.68	13.85 ± 3.97	2.37 ± 0.23	1.96 ± 0.71	51, 61
	27	13	16.3 ± 3.3	10.15 ± 3.76	2 ± 0.25	2.51 ± 0.57	51, 61
	29	4	13 ± 4	8 ± 2	1.8 ± 0.3	4.1 ± 0.7	61
Sorin Bicarbon bileaflet	19	19	29.53 ± 4.46	16.35 ± 1.99	2.5 ± 0.1	1.36 ± 0.13	25, 62, 63
	21	70	24.52 ± 7.1	12.54 ± 3.3	2.46 ± 0.31	1.46 ± 0.2	62, 63
	23	71	17.79 ± 6.1	9.61 ± 3.3	2.11 ± 0.24	1.98 ± 0.23	62, 63
	25	40	18.46 ± 3.1	10.05 ± 1.6	2.25 ± 0.19	2.39 ± 0.29	62, 63
	27	8	12 ± 3.25	7 ± 1.5	1.73 ± 0.21	3.06 ± 0.47	62
	29	4	9 ± 1.25	5 ± 0.5	1.51 ± 0.1	3.45 ± 0.02	62
Sorin Pericarbon stentless bioprosthesis	23	15	39 ± 13	25 ± 8		2.0	45
St. Jude Medical bileaflet	19	100	35.17 ± 11.16	18.96 ± 6.27	2.86 ± 0.48	1.01 ± 0.24	5, 10, 14, 34, 64–70
	21	207	28.34 ± 9.94	15.82 ± 5.67	2.63 ± 0.48	1.33 ± 0.32	5, 14, 16, 34, 63, 64, 66–72
	23	236	25.28 ± 7.89	13.77 ± 5.33	2.57 ± 0.44	1.6 ± 0.43	5, 14, 16, 34, 63, 64, 66–71
	25	169	22.57 ± 7.68	12.65 ± 5.14	2.4 ± 0.45	1.93 ± 0.45	5, 14, 16, 34, 63, 64, 66–70
	27	82	19.85 ± 7.55	11.18 ± 4.82	2.24 ± 0.42	2.35 ± 0.59	5, 14, 16, 34, 64, 66, 67, 69, 70
	29	18	17.72 ± 6.42	9.86 ± 2.9	2 ± 0.1	2.81 ± 0.57	14, 64, 70, 72
	31	4	16.0	10 ± 6	2.1 ± 0.6	3.08 ± 1.09	34, 64
St. Jude Medical HP bileaflet	19	19	25.81 ± 7.52	16.44 ± 3.57		1.65 ± 0.2	21, 25
	21	30	18.9 ± 7.31	9.62 ± 3.37		2.15 ± 0.29	71, 72
Starr–Edwards ball-and-cage	21	5	29.0			1.0	73
	22	2			4 ± 0		15
	23	22	32.6 ± 12.79	21.98 ± 8.8	3.5 ± 0.5	1.1	19, 73, 74
	24	43	34.13 ± 10.33	22.09 ± 7.54	3.35 ± 0.48		15, 19, 73, 74
	26	29	31.83 ± 9.01	19.69 ± 6.05	3.18 ± 0.35		15, 19, 73, 74
	27	14	30.82 ± 6.3	18.5 ± 3.7		1.8	19, 73
	29	8	29 ± 9.3	16.3 ± 5.5			19
Stentless Porcine **Xenografts** stentless bioprosthesis	21	3	14 ± 5	8.7 ± 3.5		1.33 ± 0.38	75
	22	3	16 ± 5.6	9.7 ± 3.7		1.32 ± 0.48	75
	23	4	13 ± 4.8	7.7 ± 2.3		1.59 ± 0.6	75
	24	3	13 ± 3.8	7.7 ± 2.2		1.4 ± 0.01	75
	25	6	11.5 ± 7.1	7.4 ± 4.5		2.13 ± 0.7	75
	26	3	10.7	7 ± 2.1		2.15 ± 0.2	75
	27	1	9.2	5.5		3.2	75
	28	1	7.5	4.1		2.3	75
Toronto Stentless **Porcine** stentless bioprosthesis	20	1	10.9	4.6		1.3	76
	21	9	18.64 ± 11.8	7.56 ± 4.4		1.21 ± 0.7	76, 77
	22	1	23.0			1.2	78
	23	84	13.55 ± 7.28	7.08 ± 4.33		1.59 ± 0.84	76–80
	25	190	12.17 ± 5.75	6.2 ± 3.05		1.62 ± 0.4	76–80
	27	240	9.96 ± 4.56	4.8 ± 2.33		1.95 ± 0.42	76–79
	29	200	7.91 ± 4.17	3.94 ± 2.15		2.37 ± 0.67	76–79

Table 5.2 Normal Doppler echocardiographic values for mitral valve prosthesis

Valve valve type	Size	n	Peak gradient (mmHg)	Mean gradient (mmHg)	Peak velocity (m/s)	Pressure half-time (ms)	Effective orifice area (cm²)	Reference
Biocor	27	3	13 ± 1					4
stentless bioprosthesis	29	3	14 ± 2.5					4
	31	8	11.5 ± 0.5					4
	33	9	12 ± 0.5					4
Bioflo Pericardial	25	3	10 ± 2	6.3 ± 1.5			2 ± 0.1	8
stented bioprosthesis	27	7	9.5 ± 2.6	5.4 ± 1.2			2 ± 0.3	8
	29	8	5 ± 2.8	3.6 ± 1			2.4 ± 0.2	8
	31	1	4.0	2.0			2.3	8
Björk–Shiley	23	1			1.7	115		13
tilting disc	25	14	12 ± 4	6 ± 2	1.75 ± 0.38	99 ± 27	1.72 ± 0.6	13, 81
	27	34	10 ± 4	5 ± 2	1.6 ± 0.49	89 ± 28	1.81 ± 0.54	13, 81
	29	21	7.83 ± 2.93	2.83 ± 1.27	1.37 ± 0.25	79 ± 17	2.1 ± 0.43	13, 17, 81
	31	21	6 ± 3	2 ± 1.9	1.41 ± 0.26	70 ± 14	2.2 ± 0.3	13, 17
Björk–Shiley Monostrut	23	1		5.0	1.9			9
tilting disc	25	102	13 ± 2.5	5.57 ± 2.3	1.8 ± 0.3			9, 11
	27	83	12 ± 2.5	4.53 ± 2.2	1.7 ± 0.4			9, 11
	29	26	13 ± 3	4.26 ± 1.6	1.6 ± 0.3			9, 11
	31	25	14 ± 4.5	4.9 ± 1.6	1.7 ± 0.3			9, 11
Carbomedics	23	2			1.9 ± 0.1	126 ± 7		22
bileaflet	25	12	10.3 ± 2.3	3.6 ± 0.6	1.3 ± 0.1	93 ± 8	2.9 ± 0.8	22, 82
	27	78	8.79 ± 3.46	3.46 ± 1.03	1.61 ± 0.3	89 ± 20	2.9 ± 0.75	22, 82, 83
	29	46	8.78 ± 2.9	3.39 ± 0.97	1.52 ± 0.3	88 ± 17	2.3 ± 0.4	22, 82, 83
	31	57	8.87 ± 2.34	3.32 ± 0.87	1.61 ± 0.29	92 ± 24	2.8 ± 1.14	22, 82, 83
	33	33	8.8 ± 2.2	4.8 ± 2.5	1.5 ± 0.2	93 ± 12		83
Carpentier–Edwards	27	16		6 ± 2	1.7 ± 0.3	98 ± 28		30, 84
stented bioprosthesis	29	22		4.7 ± 2	1.76 ± 0.27	92 ± 14		30, 84
	31	22		4.4 ± 2	1.54 ± 0.15	92 ± 19		30, 84
	33	6		6 ± 3		93 ± 12		84
Carpentier–Edwards	27	1		3.6	1.6	100		35
pericardial	29	6		5.25 ± 2.36	1.67 ± 0.3	110 ± 15		35
stented bioprosthesis	31	4		4.05 ± 0.83	1.53 ± 0.1	90 ± 11		35
	33	1		1.0	0.8	80		35
Duromedics	27	8	13 ± 6	5 ± 3	161 ± 40	75 ± 12		13, 39
bileaflet	29	14	10 ± 4	3 ± 1	140 ± 25	85 ± 22		13, 39
	31	21	10.5 ± 4.33	3.3 ± 1.36	138 ± 27	81 ± 12		13, 39
	33	1	11.2	2.5		85		39
Hancock I	27	3	10 ± 4	5 ± 2			1.3 ± 0.8	17
or not specified	29	13	7 ± 3	2.46 ± 0.79		115 ± 20	1.5 ± 0.2	17, 84
stented bioprosthesis	31	22	4 ± 0.86	4.86 ± 1.69		95 ± 17	1.6 ± 0.2	17, 84
	33	8	3 ± 2	3.87 ± 2		90 ± 12	1.9 ± 0.2	17, 84
Hancock II	27	16					2.21 ± 0.14	43
stented bioprosthesis	29	64					2.77 ± 0.11	43
	31	90					2.84 ± 0.1	43
	33	25					3.15 ± 0.22	43
Hancock pericardial	29	14		2.61 ± 1.39	1.42 ± 0.14	105 ± 36		85
stented bioprosthesis	31	8		3.57 ± 1.02	1.51 ± 0.27	81 ± 23		85

Table 5.2 *Continued*

Valve valve type	Size	n	Peak gradient (mmHg)	Mean gradient (mmHg)	Peak velocity (m/s)	Pressure half-time (ms)	Effective orifice area (cm²)	Reference
Ionescu–Shiley stented bioprosthesis	25	3		4.87 ± 1.08	1.43 ± 0.15	93 ± 11		35
	27	4		3.21 ± 0.82	1.31 ± 0.24	100 ± 28		35
	29	6		3.22 ± 0.57	1.38 ± 0.2	85 ± 8		35
	31	4		3.63 ± 0.9	1.45 ± 0.06	100 ± 36		35
Ionescu–Shiley low profile stented bioprosthesis	29	13		3.31 ± 0.96	1.36 ± 0.25	80 ± 30		85
	31	10		2.74 ± 0.37	1.33 ± 0.14	79 ± 15		85
Labcor–Santiago **Pericardial** stented bioprosthesis	25	1	8.7	4.5		97	2.2	86
	27	16	5.6 ± 2.3	2.8 ± 1.5		85 ± 18	2.12 ± 0.48	86
	29	20	6.2 ± 2.1	3 ± 1.3		80 ± 34	2.11 ± 0.73	86
Lillehei–Kaster tilting disc	18	1			1.7	140		13
	20	1			1.7	67		13
	22	4			1.56 ± 0.09	94 ± 22		13
	25	5			1.38 ± 0.27	124 ± 46		13
Medtronic Hall tilting disc	27	1			1.4	78		13
	29	5			1.57 ± 0.1	69 ± 15		13
	31	7			1.45 ± 0.12	77 ± 17		13
Medtronic Intact **Porcine** stented bioprosthesis	29	3		3.5 ± 0.51	1.6 ± 0.22			54
	31	14		4.2 ± 1.44	1.6 ± 0.26			54
	33	13		4 ± 1.3	1.4 ± 0.24			54
	35	2		3.2 ± 1.77	1.3 ± 0.5			54
Mitroflow stented bioprosthesis	25	1		6.9	2.0	90		35
	27	3		3.07 ± 0.91	1.5	90 ± 20		35
	29	15		3.5 ± 1.65	1.43 ± 0.29	102 ± 21		35
	31	5		3.85 ± 0.81	1.32 ± 0.26	91 ± 22		35
Omnicarbon tilting disc	23	1		8.0				57
	25	16		6.05 ± 1.81	1.77 ± 0.24	102 ± 16		57, 59
	27	29		4.89 ± 2.05	1.63 ± 0.36	105 ± 33		57, 59
	29	34		4.93 ± 2.16	1.56 ± 0.27	120 ± 40		57, 59
	31	58		4.18 ± 1.4	1.3 ± 0.23	134 ± 31		57, 59
	33	2		4 ± 2				57
On-X bileaflet	25	3	11.5 ± 3.2	5.3 ± 2.1			1.9 ± 1.1	60
	27–29	16	10.3 ± 4.5	4.5 ± 1.6			2.2 ± 0.5	60
	31–33	14	9.8 ± 3.8	4.8 ± 2.4			2.5 ± 1.1	60
Sorin Allcarbon tilting disc	25	8	15 ± 3	5 ± 1	2 ± 0.2	105 ± 29	2.2 ± 0.6	61
	27	20	13 ± 2	4 ± 1	1.8 ± 0.1	89 ± 14	2.5 ± 0.5	61
	29	34	10 ± 2	4 ± 1	1.6 ± 0.2	85 ± 23	2.8 ± 0.7	61
	31	11	9 ± 1	4 ± 1	1.6 ± 0.1	88 ± 27	2.8 ± 0.9	61
Sorin Bicarbon Bileaflet bileaflet	25	3	15 ± 0.25	4 ± 0.5	1.95 ± 0.02	70 ± 1		62
	27	25	11 ± 2.75	4 ± 0.5	1.65 ± 0.21	82 ± 20		62
	29	30	12 ± 3	4 ± 1.25	1.73 ± 0.22	80 ± 14		62
	31	9	10 ± 1.5	4 ± 1	1.66 ± 0.11	83 ± 14		62
St. Jude Medical bileaflet	23	1		4.0	1.5	160	1.0	87
	25	4		2.5 ± 1	1.34 ± 1.12	75 ± 4	1.35 ± 0.17	87
	27	16	11 ± 4	5 ± 1.82	1.61 ± 0.29	75 ± 10	1.67 ± 0.17	68, 84, 87
	29	40	10 ± 3	4.15 ± 1.8	1.57 ± 0.29	85 ± 10	1.75 ± 0.24	68, 84, 87
	31	41	12 ± 6	4.46 ± 2.22	1.59 ± 0.33	74 ± 13	2.03 ± 0.32	68, 84, 87

Table 5.2 Normal Doppler echocardiographic values for mitral valve prosthesis – *continued*

Valve valve type	Size	n	Peak gradient (mmHg)	Mean gradient (mmHg)	Peak velocity (m/s)	Pressure half-time (ms)	Effective orifice area (cm²)	Reference
Starr–Edwards	3	5			1.79 ± 0.26	127 ± 24		13
ball-and-cage	26	1		10.0			1.4	73
	28	27		7 ± 2.75			1.9 ± 0.57	73
	30	25	12.2 ± 4.6	6.99 ± 2.5	1.7 ± 0.3	125 ± 25	1.65 ± 0.4	73, 74
	32	17	11.5 ± 4.2	5.08 ± 2.5	1.7 ± 0.3	110 ± 25	1.98 ± 0.4	73, 74
	34	1		5.0			2.6	73
Stentless Quadrileaflet	26	2		2.2 ± 1.7	1.6	103 ± 31	1.7	88
Bovine Pericardial	28	14			1.58 ± 0.25		1.7 ± 0.6	88
stentless bioprosthesis	30	6			1.42 ± 0.32		2.3 ± 0.4	88
Wessex	29	9		3.69 ± 0.61	1.66 ± 0.17	83 ± 19		85
stented bioprosthesis	31	22		3.31 ± 0.83	1.41 ± 0.25	80 ± 21		85

drop across the prosthesis.[93,94] The range of normal Doppler velocities and gradients across bileaflet valves is large, particularly for smaller valve sizes.[64] Unfortunately, correction for the discrepancy between Doppler and catheter gradients across bileaflet valves is impossible, since the relationship between these gradients actually depends on prosthetic valve function, which is the variable that needs to be assessed with Doppler measurements. The differences between Doppler and catheter gradients decrease with restricted motion of the leaflets and eventually disappear when one leaflet gets totally stuck.[95] Thus, Doppler velocities increase less than expected from the reduction of the effective orifice area with development of obstruction.

Another caveat is the Doppler echocardiographic calculation of effective orifice areas using the continuity equation, which is significantly affected by the phenomenon of localised high velocities/gradients and pressure recovery as it occurs in bileaflet valves.[96,97] Since Doppler velocities across bileaflet valves exceed the average velocity present across the valve by far, calculated areas significantly underestimate the true effective orifice area.[14,95] These limitations have to be considered when analysing such data in order to avoid misinterpretation.

The above-mentioned problems often make it difficult to correctly interpret high Doppler gradients across bileaflet valves, even if the measured values are still in the upper range of what is reported to be normal for a given valve. In such a situation, additional fluoroscopy, which permits the assessment of the leaflet motion, should be used to clarify whether prosthetic valve function is normal or not.

Pressure half-time has been used to calculate mitral valve areas, with the simple formula stating that valve area equals 220 divided by pressure half-time. However, this equation has been empirically developed and tested for native mitral stenosis. Its application to prosthetic valves is questionable, in particular for normally functioning valves.[81,87] Therefore, only pressure half-time itself and not the calculated valve area should be reported.

Baseline Doppler echocardiographic information

Finally, the knowledge of baseline data can be very helpful. In particular when changes in clinical findings occur, they can be related to possible changes of the Doppler data. But also in the setting of a routine echo examination, interpretation of Doppler data is always easier when baseline data are available for comparison. Efforts should therefore be made to document such baseline data for each individual patient early after surgery (ideally after 3–4 weeks).

Summary

Assessment of normal and abnormal function of heart valve prostheses remains challenging. Doppler echocardiography is widely used to assess prosthetic valve function. Even normally functioning prosthetic valves are to some degree obstructive to flow and, furthermore, the normal values of gradients, pressure half-times and effective orifice areas depend on the type and size of the valve. In addition, velocities and gradients are highly flow-dependent. Appropriate Doppler echocardiographic assessment of prosthetic valve function therefore requires specification of valve type and valve size in order to allow comparison with the normal values, as well as consideration of the flow status. In order to detect changes over time, efforts should also be made to document baseline data for the individual patient.

References

1. Kirzner CF, Vinals B, Moya J, et al. Hemodynamic performance evaluation of small aortic ATS Medical valves by Doppler echocardiography. J Heart Valve Dis 1997; 6(6):661–5.

2. Karpuz H, Jeanrenaud X, Hurni M, et al. Doppler echocardiographic assessment of the new ATS medical prosthetic valve in the aortic position. Am J Card Imaging 1996; 10(4):254–60.

3. Eriksson M, Brodin LA, Ericsson A, Lindblom D. Doppler-derived pressure differences in normally functioning aortic valve prostheses. Studies in Bjork-Shiley monostrut and Biocor porcine prostheses. Scand J Thorac Cardiovasc Surg 1993; 27(2):93–7.

4. Myken PS, Berggren HE, Larsson S, et al. Long-term Doppler echocardiographic results of aortic or mitral valve replacement with Biocor porcine bioprosthesis. J Thorac Cardiovasc Surg 1998; 116(4):599–608.

5. Bech-Hanssen O, Wallentin I, Larsson S, Caidahl K. Reference Doppler echocardiographic values for St. Jude Medical, Omnicarbon, and Biocor prosthetic valves in the aortic position. J Am Soc Echocardiogr 1998; 11(5):466–77.

6. Eriksson MJ, Brodin LA, Dellgren GN, Radegran K. Rest and exercise hemodynamics of an extended stentless aortic bioprosthesis. J Heart Valve Dis 1997; 6(6):653–60.

7. Gonzalez-Juanatey JR, Garcia-Acuna JM, Vega Fernandez M, et al. Hemodynamics of various designs of 19 mm pericardial aortic valve bioprosthesis. Eur J Cardiothorac Surg 1996; 10(3):201–6.

8. Gonzalez-Juanatey JR, Garcia-Bengoechea JB, Vega M, et al. Doppler echocardiographic evaluation of the Bioflo pericardial bioprosthesis. J Heart Valve Dis 1993; 2(3):315–19; discussion 320.

9. Aris A, Padro JM, Camara ML, et al. The Monostrut Bjork-Shiley valve. Seven years' experience. J Thorac Cardiovasc Surg 1992; 103(6):1074–82.

10. Aris A, Ramirez I, Camara ML, et al. The 20 mm Medtronic Hall prosthesis in the small aortic root. Heart Valve Dis 1996; 5(4):459–62.

11. Pons-Llado G, Carreras F, Borras X, et al. Doppler-derived gradients in normally functioning Monostrut Bjork-Shiley prostheses. Am J Cardiol 1995; 76(1):100–3.

12. Kenny A, Woods J, Fuller CA, et al. Hemodynamic evaluation of the Monostrut and spherical disc Bjork-Shiley aortic valve prosthesis with Doppler echocardiography. Thorac Cardiovasc Surg 1992; 104(4):1025–8.

13. Gibbs JL, Wharton GA, Williams GJ. Doppler ultrasound of normally functioning mechanical mitral and aortic valve prostheses. Int J Cardiol 1988; 18(3):391–8.

14. Henneke KH, Pongratz G, Pohlmann M, Bachmann K. Doppler echocardiographic determination of geometric orifice areas in mechanical aortic valve prostheses. Cardiology 1995; 86(6):508–13.

15. Ramirez ML, Wong M, Sadler N, Shah PM. Doppler evaluation of bioprosthetic and mechanical aortic valves: data from four models in 107 stable, ambulatory patients. Am Heart J 1988; 115(2):418–25.

16. Habib G, Benichou M, Gisbert MP, et al. [Contribution of Doppler echocardiography in the evaluation of normal and pathologic aortic valve prosthesis]. Arch Mal Coeur Vaiss 1990; 83(7):937–45 [in French].

17. Sagar KB, Wann LS, Paulsen WH, Romhilt DW. Doppler echocardiographic evaluation of Hancock and Bjork-Shiley prosthetic values. J Am Coll Cardiol 1986; 7(3):681–7.

18. De Paulis R, Sommariva L, Russo F, et al. Doppler echocardiography evaluation of the CarboMedics valve in patients with small aortic anulus and valve prosthesis–body surface area mismatch. J Thorac Cardiovasc Surg 1994; 108(1):57–62.

19. Chakraborty B, Quek S, Pin DZ, Siong CT, Kheng TL. Doppler echocardiographic assessment of normally functioning Starr-Edwards, carbomedics and Carpentier-Edwards valves in aortic position. Angiology 1996 May; 47(5):481–9.

20. Chambers J, Cross J, Deverall P, Sowton E. Echocardiographic description of the CarboMedics bileaflet prosthetic heart valve. J Am Coll Cardiol 1993; 21(2):398–405.

21. De Paulis R, Sommariva L, De Matteis GM, et al. Hemodynamic performances of small diameter carbomedics and St. Jude valves. J Heart Valve Dis 1996; 5 (Suppl 3):S339–43.

22. Globits S, Rodler S, Mayr H, et al. Doppler sonographic evaluation of the CarboMedics bileaflet valve prosthesis: one-year experience. J Card Surg 1992; 7(1):9–16.

23. Ihlen H, Molstad P, Simonsen S, et al. Hemodynamic evaluation of the CarboMedics prosthetic heart valve in the aortic position: comparison of noninvasive and invasive techniques. Am Heart J 1992; 123(1):151–9.

24. Izzat MB, Birdi I, Wilde P, Bryan AJ, Angelini GD. Evaluation of the hemodynamic performance of small CarboMedics aortic prostheses using dobutamine-stress Doppler echocardiography. Ann Thorac Surg 1995; 60(4):1048–52.

25. Noera G, Pensa P, Lamarra M, et al. Hemodynamic evaluation of the Carbomedics R, St Jude Medical HP and Sorin-Bicarbon valve in patients with small aortic annulus. Eur J Cardiothorac Surg 1997; 11(3):473–5, discussion 475–6.

26. de Brux JL, Subayi JB, Binuani P, Laporte J. Doppler-echocardiographic assessment of the carbomedics supra-annular 'Top-Hat' prosthetic heart valve in the aortic position. J Heart Valve Dis 1996; 5 (Suppl 3):S336–8.

27. Strike PC, Edwards TJ, Gardiner D, Livesey SA, Simpson IA. Functional hemodynamic assessment of the 21–mm and 23–mm CarboMedics Top Hat aortic prosthetic valve. J Card Surg 1998; 13(2):98–103.

28. Roedler S, Moritz A, Wutte M, Hoda R, Wolner E. The CarboMedics "top hat" supraannular prosthesis in the small aortic root. J Card Surg 1995; 10(3):198–204.

29. Bojar RM, Rastegar H, Payne DD, Mack CA, Schwartz SL. Clinical and hemodynamic performance of the 19–mm Carpentier-Edwards porcine bioprosthesis. Ann Thorac Surg 1993; 56(5):1141–7.

30. Gibbs JL, Wharton GA, Williams GJ. Doppler echocardiographic characteristics of the Carpentier-Edwards xenograft. Eur Heart J 1986; 7(4):353–6.

31. McDonald ML, Daly RC, Schaff HV, et al. Hemodynamic performance of small aortic valve bioprostheses: is there a difference? Ann Thorac Surg 1997; 63(2):362–6.

32. Mullany CJ, Schaff HV, Orszulak TA, Miller FA. Early clinical and hemodynamic evaluation of the aortic intact porcine bioprosthesis. J Heart Valve Dis 1994; 3(6):641–7.

33. Wiseth R, Levang OW, Sande E, et al. Hemodynamic evaluation by Doppler echocardiography of small (less than or equal to 21 mm) prostheses and bioprostheses in the aortic valve position. Am J Cardiol 1992; 70(2):240–6.

34. Cooper DM, Stewart WJ, Schiavone WA, et al. Evaluation of normal prosthetic valve function by Doppler echocardiography. Am Heart J 1987; 114(3):576–82.

35. Lesbre JP, Chassat C, Lesperance J, et al. [Evaluation of new pericardial bioprostheses by pulsed and continuous Doppler ultrasound]. Arch Mal Coeur Vaiss 1986; 79(10):1439–48 [in French].

36. Kallis P, Sneddon JF, Simpson IA, et al. Clinical and hemodynamic

evaluation of the 19–mm Carpentier-Edwards supraannular aortic valve. Ann Thorac Surg 1992; 54(6):1182–5.

37. Hvass U, Palatianos GM, Frassani R, Puricelli C, O'Brien M. Multicenter study of stentless valve replacement in the small aortic root. J Thorac Cardiovasc Surg 1999; 117(2):267–72.

38. O'Brien MF, Gardner MA, Garlick RB, et al. The Cryolife-O'Brien stentless aortic porcine xenograft valve. J Card Surg 1998; 13(5):376–85.

39. Gioia G, Rutsch W. [Normal echo-Doppler values in Duromedics valvular prostheses]. G Ital Cardiol 1988; 18(3):213–17 [in Italian].

40. Dossche K, Vanermen H, Daenen W, Pillai R, Konertz W. Hemodynamic performance of the PRIMA Edwards stentless aortic xenograft: early results of a multicenter clinical trial. Thorac Cardiovasc Surg 1996; 44(1):11–14.

41. Jin XY, Dhital K, Bhattacharya K, et al. Fifth-year hemodynamic performance of the prima stentless aortic valve. Ann Thorac Surg 1998; 66(3):805–9.

42. Bortolotti U, Milano A, Tartarini G, et al. Hemodynamic performance of the Edwards Prima stentless valve. J Heart Valve Dis 1997; 6(2):134–7.

43. David TE, Armstrong S, Sun Z. Clinical and hemodynamic assessment of the Hancock II bioprosthesis. Ann Thorac Surg 1992; 54(4):661–7, discussion 667–8.

44. Eichinger WB, Schutz A, Simmerl D, et al. The mosaic bioprosthesis in the aortic position: hemodynamic performance after 2 years. Ann Thorac Surg 1998; 66(6 Suppl):S126–9.

45. Ius P, Totis O, Chirillo F, et al. Hemodynamic evaluation of 23 mm Pericarbon and 23 mm Hancock II bioprostheses in the aortic position at mid-term follow up. J Heart Valve Dis 1996; 5(6):656–61.

46. Bojar RM, Diehl JT, Moten M, et al. Clinical and hemodynamic performance of the Ionescu-Shiley valve in the small aortic root. Results in 117 patients with 17 and 19 mm valves. Thorac Cardiovasc Surg 1989; 98(6):1087–95.

47. O'Keefe PA, Ninan M, Ayers B, Young CP. Aortic valve replacement with the Jyros bileaflet prosthetic valve; early echocardiographic and radiological evaluation. J Heart Valve Dis 1995; 4(Suppl 1):S77–9, discussion 79–80.

48. Cartier PC, Dumesnil JG, Metras J, et al. Clinical and hemodynamic performance of the Freestyle aortic root bioprosthesis. Ann Thorac Surg 1999; 67(2):345–9, discussion 349–51.

49. Baur LH, Jin XY, Houdas Y, et al. Echocardiographic parameters of the freestyle stentless bioprosthesis in aortic position: the European experience. J Am Soc Echocardiogr 1999; 12(9):729–35.

50. Plehn JF, Arbuckle BE, Southworth J, et al. A hemodynamic comparison of Omniscience and Medtronic Hall aortic prostheses. J Heart Valve Dis 1996; 5(3):328–36.

51. Raisaro A, Caizzi V, Roda G, et al. [Doppler evaluation of the Sorin and Medtronic-Hall prostheses in the aortic position]. G Ital Cardiol 1988; 18(3):206–12 [in Italian].

52. Etienne Y, Jobic Y, Genet L, et al. [Evaluation of the normal bioprosthetic Intact aortic valve by Doppler echocardiography]. Arch Mal Coeur Vaiss 1990; 83(14):2039–44 [in French].

53. Ricou F, Brun A, Lerch R. Hemodynamic comparison of Medtronic intact bioprostheses and bileaflet mechanical prostheses in aortic position. Cardiology 1996; 87(3):212–15.

54. Jaffe WM, Barratt-Boyes BG, Sadri A, et al. Early follow-up of patients with the Medtronic Intact porcine valve. A new cardiac bioprosthesis. Thorac Cardiovasc Surg 1989; 98(2):181–92.

55. Thomson DJ, Jamieson WR, Dumesnil JG, et al. Medtronic mosaic porcine bioprosthesis satisfactory early clinical performance. Ann Thorac Surg 1998; 66(6 Suppl):S122–5.

56. Hvass U, Chatel D, Assayag P, et al. The O'Brien-Angell stentless porcine valve: early results with 150 implants. Ann Thorac Surg 1995; 60(2 Suppl):S414–17.

57. Fehske W, Kessel D, Kirchhoff PG, et al. Echocardiographic profile of the normally functioning Omnicarbon valve. J Heart Valve Dis 1994; 3(3):263–74.

58. Messner-Pellenc P, Wittenberg O, Leclercq F, et al. Doppler echocardiographic evaluation of the Omnicarbon cardiac valve prostheses. J Cardiovasc Surg (Torino) 1993; 34(3):195–202.

59. Peter M, Weiss P, Jenzer HR, et al. The Omnicarbon tilting-disc heart valve prosthesis. A clinical and Doppler echocardiographic follow-up. J Thorac Cardiovasc Surg 1993; 106(4):599–608.

60. Chambers J, Ely JL. Early postoperative echocardiographic hemodynamic performance of the On-X prosthetic heart valve: a multicenter study. J Heart Valve Dis 1998; 7(5):569–73.

61. Badano L, Bertoli D, Astengo D, et al. Doppler haemodynamic assessment of clinically and echocardiographically normal mitral and aortic Allcarbon valve prostheses. Valve Prostheses Ligurian Cooperative Doppler Study. Eur Heart J 1993; 14(12):1602–9.

62. Badano L, Mocchegiani R, Bertoli D, et al. Normal echocardiographic characteristics of the Sorin Bicarbon bileaflet prosthetic heart valve in the mitral and aortic positions. J Am Soc Echocardiogr 1997; 10(6):632–43.

63. Flameng W, Vandeplas A, Narine K, et al. Postoperative hemodynamics of two bileaflet heart valves in the aortic position. J Heart Valve Dis 1997; 6(3):269–73.

64. Chafizadeh ER, Zoghbi WA. Doppler echocardiographic assessment of the St. Jude Medical prosthetic valve in the aortic position using the continuity equation. Circulation 1991; 83(1):213–23.

65. Kadir I, Izzat MB, Birdi I, et al. Hemodynamics of St. Jude Medical prostheses in the small aortic root: in vivo studies using dobutamine Doppler echocardiography. J Heart Valve Dis 1997; 6(2):123–9.

66. Lesbre JP, Guillaumont MP, Dallocchio M, et al. [Echodoppler evaluation of the normally functioning Saint-Jude's aortic valve prosthesis]. Arch Mal Coeur Vaiss 1990; 83(10):1553–61 [in French].

67. Maribas P, Diebold B, Vanetti A, Bical O. [Evaluation of 90 normal aortic valve prosthesis of the Saint-Jude Medical type by echocardiography]. Arch Mal Coeur Vaiss 1990; 83(11):1653–8 [in French].

68. Panidis IP, Ross J, Mintz GS. Normal and abnormal prosthetic valve function as assessed by Doppler echocardiography. Am Coll Cardiol 1986; 8(2):317–26.

69. Perin EC, Jin BS, de Castro CM, Ferguson JJ, Hall RJ. Doppler echocardiography in 180 normally functioning St. Jude Medical aortic valve prostheses. Early and late postoperative assessments. Chest 1991; 100(4):988–90.

70. Ren JF, Chandrasekaran K, Mintz GS, et al. Effect of depressed left ventricular function on hemodynamics of normal St. Jude Medical prosthesis in the aortic valve position. Am J Cardiol 1990; 65(15):1004–9.

71. Carrel T, Zingg U, Jenni R, Aeschbacher B, Turina MI. Early in vivo experience with the Hemodynamic Plus St. Jude Medical heart valves in patients with narrowed aortic annulus. Ann Thorac Surg 1996; 61(5):1418–22.

72. Laske A, Jenni R, Maloigne M, et al. Pressure gradients across bileaflet aortic valves by direct measurement and echocardiography. Ann Thorac Surg 1996; 61(1):48–57.

73. Rashtian MY, Stevenson DM, Allen DT, et al. Flow characteristics of four commonly used mechanical heart valves. Am J Cardiol 1986; 58(9):743–52.

74. Lefebvre E, Isorni C, Rey JL, Lesbre JP. Echo-Doppler evaluation of normal Starr-Edwards prostheses in mitral and aortic position. Arch Mal Coeur Vaiss 1987; 80(7):1105–14 [in French].

75. Meloni L, Ricchi A, Cirio E, et al. Echocardiographic assessment of aortic valve replacement with stentless porcine xenografts. Am J Cardiol 1995; 76(4):294–6.

76. Wong K, Shad S, Waterworth PD, et al. Early experience with the Toronto stentless porcine valve. Ann Thorac Surg 1995; 60(2 Suppl):S402–5.

77. Bach DS, David T, Yacoub M, et al. Hemodynamics and left ventric-

ular mass regression following implantation of the Toronto SPV stentless porcine valve. Am J Cardiol 1998; 82(10):1214–9.

78. Goldman BS, David TE, Del Rizzo DF, Sever J, Bos J. Stentless porcine bioprosthesis for aortic valve replacement. J Cardiovasc Surg (Torino) 1994; 35(6 Suppl 1):105–10.

79. Walther T, Falk V, Autschbach R, et al. Hemodynamic assessment of the stentless Toronto SPV bioprosthesis by echocardiography. J Heart Valve Dis 1994; 3(6):657–65.

80. Walther T, Falk V, Diegeler A, et al. Stentless bioprostheses for the small aortic root. J Heart Valve Dis 1996; 5(Suppl 3):S302–7.

81. Mohan JC, Agrawal R, Arora R, Khalilullah M. Improved Doppler assessment of the Bjork-Shiley mitral prosthesis using the continuity equation. Int J Cardiol 1994; 43(3):321–6.

82. Soo CS, Ca M, Tay M, et al. Doppler-echocardiographic assessment of Carbomedics prosthetic valves in the mitral position. J Am Soc Echocardiogr 1994; 7(2):159–64.

83. Bjornerheim R, Ihlen H, Simonsen S, Sire S, Svennevig J. Hemodynamic characterization of the CarboMedics mitral valve prosthesis. J Heart Valve Dis 1997; 6(2):115–22.

84. Habib G, Benichou M, Bonnet JL, et al. [Contribution of Doppler echocardiography to the evaluation and monitoring of normal and pathologic mitral valve prostheses]. Arch Mal Coeur Vaiss 1990; 83(4):469–77 [in French].

85. Simpson IA, Reece IJ, Houston AB, et al. Non-invasive assessment by Doppler ultrasound of 155 patients with bioprosthetic valves: a comparison of the Wessex porcine, low profile Ionescu-Shiley, and Hancock pericardial bioprostheses. Br Heart J 1986; 56(1):83–8.

86. Gonzalez-Juanatey JR, Garcia-Bengoechea JB, Vega M, et al. Echocardiographic features of the normofunctional Labcor-Santiago pericardial bioprosthesis. J Heart Valve Dis 1994; 3(5):548–55.

87. Bitar JN, Lechin ME, Salazar G, Zoghbi WA. Doppler echocardiographic assessment with the continuity equation of St. Jude Medical mechanical prostheses in the mitral valve position. Am J Cardiol 1995; 76(4):287–93. Published erratum appears in Am J Cardiol 1995; 76(8):642.

88. Middlemost SJ, Manga P. The stentless quadrileaflet bovine pericardial mitral valve: echocardiographic assessment. J Heart Valve Dis 1999; 8(2):180–5.

89. Reisner SA, Meltzer RS. Normal values of prosthetic valve Doppler echocardiographic parameters: a review. J Am Soc Echocardiogr 1988; 1(3):201–10.

90. Baumgartner H, Khan S, DeRobertis M, Czer L, Maurer G. Effect of prosthetic aortic valve design on the Doppler-catheter gradient correlation: an in vitro study of normal St. Jude, Medtronic-Hall, Starr-Edwards and Hancock valves. J Am Coll Cardiol 1992; 19(2):324–32.

91. Rosenhek R, Binder T, Maurer G, Baumgartner H. Normal values for Doppler echocardiographic assessment of heart valve prostheses. J Am Soc Echocardiogr 2003; 16(11):1116–27.

92. Yoganathan AP, Chaux A, Gray RJ, et al. Bileaflet, tilting disc and porcine aortic valve substitutes: in vitro hydrodynamic characteristics. J Am Coll Cardiol 1984; 3(2 Pt 1):313–20.

93. Baumgartner H, Khan S, DeRobertis M, Czer L, Maurer G. Discrepancies between Doppler and catheter gradients in aortic prosthetic valves in vitro. A manifestation of localized gradients and pressure recovery. Circulation 1990; 82(4):1467–75.

94. Baumgartner H, Schima H, Kuhn P. Discrepancies between Doppler and catheter gradients across bileaflet aortic valve prostheses. Am J Cardiol 1993; 71(13):1241–3.

95. Baumgartner H, Schima H, Kuhn P. Effect of prosthetic valve malfunction on the Doppler-catheter gradient relation for bileaflet aortic valve prostheses. Circulation 1993; 87(4):1320–7.

96. Baumgartner H, Khan SS, DeRobertis M, Czer LS, Maurer G. Doppler assessment of prosthetic valve orifice area. An in vitro study. Circulation 1992; 85(6):2275–83.

97. Mohan JC, Bhargawa M. Doppler echocardiographic assessment of prosthetic aortic valve area: estimation with the continuity equation compared to the Gorlin formula. Int J Cardiol 1996; 55(2):177–81.

6

Problems specific to homografts, autografts and stentless valves

John R Doty and Donald B Doty

Introduction

The first cases of aortic valve replacement with the aortic homograft were published over 40 years ago, and within 5 years of these reports Donald Ross began his seminal work with the pulmonary autograft.[1–3] Persistent work and the gradual accumulation of time have resulted in several large series of patients, some exceeding 25 years of experience, who demonstrate the excellent long-term outcomes that can be achieved with human valves in the aortic position.[4–9] The aortic homograft and the pulmonary autograft provide the absolute best haemodynamic performance and are extremely resistant to infection. Although technically challenging to implant, the versatility of these valves allows for application in patients with small aortic root, left ventricular outflow tract obstruction, and reconstruction of complex root anatomy associated with aggressive infection or congenital malformation.

Stentless tissue bioprostheses are a more recent development, with the first reports published less than 20 years ago.[10] Although follow-up is not as extensive as the homograft and autograft, there are several series of patients who demonstrate very encouraging mid-term outcomes with the stentless bioprostheses.[11–14] These valves are more readily available and have a wider range of sizes, allowing for implantation in virtually any patient with aortic valve disease. The stentless bioprosthesis also has excellent haemodynamics and can be used for root reconstruction in many patients.

The natural quality of the implanted tissue is such that thromboembolism is unusual and anticoagulation is not required. These valves are also quite resistant to acquisition of bacterial endocarditis. Nevertheless, none of these valves represents the perfect prosthesis for aortic valve replacement. Each valve has unique characteristics and therefore has specific problems which have been identified from cumulative clinical experience. In addition, there are certain issues which are common to all of these 'stentless' valves.

Problems specific to homografts

Use of the aortic homograft, or allograft, began in the early 1960s by Ross in Great Britain and Barratt-Boyes in New Zealand. The method of insertion preferred by Barratt-Boyes was to use the homograft as an isolated valve replacement in the subcoronary position, removing the sinus aorta from all three sinuses of Valsalva. The valve was rotated 120° anticlockwise to place the septal myocardium above the anterior leaflet of the mitral valve. Ross, on the other hand, preferred retaining the non-coronary sinus aorta and implanting the valve in anatomical position in order to improve accuracy in proper orientation of the three commissures. This has become known as the 'modified' technique of insertion of an aortic homograft. The homograft can also be implanted as a 'mini-root' inclusion or most commonly as a full, free-standing root replacement with reimplantation of the coronary arteries on small buttons of retained aortic sinus tissue. A unique feature of the aortic homograft is that these valves are harvested with the contiguous anterior leaflet of the mitral valve. The anterior leaflet can be employed to reconstruct the recipient mitral valve in extensive annular abscess or reconstruction of complex congenital anatomy.

Initially, homografts were placed in antibiotic solution after unsterile donor harvest and refrigerated for a period of time before implantation, usually within 28 days. When the valve was implanted within 72 hours, the term 'homovital' was applied. The homovital homograft almost certainly has viable donor cells at the time of implantation. More recently, aortic homografts are cryopreserved after sterile donor harvest. Cryopreservation involves control of temperature drop during the freezing process and the addition of dimethyl sulphoxide (DMSO) to the media bathing the graft to prevent cell rupture as intracellular water converts from liquid to solid phase. Such valves can be kept frozen nearly indefinitely and provide tissue that handles naturally, but probably have few, if any, viable donor cells when implanted even though the cell matrix is well preserved.

Both homovital and cryopreserved homografts are subject to gradual calcification, which can result in leaflet immobility, aortic wall rigidity, or both. This calcification is probably the result of a continuous low-grade immune response to the foreign homograft, typically occurs over several years and is the most common cause of regurgitation. As the homograft calcifies, leaflet motion is restricted and the valve becomes insufficient. The calcification process can also render the commissures and retained non-coronary sinus stiff and inflexible. When the homograft is used for full root replacement, the entire homograft can become a rigid tube. The calcification also affects the contiguous anterior leaflet of the mitral valve if this portion was used in the original implantation. The calcification process usually progresses gradually, although the degenerative process in the tissue may result in cusp rupture with sudden onset of severe valve insufficiency. Younger patients appear to exert a more robust immune response and are therefore more likely to calcify the homograft, particularly children and young adolescents.[15] The immune response in children persists for many years, as measured by panel-reactive antibodies.[16]

Various strategies have been employed in attempts to reduce antigenicity of the homograft in order to delay this calcification process. To date, there has been no evidence that the use of immunosuppressive medication affects the development of progressive calcification.[17] Likewise, blood type mismatch does not appear to have a significant impact on the long-term development of calcification or homograft function.

The long-term data from Yacoub suggest that the most favourable combination is an older recipient with a young homograft.[18] This approach is more feasible in Great Britain where the appropriate patient can be selected from a waiting list when a suitable homograft becomes available. The limited availability of cryopreserved homografts in North America renders this situation unlikely, and the surgeon is usually restricted by homograft size issues in choosing a valve for the patient.

Size discrepancy is typically not a major problem as the aortic homograft has excellent haemodynamics even in very small sizes. However, if there is a size mismatch exceeding 2–3 mm between the homograft and the native aortic root, the native root must be altered to match the size of the homograft. If the left ventricular outflow tract is small and restrictive, it should be enlarged to the appropriate size. Several manoeuvres are available for root enlargement, ranging from simple mobilisation of the interleaflet triangles to more extensive procedures involving division of the aortic annulus and widening of the left ventricular outflow tract. Our preferred approach in the small, restrictive aortic root is to extend an incision into the commissure

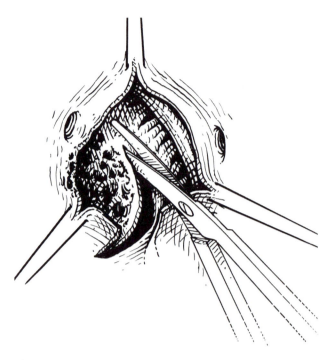

Figure 6.1
If greater root enlargement is necessary or if there is subvalvular pathology (as shown in this figure), demonstrating annular abscess that involves the mitral valve and requires debridement, the incision is carried across the mitral annulus into the anterior leaflet of the mitral valve. Reproduced from Kouchoukos et al, Cardiac surgery, Churchill Livingstone, 2003: 573, with permission from Elsevier.

between the left and non-coronary sinuses, between the fibrous attachment of the aortic annulus, down to the upper edge of the anterior leaflet of the mitral valve. If still greater enlargement is necessary or if there is subvalvular pathology, the incision is carried across the mitral annulus into the middle of the anterior leaflet (Figure 6.1). The attached anterior leaflet of the homograft mitral valve is then used to repair the anterior leaflet of the mitral or to widen the left ventricular outflow tract. The defect in the roof of the left atrium is repaired with a patch or either a piece of homograft aorta or pericardium (Figure 6.2).

Imperfect technical implantation of a subcoronary homograft can result from improper positioning of the commissures or distortion of the valve during closure of the aortotomy. Such asymmetric implantation results in uneven stress and strain on the leaflets and predisposes the homograft to rupture, tearing and early development of insufficiency. Dividing the aorta above the sinotubular junction or using a long transverse aortotomy provides the best opportunity for symmetric implantation of the valve and completely avoids distortion during closure of a typical oblique aortotomy. These events are more likely to occur in a dilated aortic root, which overstretches the homograft leaflets and is of particular concern when the annulus

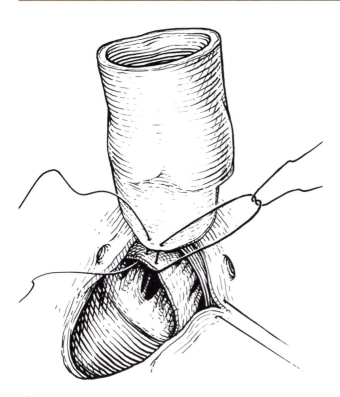

Figure 6.2
The attached anterior leaflet of the homograft mitral valve is used to repair the anterior leaflet of the mitral valve or to widen the left ventricular outflow tract. Reproduced from Kouchoukos et al, Cardiac surgery, Churchill Livingstone, 2003: 573, with permission from Elsevier.

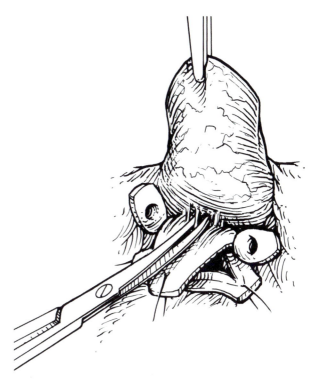

Figure 6.3
The pulmonary artery is carefully dissected off the aorta and top of the right ventricle until muscle fibres in the ventricular infundibulum are identified running in a perpendicular orientation. Reproduced from Kouchoukos et al, Cardiac surgery, Churchill Livingstone, 2003: 580, with permission from Elsevier.

exceeds 30 mm in diameter. Subcoronary homograft implantation is best reserved for patients with small, symmetric aortic root and should be avoided in patients with an enlarged aortic root. Such patients are ideally treated by reducing and stabilising the annulus with a circumferential non-absorbable suture and then implanting an appropriately sized homograft as a free-standing full root replacement.[19]

Problems specific to autografts

The pulmonary autograft (Ross procedure) was introduced in 1967, and, like the aortic homograft, was initially implanted as an isolated subcoronary valve. More widespread use of the operation gradually evolved into implantation of the autograft as a full root to avoid the same technical challenges of the subcoronary homograft: namely, avoidance of asymmetric implantation and distortion of the valve. The right ventricular outflow tract is replaced with a pulmonary homograft in the vast majority of cases.

The Ross procedure carries an inherent risk to the patient by virtue of the harvesting technique for the pulmonary autograft. Extreme care must to taken to avoid injury to the pulmonary valve and to the surrounding structures during the dissection of the right ventricular outflow tract. Common problem areas include thinning or perforation of the pulmonary sinuses during dissection behind the pulmonary artery, injury to the pulmonary valve leaflets while dividing the free wall of the right ventricle and damage to the first septal branch of the left anterior descending coronary artery during dissection of the septal portion of the pulmonary trunk.

The pulmonary artery should be divided near its bifurcation to avoid entering the pulmonary sinuses or encroaching upon the sinotubular junction. Next, the pulmonary artery is carefully dissected off the aorta and top of the right ventricle until the ventricular muscle fibres are identified running in a perpendicular orientation (Figure 6.3). The pulmonary valve is carefully inspected and a small right angle clamp is passed well below the pulmonary annulus along a line with the anterior commissure. The clamp is pushed out through the right ventricular free wall and the right ventricle is divided well below the pulmonary annulus

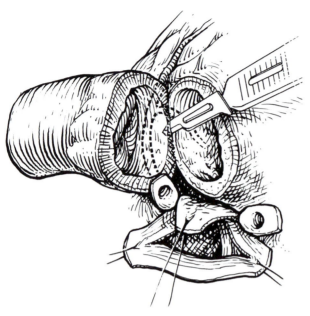

Figure 6.4
Sharp dissection of the ventricular septum with a knife is used to separate the pulmonary trunk from the right ventricle in order to protect the first septal perforating coronary artery. Reproduced from Kouchoukos et al, Cardiac surgery, Churchill Livingstone, 2003: 581, with permission from Elsevier.

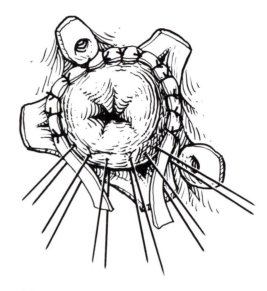

Figure 6.5
Annular dilation can be prevented by using the free-standing root technique for the pulmonary autograft and supporting the autograft annulus with a thin strip of felt, polyester fabric, or autologous pericardium within the proximal suture line. Interrupted sutures are tied over the support ring with the autograft partially inverted into the left ventricular outflow tract to assure accurate approximation of the autograft to the aortic wall. Reproduced from Kouchoukos et al, Cardiac surgery, Churchill Livingstone, 2003: 582, with permission from Elsevier.

with direct visualisation of the pulmonary valve leaflets. Sharp dissection of the ventricular septum with a knife is used to separate the pulmonary trunk from the right ventricle in order to protect the first septal branch of the left anterior descending coronary artery (Figure 6.4).

Unlike the aortic homograft, the pulmonary autograft has shown remarkable resistance to calcification. The pulmonary leaflets may thicken with time, but remain pliable and mobile. Likewise, the autograft sinuses and commissures also do not generally become calcified. In contrast to the homograft root, which can become a rigid, calcified tube, the autograft root can undergo progressive dilation of the aortic annulus or sinotubular junction.[20,21] These developments can render the autograft incompetent, as annular dilation stretches the leaflets and sinotubular junction dilation separates the commissures, resulting in lack of central coaptation and regurgitation. In most larger series of patients, this is an uncommon event, with about 80–90% of patients free from autograft insufficiency or reoperation at 10 years. It is this process that has led to the general abandonment of the subcoronary technique.

Annular dilation can be prevented by using the free-standing root technique for the pulmonary autograft and supporting the autograft annulus with a thin strip of felt, polyester fabric, or autologous pericardium within the proximal suture line (Figure 6.5).[22] Dilation of the sinotubular junction can also be prevented by placing a collar

of polyester graft size matched to the autograft diameter around the outside of the autograft at the top of the commissures (Figure 6.6). These two measures fix the inflow and outflow diameters of the autograft, ensuring that no distortion of the leaflets or commissures can occur over time.

Although the autograft leaflets have been shown to tolerate the higher pressures of the systemic circulation, the autograft sinuses can also become markedly enlarged and even aneurysmal. At this time, there is no universally accepted method for preventing the development of autograft sinus enlargement. In our opinion, reoperation in such a patient is only indicated if the sinuses become markedly enlarged or if the patient develops concomitant progressive autograft regurgitation. At surgery, a valve-sparing operation (Yacoub type) can be employed if the autograft is competent and the leaflets are acceptable.[23–26] If the autograft has become regurgitant, a valve-sparing operation is unlikely to be successful and the autograft should be replaced with an alternative valve prosthesis.

A small subset of patients with a pulmonary autograft will develop regurgitation in the absence of autograft dilation. This regurgitation generally remains stable and has little if any impact on the patient's quality of life and

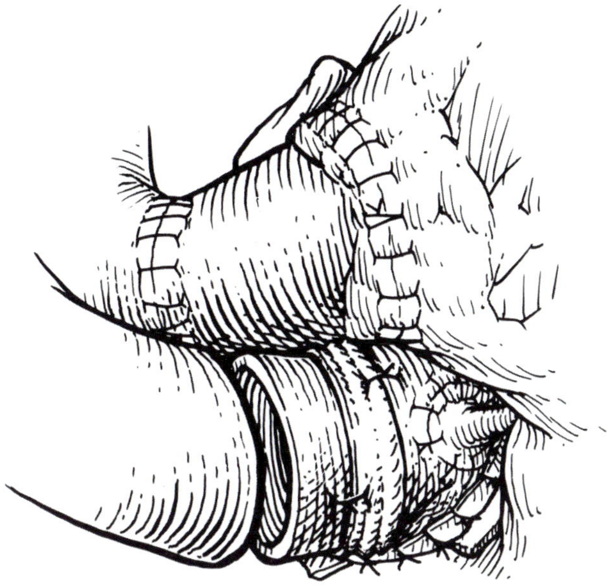

Figure 6.6

Dilation of the sinotubular junction can be prevented by placing a collar of polyester graft size matched to the autograft diameter around the outside of the autograft at the top of the commissures. Position of the retention collar is assured by placing sutures at the top of the three commissures passed to the outside and through the graft. Reproduced from Kouchoukos et al, Cardiac surgery, Churchill Livingstone, 2003: 587, with permission from Elsevier.

well-being. Surveillance echocardiography can identify those few patients who have progressive autograft insufficiency, and we recommend reoperation only when the regurgitation is severe.

Patients with underlying aortic disease such as Marfan syndrome, Ehlers–Danlos syndrome or other connective tissue disorders should not undergo the pulmonary autograft operation. In these patients, the pulmonary trunk may also be affected by the connective tissue disorder and be at risk for accelerated dilation or dissection after implantation in the aortic position. In patients with other forms of annular dilation who are otherwise candidates for the pulmonary autograft operation, it is imperative that the aortic annulus be reduced to match the pulmonary autograft.[27] Any discrepancy will tend to stretch the autograft and result in early regurgitation and failure of the autograft. Reduction of the aortic annulus is performed in the same manner as with homograft root replacement.

The pulmonary homograft implanted in the right ventricular outflow tract is subject to a similar process of calcification as the aortic homograft.[28,29] As with the aortic homograft, the pulmonary homograft can be antibiotic preserved, homovital or cryopreserved, and there is little to suggest the superiority of one preservation technique over another. As the calcification progresses, the pulmonary homograft leaflets become thickened and restricted, resulting in pulmonary insufficiency. Calcification can also affect the inflow or outflow suture lines, creating a localised stenosis, or the entire homograft can become a long, stenotic, thickened and calcified tube with an incompetent valve. It is this gradual degeneration of the homograft that is the source of most reoperations, with up to 25% of patients requiring replacement of the pulmonary homograft in long-term follow-up.

Although the calcification process typically occurs over an extended period of time, a smaller subset of patients (5%) will develop early and rapid calcification and stenosis of the pulmonary homograft. Such patients present with a harsh systolic murmur and are not usually symptomatic. Echocardiography will often demonstrate a substantial gradient across the right ventricular outflow tract. Attempts have been made to perform percutaneous pulmonary valvotomy with limited success. In general, an operation is not indicated unless the patient becomes symptomatic or the right ventricle becomes dilated and has reduced contractile function.

Problems specific to stentless bioprostheses

Limited availability of homografts and limited durability of stented bioprostheses led to the development of stentless porcine bioprostheses in the late 1980s.[10] There are now several stentless devices available with some variation in the individual designs, but the distinguishing feature in all of these valves is the absence of a rigid supporting stent for the commissures or annulus. Many of the stentless bioprostheses have a thin layer of polyester fabric or pericardium to assist in suturing the valve, but such material adds little support to the prosthesis itself.

Stentless bioprostheses offer several potential advantages over other valve replacement devices. These valves are readily available in a wide range of sizes and can therefore be easily matched to the native aortic annulus. The absence of a rigid supporting stent allows for a comparatively larger device to be inserted into patients with a small aortic annulus, so that these valves exhibit excellent haemodynamics even in the smaller size ranges.[30–35] Although more challenging to implant than a stented prosthesis, these valves are technically easier to use than either homografts or autografts because they are glutaraldehyde-fixed and tend to retain their inherent configuration during implantation and conforming to the native aortic root. Lastly, the full aortic root models are quite versatile, allowing implantation as a full root, inclusion root or modified subcoronary technique.

Despite these advantages, all tissue bioprostheses are subject to eventual calcification and degeneration. New anticalcification and preservation techniques, combined with flexibility and the absence of stent-related stress and strain, may offer improved resistance to calcification and long-term degeneration. The most recent reports suggest that stentless bioprostheses are performing very well at the 10-year interval after implantation.[11–14]

Subcoronary implantation of a stentless bioprosthesis is more reproducible than a homograft and autograft, but can be problematic in two specific situations. Technical inaccuracy in commissural alignment is the first problem. In those prostheses in which there is no retained sinus tissue, the valve is implanted as a completely freehand subcoronary valve. Care must be taken to precisely align all three commissures, as distortion will result in failure of leaflet coaptation and early valve failure. This is somewhat easier to avoid if the prosthesis can be used with the retained non-coronary sinus, as this effectively fixes the relationship between two of the commissures and the surgeon need only ensure correct alignment of the commissure between the left and right sinuses. In addition, the tops of the commissures must be placed at the natural level of the bioprosthesis, which may or may not correlate with the level of the native commissures. If the bioprosthesis is forced out of its natural configuration in an attempt to mould it to the native commissures, it can become distorted. This is particularly evident in the patient with a bicuspid valve, as the sinuses are not symmetric and will not align exactly with the bioprosthesis. Rather, the stentless valve should be allowed to assume its natural contours and the distal suture line carried along the native aortic wall in this position (Figure 6.7).

The second problem in subcoronary implantation occurs with abnormal positioning of the native coronary arteries.[36] Occasionally a patient will have widely spaced coronary ostia and one or both may become obstructed during standard subcoronary implantation. In this setting, the valve should be slightly rotated in one direction or the other prior to annular attachment to ensure that the distal suture line can be safely completed below each coronary ostium. This usually involves placing one ostium in a relatively normal position at the nadir of its sinus with the other coronary ostium off to one side along the bioprosthesis commissure. If it is apparent that one or both coronary ostium may be impaired in any manner, the subcoronary technique should be abandoned and the entire root replaced to ensure satisfactory coronary perfusion.

When the stentless bioprosthesis is used as a root replacement device, it is more often the case that the native coronary buttons do not align exactly with the porcine coronary ostia. The porcine coronary arteries arise at a more acute angle than the human coronary arteries. Typically, one coronary button will line up evenly with one

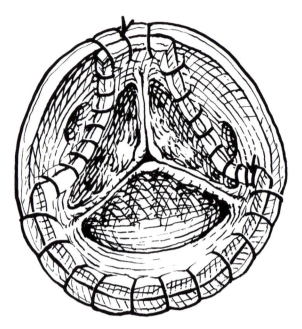

Figure 6.7
Proper alignment of a stentless bioprosthesis with intact non-coronary sinus and distal suture line. Performing the implantation within the intact aortic root provides accurate alignment of the commissures of the graft. Reproduced from Kouchoukos et al, Cardiac surgery, Churchill Livingstone, 2003: 578, with permission from Elsevier.

porcine ostium, and this is easily implanted. The second coronary button is then carefully aligned and a separate incision made for implantation. Extensive mobilisation of the native coronary arteries and undue tension on the coronary anastomoses should be avoided to prevent coronary insufficiency.

Problems common to all

Regardless of whether a homograft, autograft or stentless bioprosthesis is used, there are a few common situations that can present a unique problem. The patient with a bicuspid valve is at increased risk for concomitant or late development of aneurysm of the ascending aorta. Failure to address this disease process can result in late rupture of the aneurysm, aortic dissection or dilation of the sinotubular junction and progressive valvular insufficiency.[37–39] We recommend resection of the ascending aorta and replacement with a prosthetic polyester graft if the aorta exceeds 40 mm. This adds minimal risk to the operation, with great added long-term benefit to the patient.

A second potential problem is the development of coronary insufficiency during aortic root replacement.[40] This can be minimised by retaining large buttons of aortic sinus

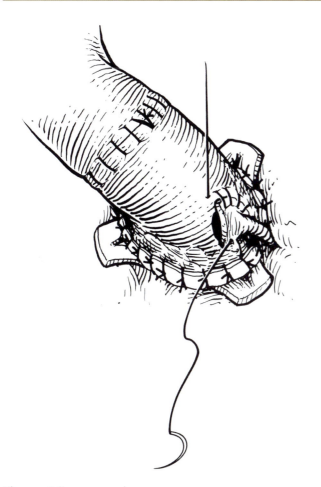

Figure 6.8
Proper alignment of the right coronary artery to the xenograft aortic root is aided by temporarily filling the right ventricle to estimate the natural position of the right coronary artery relative to the xenograft aorta. Reproduced from Kouchoukos et al, Cardiac surgery, Churchill Livingstone, 2003: 583, with permission from Elsevier.

tissue to avoid narrowing the coronary anastomosis. Extensive mobilisation is not typically necessary and may result in kinking of the native coronary artery after reimplantation. Proper alignment of the right coronary artery is aided by filling the right heart to estimate a more natural position of the right ventricle and temporary distension of the aortic root (Figure 6.8).

Conclusion

The collective long-term experience with aortic valve replacement using aortic homografts, pulmonary autograft and stentless bioprostheses has demonstrated excellent performance of these valves. All show superior haemo-

dynamic profiles, do not require anticoagulation, provide excellent quality of life and can be used to address simple as well as complex forms of aortic valve and left ventricular outflow tract pathology. Each valve has specific areas of concern, some of which can be minimised with careful surgical technique and patient selection.

References

1. Ross DN. Homograft replacement of the aortic valve. Lancet 1962; 2:487.
2. Barratt-Boyes BG. Homograft aortic valve replacement in aortic incompetence and stenosis. Thorax 1968; 19:131–50.
3. Ross DN. Replacement of aortic and mitral valves with pulmonary autograft. Lancet 1967; 2:956–8.
4. Doty JR, Salazar JD, Liddicoat JR, Flores JH, Doty DB. Aortic valve replacement with cryopreserved aortic allograft: ten-year experience. J Thorac Cardiovasc Surg 1998; 115:371–80.
5. Lund O, Chandrasekaran V, Grocott-Mason R, et al. Primary aortic valve replacement with allograft over twenty-five years: valve-related and procedure-related determinants of outcome. J Thorac Cardiovasc Surg 1999; 117:77–91.
6. Palka P, Harrocks S, Lange A, Burstow DJ, O'Brien MF. Primary aortic valve replacement with cryopreserved aortic allograft. Circulation 2002; 105:61–6.
7. Kouchoukos NT, Masetti P, Nickerson NJ, et al. The Ross procedure: long-term clinical and echocardiographic follow-up. Ann Thorac Surg 2004; 78:773–81.
8. Stelzer P, Weinrauch S, Tranbaugh RF. Ten years of experience with the modified Ross procedure. J Thorac Cardiovasc Surg 1998; 115:1091–100.
9. Al-Halees Z, Pieters F, Qadoura F, et al. The Ross procedure is the procedure of choice for congenital aortic stenosis. J Thorac Cardiovasc Surg 2002; 123:437–42.
10. David TE, Pollick C, Boss J. Aortic valve replacement with stentless porcine aortic bioprosthesis. J Thorac Cardiovasc Surg 1990; 99:113–18.
11. Bach DS, Kon ND, Dumesnil JG, Sintek CF, Doty DB. Eight-year results after aortic valve replacement with the Freestyle stentless bioprosthesis. J Thorac Cardiovasc Surg 2004; 127:1657–63.
12. Desai ND, Merin O, Cohen GN, et al. Long-term results of aortic valve replacement with the St. Jude Toronto stentless porcine valve. Ann Thorac Surg 2004; 78:2076–83.
13. Luciani GB, Santini F, Auriemma S, et al. Long-term results after aortic valve replacement with the Biocor PSB stentless xenograft in the elderly. Ann Thorac Surg 2001; 71:S306–10.
14. O'Brien MF, Gardner MAH, Garlick B, et al. Cryolife-O'Brien stentless valve: 10-year results of 402 implants. Ann Thorac Surg 2005; 79:757–66.
15. Pompilio G, Polvani G, Piccolo G, et al. Six-year monitoring of the donor-specific immune response to cryopreserved aortic allograft valves: implications with valve dysfunction. Ann Thorac Surg 2004; 78:557–63.
16. Hooper DK, Hawkins JA, Fuller TC, Profaizer T, Shaddy RE. Panel-reactive antibodies late after allograft implantation in children. Ann Thorac Surg 2005; 79:641–5.
17. Shaddy RE, Lambert LM, Fuller TC, et al. Prospective randomized trial of azathioprine in cryopreserved valved allografts in children. Ann Thorac Surg 2001; 71:43–8.
18. Yacoub M, Rasmi NRH, Sundt T, et al. Fourteen-year experience with homovital homografts for aortic valve replacement. J Thorac Cardiovasc Surg 1995; 110:186–94.

19. Elkins RC, Knott-Craig CJ, Howell CE. Pulmonary autografts in patients with aortic annulus dysplasia. Ann Thorac Surg 1996; 61:1141–5.

20. Luciani GB, Casali G, Favaro A, et al. Fate of the aortic root later after Ross operation. Circulation 2003; 108(Suppl II):II61–7.

21. David TE, Omran A, Ivanov J, et al. Dilation of the pulmonary autograft after the Ross procedure. J Thorac Cardiovasc Surg 2000; 119:210–20.

22. Oswalt JD, Dewan SJ, Mueller MC, Nelson S. Highlights of a ten-year experience with the Ross procedure. Ann Thorac Surg 2001; 71:S332–5.

23. Ishizaka T, Devaney EJ, Ramsburgh SR, et al. Valve sparing aortic root replacement for dilatation of the pulmonary autograft and aortic regurgitation after the Ross procedure. Ann Thorac Surg 2003; 75:1518–22.

24. Leyh RG, Kofidis T, Fischer S, et al. Aortic root reimplantation for successful repair of an insufficiency pulmonary autograft valve after the Ross procedure. J Thorac Cardiovasc Surg 2002; 124:1048–9.

25. Luciani GB, Favaro A, Viscardi F, Bertolini P, Mazzucco A. Valve-sparing root replacement for pulmonary autograft dissection late after the Ross operation. J Thorac Cardiovasc Surg 2004; 128:753–6.

26. Masetti P, Davila-Roman VA, Kouchoukos NT. Valve-sparing procedure for dilatation of the autologous pulmonary artery and ascending aorta after the Ross operation. Ann Thorac Surg 2003; 76:915–16.

27. David TE, Omran A, Webb G, Rakowski H, Armstrong S, Sun Z. Geometric mismatch of the aortic and pulmonary roots causes aortic insufficiency after the Ross procedure. J Thorac Cardiovasc Surg 1996; 112:1231–9.

28. Niwaya K, Knott-Craig CJ, Lane MM, et al. Cryopreserved homograft valves in the pulmonary position: risk analysis for intermediate-term failure. J Thorac Cardiovasc Surg 1999; 117:141–7.

29. Raanani E, Yau TM, David TE, et al. Risk factors for late pulmonary homograft stenosis after the Ross procedure. Ann Thorac Surg 2000; 70:1953–7.

30. Cohen G, Christakis GT, Joyner CD, et al. Are stentless valves hemodynamically superior to stented valves? A prospective randomized trial. Ann Thorac Surg 2002; 73:767–8.

31. David TE, Puschmann R, Ivanov J, et al. Aortic valve replacement with stentless and stented porcine valves: a case-matched study. J Thorac Cardiovasc Surg 1998; 116:236–41.

32. Jin XY, Westaby S. Pericardial and porcine stentless aortic valves: are they hemodynamically different? Ann Thorac Surg 2001; 71:S311–14.

33. Hvass U, Palatianos GM, Frassani R, Puricelli C, O'Brien M. Multicenter study of stentless valve replacement in the small aortic root. J Thorac Cardiovasc Surg 1999; 117:267–72.

34. Rao V, Christakis GT, Sever J, et al. A novel comparison of stentless versus stented valves in the small aortic root. J Thorac Cardiovasc Surg 1999; 117:431–8.

35. Sintek CF, Fletcher AD, Khonsari S. Stentless porcine aortic root: valve of choice for the elderly patient with small aortic root? J Thorac Cardiovasc Surg 1995; 109:871–6.

36. Kalangos A, Trigo-Trindade P, Vala D, Panos A, Faidutti B. Aortic valve replacement with the Freestyle stentless bioprosthesis with respect to spacial orientation of patient coronary ostia. J Thorac Cardiovasc Surg 2000; 119:1185–93.

37. de Sa M, Moshkovitz Y, Butany J, David TE. Histologic abnormalities of the ascending aorta and pulmonary trunk in patients with bicuspid aortic valve disease: clinical relevance to the Ross procedure. J Thorac Cardiovasc Surg 1999; 118:588–96.

38. Luciani GB, Barozzi L, Tomezzoli A, Casali G, Mazzucco A. Bicuspid aortic valve disease and pulmonary autograft root dilatation after the Ross procedure: a clinicopathologic study. J Thorac Cardiovasc Surg 2001; 122:74–9.

39. Schmidtke C, Bechtel M, Hueppe M, Sievers HH. Time course of aortic valve function and root dimensions after subcoronary Ross procedure for bicuspid versus tricuspid aortic valve disease. Circulation 2001; 104(Suppl I):I21–4.

40. Koh TW, Ferdinand FD, Jin XY, Gibson DG, Pepper JR. Coronary artery problems during homograft aortic valve replacement: role of transesophageal echocardiography. Ann Thorac Surg 1997; 64:533–5.

7

Management after valve repair

Manuel J Antunes

Valve repair has many advantages over valve replacement, including avoidance of long-term anticoagulation if there are no other indications for anticoagulation, larger effective valve area, better preservation of left ventricular function and a lower risk of endocarditis. However, close follow-up of these patients is important in order to detect recurrence of regurgitation or stenosis, to detect the onset of atrial fibrillation and to monitor left ventricular function.

Mitral valvuloplasty

Since the late 1970s and early 1980s, when it was developed by Carpentier, Duran and others, mitral valve repair has become a generally accepted alternative to prosthetic replacement for the surgical treatment of mitral valve disease in suitable patients. Although the feasibility of mitral valvuloplasty varies with the different types of pathology (Figure 7.1) and from centre to centre, most surgeons now recognise its superiority, in terms of both early and late results.[1–7]

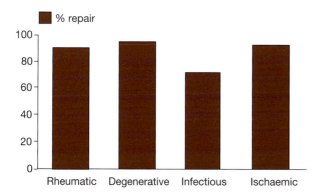

Figure 7.1
Feasibility of mitral valvuloplasty according to pathology, in more than 2500 patients in Coimbra in the last 16 years.

However, mitral valvuloplasty rarely cures the underlying pathological process in the valve, which usually continues to evolve after surgical treatment, especially in rheumatic cases.[8,9] The continued competence of the repaired valve is also significantly dependent on the geometry of the left heart cavities, especially the ventricle. Reverse remodelling of the left ventricle is essential after mitral valvuloplasty for the stability and durability of a good repair. A dilated or dilating left ventricle predisposes to recurrence of mitral regurgitation because of malalignment of the papillary muscles.

Finally, the evolution of a repaired mitral valve depends on the prior pathophysiology, whether stenosis or regurgitation, on the techniques used for repair (usually multiple, sometimes very complex) and the utilisation of foreign materials, such as sutures, artificial chordae, prosthetic rings, etc., which may influence the incidence of thromboembolic complications and infective endocarditis.

Cerfolio et al[10] found that original repairs were intact in over half of patients undergoing reoperation, late valve dysfunction often being due to new degenerative lesions, and this finding is similar to that reported by Marwick and colleagues.[11]

For these reasons, the incidence of reoperation after mitral valvuloplasty may be at least as frequent, if not more frequent, than after valve replacement, and this has been considered its major drawback.[10,12–13] Although there have been no randomised studies comparing mitral valvuloplasty and replacement, patient survival after mitral valve repair has been in the experience of many authors superior to that of valve replacement, independently of the prosthesis used.[14–17] In a detailed multivariate analysis, after statistical allowance for multiple variables, including year of surgery, preoperative ejection fraction, age, sex, preoperative New York Heart Association classification, presence of congestive heart failure, atrial fibrillation, renal status, blood pressure and concomitant coronary artery bypass surgery, Enriquez-Sarano and his colleagues at the Mayo Clinic[5] found that mitral valve repair is an independent predictor of improved operative and long-term mortality, ejection fraction and functional result. Their findings dispel the suspicion that mitral valve repair produces better results solely because patients undergoing repair have better functional status before surgery. After statistically accounting for the bias favouring repair, the 10-year overall survival rate was better for valve repair (68%) than for replacement (52%) and approaches that expected in the normal population. Nevertheless, it must be acknowledged that many of the prostheses used in this series were first-generation (Starr–Edwards) prostheses with intrinsically high gradients and that anticoagulation control was in the pre-INR (international normalised ratio) era.

Although the incidence of valve-related mortality is much lower than in valve replacement and the functional condition of most patients remains very good, even in the presence of mild-to-moderate valve dysfunction, mitral valvuloplasty is nevertheless a palliative procedure and follow-up of the patients is essential. Some prophylactic measures may be warranted.

Anticoagulation and prophylaxis of endocarditis

The incidence of thromboembolism after mitral valve repair is low, especially after the first 6 months, and is probably not higher than that observed preoperatively. Hence, in the majority of cases there is no indication for long-term anticoagulation, unless there is another reason for it, such as atrial fibrillation, impaired left ventricular function or a large left atrium. This is also the case after mitral commissurotomy, be it surgical- or catheter-based, especially in patients with known or previous atrial thrombi.[18] Nevertheless, some authors have recommended oral anticoagulation for 3–6 months, which is the period estimated for complete endothelialisation of the ring and other foreign material to occur. Even in this case, the intensity of anticoagulation should be significantly lower than that suggested for patients with valve prostheses, and an INR of 2–2.5 is probably more than adequate, in order to minimise the occurrence of bleeding complications.

However, there is no evidence that the use of oral anticoagulants in the early postoperative period leads to a decrease in the incidence of thromboembolic complications. Hence, many surgeons are now using antiplatelet agents alone for a similar period of time (see also Chapter 8). In a small non-randomised study involving 162 patients who underwent either valve repair (59 patients) or replacement with a bioprosthesis (103 patients, predominantly aortic valve replacement (AVR)), Aramendi et al[19] found that ticlopidine was associated with less thromboembolism than conventional therapy with oral anticoagulants, but the incidence of haemorrhage was the same.

Anticoagulation or antiplatelet therapy should be avoided if possible in patients with bleeding disorders. In

an experience with rheumatic mitral valve repair in the rather special circumstances of a young, underdeveloped population group, characteristically non-compliant, in Johannesburg, South Africa, neither of these two groups of drugs was utilised and there was no evidence of an increased incidence of thromboembolic events.[8]

Endocarditis after mitral valve repair is also rare and the incidence is probably not significantly higher than the baseline for valves that are affected by the primary pathology. Karavas et al[20] found that the incidence of (non-recurrent) endocarditis after mitral valve repair requiring surgical intervention was infrequent in 1275 patients who had mitral valve repair at the Brigham and Women's Hospital, Boston, in a 10-year period. Ten-year freedom from endocarditis after mitral valve repair averages 95–99%.[21–25] In patients who develop endocarditis, leaflet vegetations are a common finding, resembling the pathology of native valve endocarditis, but the organisms identified are usually staphylococcal species, similar to those causing prosthetic valve endocarditis.[24]

However, the annuloplasty ring, used in a large number of cases, is susceptible to colonisation by bacteria and other infecting microorganisms. Consequently, perioperative antibiotic prophylaxis is justified, as in the case of other prostheses (see Chapter 12). Secondary prophylaxis should also be utilised during the first 6–12 months after surgery. Further prophylaxis depends on the residual valve dysfunction. If the valve is anatomically normal and has near normal function, prophylaxis may not be necessary.

Treatment for endocarditis occurring after mitral valve repair begins with antibiotic therapy. The majority of patients eventually require operation for severe mitral valve dysfunction, and this usually entails valve replacement. However, an operation is rarely required as an emergency. Antibiotic therapy alone can successfully sterilise many valves in which the only pathology is a leaflet vegetation.[21]

Function of the repaired mitral valve

Immediately after repair the mitral valve should be competent and look anatomically 'normal' (Figure 7.2), although this is not always possible. In most surgeons' experience, more than trivial residual regurgitation already present at the end of repair tends to progress rapidly and should be corrected by further surgical manoeuvres or, if this proves impossible, by valve replacement.

Persistence or early recurrence of regurgitation after mitral valve repair is usually of technical origin and is reported to occur in 2–5% of the cases. It is the most important reason for reoperations in the first year after repair.[10–12] In my own experience in South Africa, with a rheumatic population, it accounted for two-thirds of the

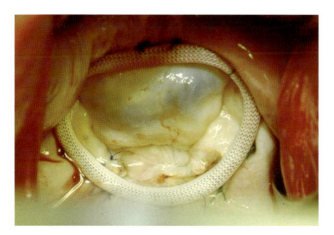

Figure 7.2
Intraoperatve photograph taken immediately after repair of mitral regurgitation due to isolated posterior leaflet prolapse. The valve is being tested by intraventricular injection of saline and is fully competent, with good apposition of the leaflets.

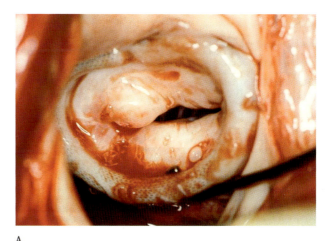

A

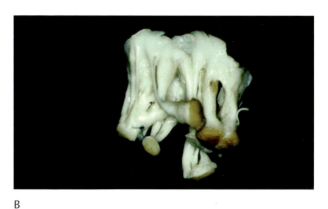

B

Figure 7.3
Intraoperative photograph during reoperation for recurrent mitral regurgitation, 4 years after valvuloplasty in a young patient. Continued rheumatic activity caused thickening and retraction of the leaflets (A). The subvalvar apparatus was grossly fibrotic and distorted (B).

reoperations required in the first 5 years and occurred at a mean of 9 months after the procedure.[8] Residual and/or recurrent leaflet prolapse, ruptured chordae tendineae and partial dehiscence of the annuloplasty ring were the most common occurrences. Occasionally, severe haemolysis also required reintervention. Patients with haemolysis generally present within 3 months of mitral valve repair. Although echocardiographic features vary, most patients have high-grade mitral regurgitation and regurgitant jets.[26] In the majority of the cases valve replacement is required at reoperation, but in approximately one-quarter of the patients re-repair is possible.[26]

By contrast, late recurrence of regurgitation is associated with many different factors. As referred to above, mitral valvuloplasty is essentially a palliative procedure. A repaired mitral valve is never a normal mitral valve. The evolution of its function depends on the initial pathology and on the type of repair.[27] Whereas in the typical case of isolated mid-scallop prolapse of the posterior leaflet (P2), the classical quadrangular resection restores the anatomy close to normal, the progression of disease in rheumatic cases and Barlow's disease make progressive valve dysfunction very likely after repair. Hence, regular and frequent clinical and echocardiographic follow-up is essential in these patients, to detect early signs of dysfunction which may be reversible with adequate medical therapy or, eventually, with surgical reintervention.

Experience with rheumatic mitral valve regurgitation in young patients demonstrates that about 15% of the patients who have good valve function early after surgery develop significant valve dysfunction at the 6-year follow-up,[8,9] probably due to evolution of the rheumatic process, which makes it mandatory to initiate or continue penicillin prophylaxis for rheumatic fever in patients younger than 30–35 years of age (Figure 7.3) – see also Chapter 17.

However, other factors may play a significant role in the onset or progression of valve dysfunction. Remodelling of the left ventricle is now recognised as an important factor in the genesis and perpetuation of mitral regurgitation.[28] Normal function of the mitral valve apparatus depends on the correct alignment of the papillary muscles, which is in turn influenced by the geometry of the left ventricular walls.[29] The posterior wall is particularly important, since when it bulges it stretches the chordae tendineae and tends to pull back and immobilise the posterior leaflet. Hence, adequate reverse remodelling, with restoration of the geometry of the ventricle, is a major factor for maintaining the stability after repair.

With abolition of mitral regurgitation, a significant decrease in the size of the left ventricle is to be expected and the repair itself has to take account of this, especially when the chordae tendineae need to be shortened or replaced.

Short- to medium-term persistence of medical therapy (diuretics and/or vasodilators) used in the preoperative management of mitral regurgitation may be useful postoperatively in preserving left ventricular function and valve competence, although there are no trials on which to base firm recommendations.

Echocardiographic evaluation and follow-up (see also Chapter 4)

Echocardiographic examination has two important aims: evaluation of the morphology and physiology of the valve and of the left ventricle.[11,30,31] A baseline echocardiogram should be performed at the time of discharge from hospital to facilitate subsequent follow-up comparisons.

Even in the absence of a prosthetic ring, the anatomy of the repaired mitral valve often differs considerably from that of the normal valve. One of the most important features is the immobility of the posterior leaflet which is observed both after open commissurotomy and after ring annuloplasty. Essentially, the valve becomes functionally unicuspid and the posterior leaflet becomes a mere support for closure of the anterior leaflet. Hence, assessment of the mobility of the anterior leaflet is of paramount importance. Characterisation of the mobility, degree of thickening and length of the chordae tendineae is also important.

Dehiscence of the annuloplasty ring, one of the causes of failure of the repair, can be easily diagnosed by echocardiography, especially by comparing the images with those obtained in the immediate postoperative period.

Assessment of valve dysfunction, whether regurgitation or stenosis, is carried out by standard means but under these circumstances jets of incompetence are characteristically more asymmetrical and need to be sought more thoroughly as they often run tangentially to the atrial walls.

Finally, as indicated above, ventricular function is intimately related to valve function. Dyskinesia of the left ventricular free wall results in tethering of the chordae tendineae that attach to the posterior leaflet, thus compromising coaptation with the anterior leaflet. Volume overload of the ventricle aggravates this mechanism. Hence, the need to maintain the size of the ventricle as small as possible. Echocardiographic assessment of ventricular function, both global and segmental, is an invaluable tool in the follow-up of patients after mitral valve repair, to control the need for antifailure medication.

Reoperation

The main disadvantage of mitral valve reconstruction over mitral valve replacement is the incidence of late reoperation, which is similar after the two procedures.[5,14–17,32] Mitral valve reconstruction is followed by a high initial instantaneous risk of valve failure and a subsequent low constant risk of late valve failure. Most authors report a 5-year freedom from reoperation from 85% to 90%.[4,6,12,18,19]

Depending on the series, the need for reoperation averages 0.5–2.5% per patient-year.[1–5,9,12,13,27] The highest rates are observed in rheumatic series, followed by ischaemic regurgitation and Barlow's disease, and are lowest for isolated mid-scallop posterior leaflet prolapse. Most reoperations are required in the first year after the valvuloplasty, mostly as a result of technical errors.[27] Hence, more frequent follow-up should be observed in the early period. Late valve dysfunction is often due to new degenerative lesions.[10]

Patients with severe valve dysfunction should be treated as in the primary disease and the indications for reintervention are the same, bearing in mind that reoperation means valve replacement in the majority of cases. Nevertheless, experience indicates that residual or recurrent valve dysfunction is not necessarily equivalent to significant functional disability of the patient. Even with severe regurgitation, patients are often symptomatically better than before surgery, simply because the regurgitant fraction is much lower. Thus, repeat surgery may be delayed for quite a long time under protection of antifailure therapy, monitoring the size of the left ventricle in order to avoid development of dysfunction.

Timing of reoperation is dependent on the mechanism of repair failure. In my experience with rheumatic patients, the mean interval to reoperations was 9.9 months and more than 80% of reoperations were required in the first year after repair, which clearly indicates a predominance of technical failures. In the experience of Gillinov et al,[27] the mean time interval between initial mitral valvuloplasty and reoperation was 22.5 ± 4.5 months for patients with valve-related failure versus 12.8 ± 3.2 months for patients with procedure-related failure. In addition, there was a trend toward longer time to reoperation in patients with rheumatic valvular disease than in patients with degenerative valvular disease (median time intervals of 14 months and 6.5 months, respectively).

Surgical technique

When reoperation is eventually undertaken, a similar technique as for primary interventions is usually followed. The only special care required is in the re-sternotomy, which, however, is usually simple in cases where the pericardium was closed after the original operation. Dissection of the intrapericardial adhesions requires accurate technique but is usually uncomplicated. Alternatively, when a complicated re-entry is expected, cardiopulmonary bypass may be instituted by femoral vessel cannulation before sternotomy, but this is seldom necessary.

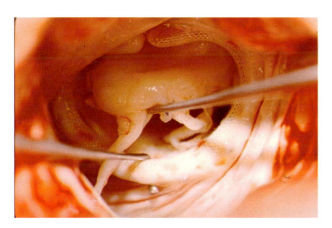

Figure 7.4
Chordal rupture occurred in this patient 2 years after initial repair. Another conservative procedure was possible using chordal replacement with polytetrafluoroethylene (PTFE) sutures.

In some cases, it may be possible to re-repair the valve, especially in the presence of a clearly identifiable technical error from the previous surgery, or in the rare cases of ring dehiscence or of isolated rupture of a chorda tendinea (Figure 7.4).[10] Karavas et al[20] found that attempts at re-repair may be successful only in selected patients with infective endocarditis. Even in these cases, reoperation was accomplished with acceptable morbidity and mortality, and often required mitral valve replacement; despite this, there was no subsequent prosthetic valve endocarditis.

In the majority of cases of failed valve repair, it is necessary to replace the valve. This is usually performed easily in much the same way as in primary valve replacement, once a previously implanted ring has been removed. Mitral valve replacement after a previous valvuloplasty usually carries a much lower morbidity and mortality than reoperations for prosthetic dysfunction, and almost as low as for primary replacements.[10] Jones et al[33] reviewed their experience with first heart valve reoperations involving 671 patients between 1969 and 1998. Their overall operative mortality for first-time heart valve reoperation was 8.6%, which increased from 3.0% for reoperation on a failed repair or reoperation at a new valve site to 10.6% for prosthetic valve dysfunction or periprosthetic leak and to 29.4% for associated endocarditis or valve thrombosis.

Aortic valvuloplasty

Conservative aortic procedures are being performed with increasing frequency.[34–39] The arguments in favour of this approach are identical to those used for mitral valvuloplasty and the same imperatives apply with regard to follow-up. The need for close follow-up or otherwise depends on the result obtained and on the degree of residual dysfunction. Because there is usually no foreign material, the routine use of anticoagulants or antiplatelet agents is unnecessary unless there is another indication, such as atrial fibrillation or very poor left ventricular function. Here also, the incidence of infective endocarditis is low, probably not higher than the baseline. However, prophylaxis is necessary in these patients, as the valve is not normal.

Generally speaking, especially in the cases where the primary lesion was aortic regurgitation, the evolution of the disease is towards regurgitation, which in the long-term has potential deleterious effects on the function of the left ventricle. Hence, close and careful follow-up is also essential in these patients to detect early signs of progressive ventricular dilatation and dysfunction, which constitute absolute indications for reoperation.

When surgery is again required, reoperation should be as simple as the first procedure, because there is usually no prosthetic material to be removed. The results are similar to those of the primary operation. By contrast with the mitral valve, aortic valve replacement is almost always required at reoperation.

Late-occurring tricuspid regurgitation

One of the emerging complications after valve surgery is late appearance of tricuspid regurgitation (TR), which is exemplified by a patient who has been subjected to mitral valve or, infrequently, aortic valve surgery and presents later with symptoms and signs of right heart failure and significant TR.

Persisting or worsening TR results from several mechanisms. First, persisting or recurrent mitral valve disease predisposes to tricuspid dysfunction. Although late TR may occur after mitral valve replacement, it is more frequent after conservative mitral valve surgery. The more severe the TR already present at the time of the first surgery, the more likely it is to persist or to increase late after mitral valve surgery. Mild TR rarely persists or progresses, whereas moderate or severe TR usually does. On the other hand, long-standing, perhaps irreversible, right ventricular dilatation secondary to mitral valve or pulmonary vascular disease probably also predisposes to persistent TR. All these factors take part in the restriction-dilatation syndrome described by Barlow and co-workers in 1987.[40]

Late TR appears to be more frequently associated with rheumatic heart disease. In a study performed at Papworth Hospital with 264 patients following mitral valve repair, where just over 80% had had degenerative mitral regurgitation, significant TR was not detected clinically 1–11 years after mitral valve repair.[41] Hence, it would seem that the development of significant TR is rare after mitral valve surgery for degenerative disease.

Follow-up and diagnosis

Patients who had mitral valve surgery are routinely subject to close follow-up. The details and methodology of this follow-up and the complications which may be experienced are the subject of this book, and each aspect is the subject of detailed discussion in the various chapters. Patients who had tricuspid valve surgery, or have TR which has not completely resolved after left-sided valve surgery, require no special considerations, but should be followed more closely.

Clinical detection of tricuspid regurgitation is simple and accurate.[42,43] Raised jugular venous pressure, hepatomegaly, pulsatile liver and hepatojugular reflux are followed by ankle swelling and, later, by ascites and generalised oedema. The characteristic systolic wave is both visible and palpable in the neck veins. On auscultation, a systolic murmur, variable with respiration, is usually present. Echocardiographic examination confirms the diagnosis and is useful to assess the size of the right cardiac chambers and right ventricular function. In severe TR there is usually dilatation of both the right atrium and ventricle. Retrograde flow in the vena cavae is characteristic of severe TR.

Once the patient becomes symptomatic, aggressive antifailure therapy with furosemide is indicated. Spironolactone appears especially indicated in patients with TR and in right ventricular failure. Diuretic therapy may reduce the haemodynamic severity of tricuspid regurgitation by relieving right ventricular distension and hence lowering right atrial pressure. If this is not sufficient, consideration must be given to tricuspid valve surgery.

Surgery

Reoperation for late TR, whether isolated or in conjunction with repeat surgery of another valve, has an operative risk which is higher than that which occurs after other redo valve surgery and may reach 10–20%.[44] Preoperative preparation to reduce cardiac failure, physiotherapy and good anaesthesia and surgical technique contribute to reduce the risk. Special attention must be given to renal function, as significant renal failure dramatically increases the surgical risk. Because surgery is rarely required on an emergency basis, all measures that may improve the patient's condition before surgery are justified.

In most repeat operations, morbidity and even mortality is often related to the re-entry. Classical median sternotomy may be used, but a right thoracotomy may be advantageous for a second and third reoperation. However, pericardial adhesions, together with extreme dilatation of the right atrium and ventricle, may dictate the need for femoral cannulation in some cases, especially in multiple reoperations. Median sternotomy and the classical vena cavae – aortic cardiopulmonary bypass is still preferred in the majority of cases.

In the tricuspid position, prosthetic valve substitutes have at least the same type and degree of complications as in the aortic and the mitral positions. However, only exceptionally does the tricuspid valve need to be replaced as a first procedure, because the valve is tolerant of a less than perfect repair, in contrast to the aortic and the mitral valves where complete competence is of paramount importance. Hence, annuloplasty is the surgery of choice when dealing with most forms of TR.

In the early 1970s, Deloche et al, from Carpentier's group,[45] found that dilatation of the tricuspid annulus occurs almost entirely in the mural portion of the annulus and, based also on his own findings, DeVega[46] developed his very well-known procedure, which consists of plication of the portion of the annulus corresponding to the posterior and anterior leaflets, preserving the septal portion, with a double continuous suture. This procedure has since been used in tens of thousands of cases by most surgeons throughout the world and it appears to be safe and efficacious. Sometimes, however, the sutures may pull out of the tissues and the guitar-string syndrome occurs. In order to avoid this type of complication, in 1983 Antunes and Girdwood[47] described a modification of the procedure, which consisted of the interposition of Teflon pledgets in each bite of the suture, but the concept remains exactly the same (Figure 7.5).[48] Other methods of suture annuloplasty have been described and used by some groups, but the DeVega annuloplasty or its modifications have gained wider acceptance.

The routine use of an annuloplasty ring, whether pre-shaped or flexible, has been suggested by others.[49] However, the implantation of a ring is only specifically indicated when there is organic involvement of the tricuspid valve (usually with stenosis, where commissurotomy is also necessary), or in the case of reoperation, in which the greater tendency for deformity of the whole valve mechanism, rather than isolated annular dilatation, may dictate the use of a prosthetic ring. In these circumstances, the Carpentier ring is preferred.

Advanced functional class, severe right heart failure, low right ventricular ejection fraction, high pulmonary pressure and pulmonary arterial resistance are important risk factors for repeat tricuspid surgery. Enlargement of the right ventricle increases the risk of sternal re-entry, but this may be reduced by careful surgical technique.

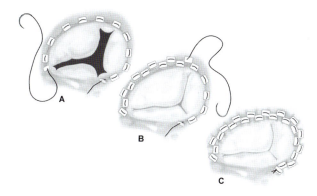

Figure 7.5
Antunes and Girdwood modification of the DeVega annuloplasty.

Conclusion

Valvuloplasty, especially of the mitral valve, is becoming increasingly used, but these interventions are seldom curative (inasmuch as the abnormal tissues are preserved) and patients therefore require continued vigilance. Because there is no significant amount of foreign material, the valve remains structurally very natural and the follow-up and indications for reoperation are similar to those of untouched valves. However, even in cases of significant residual or recurrent valve dysfunction, patients may remain in good functional condition. Particular care must therefore be exercised to avoid the development of left ventricular dysfunction. Early reoperations may be required to avoid irreversible damage to the ventricle. Optimally timed reoperations should have low mortality and morbidity rates, similar to those observed in primary operations. If tricuspid regurgitation occurs or progresses late after valve surgery, aggressive medical therapy is indicated but surgery of the tricuspid valve may be required. Although it carries a higher operative risk, patients usually show significant clinical improvement.

References

1. Carpentier A. Cardiac valve surgery – the 'French correction'. J Thorac Cardiovasc Surg 1983; 86:323–37.
2. Spencer FC, Colvin SB, Culliford AT, Isom OW. Experiences with the Carpentier techniques of mitral valve reconstruction in 103 patients (1980–1985). J Thorac Cardiovasc Surg 1985; 90:341–50.
3. Cosgrove DM, Chavez AM, Lytle BW, et al. Results of mitral valve reconstruction. Circulation 1986; 74:I82–7.
4. Deloche A, Jebara VA, Relland JY, et al. Valve repair with Carpentier techniques: the second decade. J Thorac Cardiovasc Surg 1990; 99:990–1001.
5. Enriquez-Sarano M, Schaff HV, Orszulak TA, et al. Valve repair improves the outcome of surgery for mitral regurgitation: a multivariate analysis. Circulation 1995; 91:1022–8.
6. Braunberger E, Deloche A, Berrebi A, et al. Very long-term results (more than 20 years) of valve repair with Carpentier's techniques in nonrheumatic mitral valve insufficiency. Circulation 2001; 104:I8–11.
7. Gillinov AM, Cosgrove DM. Mitral valve repair for degenerative disease. J Heart Valve Dis 2002; 11:S15–20.
8. Antunes MJ, Magalhaes MP, Colsen PR, Kinsley RH. Valvuloplasty for rheumatic mitral valve disease. A surgical challenge. J Thorac Cardiovasc Surg 1987; 94:44–56.
9. Skoularigis J, Sinovich V, Joubert G, Sareli P. Evaluation of the long-term results of mitral valve repair in 254 young patients with rheumatic mitral regurgitation. Circulation 1994; 90:II167–74.
10. Cerfolio RJ, Orzulak TA, Pluth JR, Harmsen WS, Schaff HV. Reoperation after valve repair for mitral regurgitation: early and intermediate results. J Thorac Cardiovasc Surg 1996; 111:1177–84.
11. Marwick TH, Stewart WJ, Currie PJ, Cosgrove DM. Mechanisms of failure of mitral valve repair: an echocardiographic study. Am Heart J 1991; 122:149–56.
12. David TE, Armstrong S, Sun Z, Daniel L. Late results of mitral valve repair for mitral regurgitation due to degenerative disease. Ann Thorac Surg 1993; 56:7–12.
13. Grossi EA, Galloway AC, Steinberg BM, et al. Severe calcification does not affect long-term outcome of mitral valve repair. Ann Thorac Surg 1994; 58:685–7.
14. Perier P, Deloche A, Chauvaud S, et al. Comparative evaluation of mitral valve repair and replacement with Starr, Björk, and porcine valve prostheses. Circulation 1984; 70(Suppl):I187–92.
15. Akins CW, Hilgenberg AD, Buckley MJ, et al. Mitral valve reconstruction versus replacement for degenerative or ischemic mitral regurgitation. Ann Thorac Surg 1994; 58:668–76.
16. Galloway AC, Colvin SB, Baumann FG, et al. A comparison of mitral valve reconstruction with mitral valve replacement: intermediate-term results. Ann Thorac Surg 1989; 47:655–62.
17. Sand ME, Naftel DC, Blackstone EH, Kirklin JW, Karp RB. A comparison of repair and replacement for mitral valve incompetence. J Thorac Cardiovasc Surg 1987; 94:208–19.
18. Kang DH, Song JK, Chae JK, et al. Comparison of outcomes of percutaneous mitral valvuloplasty versus mitral valve replacement after resolution of left atrial appendage thrombi by warfarin therapy. Am J Cardiol 1998; 81:97–100.
19. Aramendi JL, Agredo J, Llorente A, Larrarte C, Pijoan J. Prevention of thromboembolism with ticlopidine shortly after valve repair or replacement with a bioprosthesis. J Heart Valve Dis 1998; 7:610–14.
20. Karavas AN, Filsoufi F, Mihaljevic T, et al. Risk factors and management of endocarditis after mitral valve repair. J Heart Valve Dis 2002; 11:660–4.
21. Gillinov M, Faber CN, Sabik JF, et al. Endocarditis after mitral valve repair. Ann Thorac Surg 2002; 73:1813–16.
22. Gillinov AM, Cosgrove DM, Blackstone EH, et al. Durability of mitral valve repair for degenerative disease. J Thorac Cardiovasc Surg 1998; 116:734–43.
23. Alvarez JM, Deal CW, Loveridge K, et al. Repairing the degenerative mitral valve: ten- to fifteen-year follow-up. J Thorac Cardiovasc Surg 1996; 112:238–47.
24. Kuwaki K, Kiyofumi M, Tsukamoto M, Abe T. Early and late results of mitral valve repair for mitral valve regurgitation. Significant risk factors of reoperation. J Cardiovasc Surg (Torino) 2000; 41:187–92.
25. Pettersson G, Carbon C, Al-Hallees Z, et al. Recommendations for the surgical treatment of endocarditis. Clin Microbiol Infect 1998; 4(Suppl 3):S34–6.
26. Lam BK, Cosgrove DM, Bhudia SK, Gillinov AM. Hemolysis after mitral valve repair: mechanisms and treatment. Ann Thorac Surg 2004; 77:191–5.
27. Gillinov AM, Cosgrove DM, Lytle BW, et al. Reoperation for failure of mitral valve repair. J Thorac Cardiovasc Surg 1997; 113:467–75.
28. Hueb AC, Jatene FB, Moreira LF, et al. Ventricular remodeling and

mitral valve modifications in dilated cardiomyopathy: new insights from anatomic study. J Thorac Cardiovasc Surg 2002; 124:1216–24.

29. Otsuji Y, Handschumacher MD, Liel-Cohen N, et al. Mechanism of ischemic mitral regurgitation with segmental left ventricular dysfunction: three-dimensional echocardiographic studies in models of acute and chronic progressive regurgitation. J Am Coll Cardiol 2001; 37:641–8.

30. Enriquez-Sarano M, Tajik AJ, Schaff HV, et al. Echocardiographic prediction of survival after surgical correction of organic mitral regurgitation. Circulation 1994; 90:830–7.

31. Freeman WK, Schaff HV, Khandheria BK, et al. Intraoperative evaluation of mitral valve regurgitation and repair by transesophageal echocardiography: incidence and significance of systolic anterior motion. J Am Coll Cardiol 1992; 20:599–609.

32. Mohty D, Orszulak TA, Schaff HV, et al. Very long-term survival and durability of mitral valve repair for mitral valve prolapse. Circulation 2001; 104:12(Suppl 1):I1–17.

33. Jones JM, O'Kane H, Gladstone DJ, et al. Repeat heart valve surgery: risk factors for operative mortality. J Thorac Cardiovasc Surg 2001; 122:913–18.

34. Grinda JM, Latremouille C, Berrebi AJ, et al. Aortic cusp extension valvuloplasty for rheumatic aortic valve disease: midterm results. Eur J Cardiothorac Surg 1999; 15:302–8.

35. van Son JAM, Reddy VM, Black MD, et al. Morphologic determinants favoring surgical aortic valvuloplasty versus pulmonary autograft aortic valve replacement in children. Thorac Cardiovasc Surg 1996; 111:1149–57.

36. Cosgrove DM, Rosenkranz ER, Hendren WG, Bartlett JC, Stewart WJ. Valvuloplasty for aortic insufficiency. J Thorac Cardiovasc Surg 1991; 102:571–6.

37. Haydar HS, He GW, Hovaguimian H, et al. Valve repair for aortic insufficiency: surgical classification and techniques. Eur J Cardiothorac Surg 1997; 11:258–65.

38. Hyuk Ahn, Kyung-Hwan Kim, Yong Jin Kim. Midterm result of leaflet extension technique in aortic regurgitation. Eur J Cardiothorac Surg 2002; 21:465–9.

39. Casselman FP, Gillinov AM, Akhrass R, et al. Intermediate-term durability of bicuspid aortic valve repair for prolapsing leaflet. Eur J Cardiothorac Surg 1999; 15:302–8.

40. Barlow JB, Pocock WA, Antunes MJ, Sareli P, Meyer TE. Surgical aspects of mitral valve disease. 2. Late postoperative course and complications: emphasis on the 'Restriction-dilatation syndrome'. In: Barlow JB, ed. Perspectives on the mitral valve. Philadelphia: FA Davis, 1987: 270–88.

41. Lim E, Ali ZA, Barlow CW, et al. Determinants and assessment of regurgitation after mitral valve repair. J Thorac Cardiovasc Surg 2002; 124: 911–17.

42. Barlow JB. Aspects of mitral and tricuspid regurgitation. J Cardiol 1991; 21:3–33.

43. Barlow JB. Aspects of tricuspid valve disease, heart failure and the 'Restriction-dilatation syndrome'. Rev Port Cardiol 1995; 14(12):991–1004.

44. Hornick P, Harris PA, Taylor KM. Tricuspid valve replacement subsequent to previous open heart surgery. J Heart Valve Dis 1996; 5:20–5.

45. Deloche A, Guerinon J, Fabiani JN, et al. Anatomical study of rheumatic tricuspid valve diseases: application to the study of various valvuloplasties. Ann Chir Thorac Cardiovasc 1973; 12:343–9.

46. DeVega NG. La anuloplastia selectiva, reguable y permanente. Rev Esp Cardiol 1972; 25:6–9.

47. Antunes MJ, Girdwood RW. Tricuspid annuloplasty: a modified technique. Ann Thorac Surg 1983; 35:676–8.

48. Antunes MJ. Segmental tricuspid annuloplasty revisited (letter). J Thorac Cardiovasc Surg 1992; 103:1025.

49. McCarthy PM, Bhudia SK, Rajeswaran J, et al. Tricuspid valve repair: durability and risk factors for failure (see also discussion). J Thorac Cardiovasc Surg 2004; 127:674–85.

8

Antithrombotic management

Eric G Butchart, Christa Gohlke-Bärwolf, Giulia Renda and Raffaele De Caterina

As valve thrombosis, thromboembolism and anticoagulant-related bleeding together account for about 75% of complications encountered by patients with prosthetic valves, and because each of these complications can have devastating consequences, their prevention by optimising antithrombotic management is arguably the most important aspect of postoperative and long-term care. Antithrombotic management after heart valve surgery should therefore be individualised for each patient, depending on the type of surgery (repair or replacement), the type of prosthesis and the patient's own risk factors (see Box 8.1), bearing in mind that thrombosis and embolism may have other sources in addition to a repaired or replaced valve, and that some patients may be more prone to thrombosis or more prone to bleeding. This concept of patient-specific and prosthesis-specific antithrombotic management requires an understanding of the basic mechanisms of thrombosis and embolism in valve surgery patients, the limitations of anticoagulation and antiplatelet therapy and the subtle differences between one prosthesis and another, even within a broad design category. It thus involves much more detailed patient assessment and prosthesis evaluation than contained in previously published guidelines.[1,2] Whereas a uniform approach, categorising patients only according to the position of the prosthesis within the heart and its broad design category (caged-ball, tilting-disc, bileaflet or bioprosthesis) may be more convenient for anticoagulation clinics and those supervising the care of large numbers of valve surgery patients, it may not benefit the individual patient, who may be under-anticoagulated or over-anticoagulated for his/her risk factors and particular type of prosthesis. Unfortunately, not all prostheses within a particular design category have the same thrombogenicity.

An inappropriately high intensity of anticoagulation or the unnecessary addition of aspirin to anticoagulation in patients with low thrombogenicity mechanical valves and no risk factors for thromboembolism will increase the incidence of major bleeding without conferring any additional antithrombotic protection. This also has an important bearing on the mechanical versus bioprosthesis debate, as anticoagulant-related bleeding is perceived as the major disadvantage of a mechanical valve and reported series with unnecessarily high rates of major bleeding strongly influence the balance of the debate.

Box 8.1 Patient factors to consider in determining antithrombotic management

Age, mental capacity, social circumstances, family support

Risk factors for bleeding:
- Previous history of gastrointestinal bleeding or other bleeding source
- Peptic ulcer history
- Systemic hypertension
- Renal failure
- New York Health Association (NYHA) class III/IV, multiple medications

Thrombotic risk factors associated with low-flow conditions:
- Atrial fibrillation
- Left atrial enlargement (>5.0 cm)
- Impaired left ventricular (LV) function (ejection fraction <30%)
- NYHA class IV

Thrombotic risk factors associated with arterial disease or endothelial dysfunction:
- Systemic hypertension
- Diabetes
- Aortic and/or carotid atheroma

Thrombotic risk factors associated with increased coagulability and/or platelet aggregability:
- Diabetes
- Cigarette smoking
- Hyperlipidaemia
- Chronic inflammation/infection
- Chronic haemolysis

(cont'd)

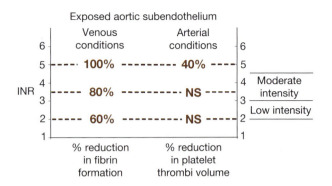

Figure 8.1

In this experimental study,[7] human blood at different INRs was drawn over rabbit aortic subendothelium (a thrombogenic surface) at simulated venous and arterial flow conditions and the volume of fibrin or platelet thrombus deposition measured. Total abolition of fibrin deposition under 'venous' conditions required an INR of 5.0. No significant reduction in platelet thrombus deposition under 'arterial' condition occurred until an INR of 5.0 was reached and then the reduction was only 40%.

Mechanisms of thrombosis and embolism

The pathogenetic mechanisms involved in thrombosis and embolism in valve surgery patients are complex and often interactive. Even optimum anticoagulation control does not prevent all 'thromboembolism'. There are three principal reasons for this apparent 'treatment failure':

1. Many events are part of the background incidence of stroke and transient ischaemic attack (TIA) in the general population, which varies considerably with age,[3] with geography (highest in Eastern Europe)[4] and even within different regions of the same country.[5]
2. Many risk factors such as hypertension and diabetes exert their effects through mechanisms uninfluenced or little influenced by anticoagulation.[6]
3. Total prevention of thrombosis on very thrombogenic surfaces requires anticoagulation at such a high international normalised ratio (INR)[7] that its efficacy is outweighed by the risk of serious bleeding (Figure 8.1).

The presence of coronary disease increases the risk of stroke two- to three-fold depending on age,[8] whereas carotid disease and aortic atheroma increase the risk still further.[9] In addition, hypertension, diabetes, increased left ventricular mass and cigarette smoking each act as major independent stroke risk factors.[10–14]

Following aortic valve replacement (AVR) in a middle-aged and elderly population, the incidence of cerebrovascular events has been shown to be predominantly associated with established stroke risk factors, particularly hypertension and continued cigarette smoking[6] and to be relatively little influenced by differences in anticoagulation intensity.[15] In a series based on the Medtronic Hall tilting-disc valve, patients who were normotensive, in sinus rhythm, non-diabetic and non-smokers with no evidence of arterial disease suffered no cerebrovascular events during a 13-year follow-up period.[6] Although it may not be possible to extrapolate these data to other types of prosthesis, this series serves to underline the importance of taking stroke risk factors into account when planning antithrombotic management. The mechanism of cerebrovascular events in this series of patients after AVR remains speculative. The overall incidence is in keeping with epidemiological data on stroke in the age- and sex-matched general population without prosthetic valves (Figure 8.2), although the possibility of some interaction between the prosthesis and stroke risk factors remains.

In patients with prosthetic heart valves, abnormal flow conditions imposed by the prosthesis coexist with disturbed flow conditions due to abnormal cardiac function and/or with irregular roughened arterial surfaces due to atheromatous plaques. The latter and the prothrombotic endothelial dysfunction which accompanies them[16,17] are in turn associated with well-established risk factors for arterial disease: hypertension, cigarette smoking, diabetes and hyperlipidaemia.[18]

The abnormal flow conditions caused by prosthetic valves are of two types: relative stagnation and high-velocity disturbed flow causing high shear stress.[19] Relative

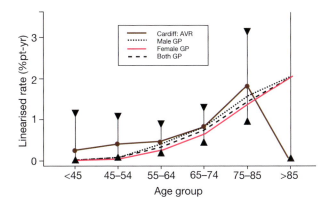

Figure 8.2

Incidence of stroke (% per year with 95% confidence intervals) following aortic valve replacement (AVR) in a large prosthetic series based on the Medtronic Hall valve[150] (Cardiff: AVR line) in comparison to the expected stroke incidence (Both GP line) for the age- and sex-matched general population. Data from the Oxford Community Stroke Project.[3]

stagnation exists in areas of very low flow or even reversed flow adjacent to certain parts of the prosthesis according to its particular design (e.g. the hinge pockets of a bileaflet valve and the concave outflow surfaces of a bioprosthe-

sis).[20] High shear stress occurs during forward flow and in mechanical valves during regurgitant flow when high-velocity jets of blood are forced through narrow gaps in the mechanism with the prosthesis in a closed position. The degree of shear stress also varies according to valve design.[19] Relative stagnation in any part of the circulation increases the risk of thrombosis[21] but is particularly dangerous in proximity to an artificial surface.[22] High shear stress is also deleterious in that it induces platelet activation.[23–25] Activated platelets may subsequently adhere to a prosthetic surface[26] or to an abnormal surface downstream from the prosthesis, e.g. an aortic atheromatous plaque, with subsequent microembolism[27] (Figure 8.3).

Prostheses in different positions within the heart impose and are associated with different flow conditions that have implications for the mechanisms of thrombosis and embolism and for antithrombotic therapy. Aortic prostheses are associated with relatively little stagnation unless of inferior design or incorrectly implanted; the dominant feature, rather, is high shear stress.[19] In addition, many aortic valves are implanted within aortas scarred by atherosclerosis. Mitral prostheses, in contrast, are associated with much more stagnation,[20] not only because the velocity of forward flow is much lower, especially in atrial fibrillation, but also because they are situated facing into the left atrium, which is itself an area of relative stagnation in many cases of

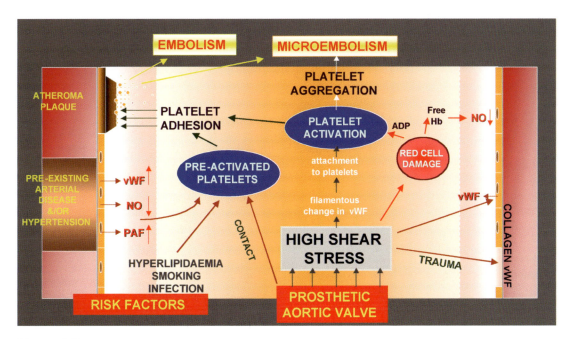

Figure 8.3

Diagrammatic representation of the interaction between an aortic prosthesis and risk factors through the effects of higher shear stress, which activates platelets directly and indirectly by liberating adenosine diphosphate (ADP) from damaged red cells. Free haemoglobin (Hb) from damaged red cells also inactivates nitric oxide (NO) in plasma, one of the defence mechanisms against thrombus deposition on the endothelial surface. High shear stress also liberates von Willebrand factor (vWF) from endothelium and physical damage to the endothelium exposes subendothelial collagen which is thrombogenic. PAF = platelet activating factor.

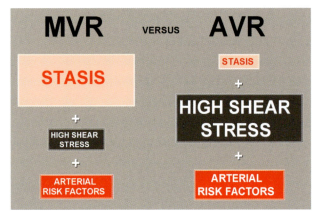

Figure 8.4
Mitral valve replacement (MVR) versus aortic valve
replacement (AVR).

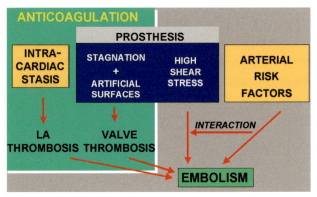

Figure 8.5
Embolism and prosthetic valves.

mitral valve disease as a result of chamber enlargement and
atrial fibrillation.[21] Mitral valve disease, particularly
rheumatic disease, is also usually associated with less arterial disease than aortic valve disease.[6,28]

These fundamental differences result in a higher incidence of both valve thrombosis and embolism after mitral
valve replacement (MVR) than after AVR (Figure 8.4).[29]
Because these complications are related to blood stagnation both in the left atrium and adjacent to the prosthesis
and because anticoagulation is particularly useful for
reducing thrombosis under these conditions, a
dose–response effect can be demonstrated with increasing
intensity of anticoagulation.[15] In contrast, embolism after
AVR appears to be less influenced by the intensity of anticoagulation,[15] suggesting a dominant effect of either
platelet activation or coexisting stroke risk factors.[6] Several
randomised trials have failed to detect any significant difference in embolic incidence with different intensities of
anticoagulation in populations in which AVR and sinus
rhythm predominated.[30–34]

Thus, in patients with prosthetic valves, anticoagulation
is of most value in preventing thrombosis on the prosthesis
itself and within the left atrium, and the embolism which
arises from these sites, but is of much less value in preventing 'embolism' arising as the result of high shear stresses or
arterial disease or any interaction between the two (Figure
8.5).

Antithrombotic management should therefore encom-
pass other strategies in addition to anticoagulation to
reduce the risk of thromboembolism. A recent prospective
observational study of patients undergoing valve replacement, based on factors at the time of surgery, identified
several risk factors predictive of future thromboembolism
during follow-up on multivariate analysis.[35] These risk factors were additive in their effect, enabling a scoring system
to be developed: the greater the number of risk factors, the

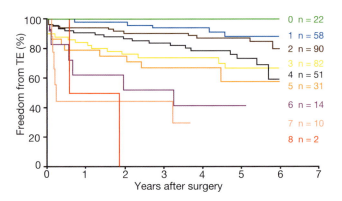

Figure 8.6
Freedom from thromboembolism (TE) following valve
replacement, according to the number of risk factors present
at the time of surgery. Patients with no risk factors suffered
no events. The greater the number of risk factors, the greater
the risk of TE during follow-up. Reprinted from Reference 35,
with permission.

higher the risk (Figure 8.6). The clinical and laboratory risk
factors which were identified are shown in Box 8.2,
together with the valve position in which each risk factor
exerted its greatest effect.

The measures that can be undertaken to reduce the effect
of those risk factors which can be modified are shown in
Box 8.3. Risk factors identified in other studies have also
been included in the lower part of this panel. It should be
stressed, however, that no studies have yet been conducted
to assess the effect of risk factor modification in patients
with prosthetic heart valves.

Many of the modifiable risk factors in Box 8.3 are also
acknowledged independent risk factors for stroke in the
general population and their control is equally as

Box 8.2 Risk factors increasing the risk of thromboembolism

Risk factor	Valve position
Clinical	
Previous TE event	AVR
Systemic hypertension	AVR
Previous cancer history	AVR
Previous mitral valvotomy	MVR
Postoperative infection	AVR
Laboratory	
Chronic *Chlamydia pneumoniae* infection	MVR, AVR
Increased mean platelet volume	MVR
Raised eosinophil count	AVR
Factor VII 'resistance' to warfarin	MVR
Raised fibrinogen	MVR
Raised reticulocyte count	MVR

AVR = aortic valve replacement, MVR = mitral valve replacement, TE = thromboembolism.
The higher the number of risk factors, the greater the risk.
Reproduced from Reference 35.

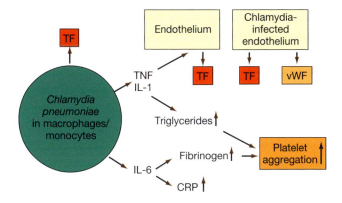

Figure 8.7
Diagrammatic representation of the prothrombotic effects of infection with *Chlamydia pneumoniae*. Circulating monocytes infected with *C. pneumoniae* express tissue factor (TF), and liberate the cytokines, tumour necrosis factor (TNF), interleukin-1 (IL-1) and interleukin-6 (IL-6). Endothelium infected with *C. pneumoniae* also expresses TF and liberates von Willebrand factor (vWF). CRP = C-reactive protein.

important in patients with heart valve disease.[11,14,36–39] Diabetes enhances the effect of other risk factors,[40] and the effect of atrial fibrillation is magnified by other factors which contribute to low intracardiac flow conditions, such as left atrial enlargement and impaired left ventricular function.[41] Obesity is associated with a prothrombotic state[42] and is an independent risk factor for stroke in both men[43,44] and women.[45]

Increased mean platelet volume has been identified as an independent risk factor for stroke in patients with known cerebrovascular disease.[46] It is also associated with diabetes.[47] In the absence of rare congenital platelet abnormalities associated with large size, increased platelet size is usually associated with greater than normal platelet turnover consequent upon excessive platelet consumption.[48] Thus, increased platelet size as a marker of thromboembolic risk after MVR[35] may indicate a prothrombotic milieu within the left atrium and the necessity for further investigation with transoesophageal echocardiography (TOE). If no modifiable abnormalities are found on TOE (e.g. left atrial or prosthetic thrombus or spontaneous echocardiographic contrast (SEC) secondary to a high transprosthetic gradient), consideration should be given to prescribing antiplatelet therapy in addition to anticoagulation, particularly if the patient has already experienced a thromboembolic event, because larger than normal platelets are more reactive and therefore more 'sticky'.[49] (See section on Antiplatelet Therapy.)

Raised levels of fibrinogen elevate thrombotic risk by increasing platelet activation and by raising plasma viscosity.[36] High plasma viscosity and areas of sluggish flow adjacent to a prosthesis are additive in their prothrombotic effect. Causes of hyperfibrinogenaemia should be sought and treated if possible.[50] Dehydration, which also raises plasma viscosity, should be particularly avoided in the presence of hyperfibrinogenaemia.

In the risk factor study referred to above, chronic infection with *Chlamydia pneumoniae* was the strongest overall predictor of stroke, the effect occurring after both AVR and MVR.[35] This new finding is in keeping with similar data for stroke in the general population.[51,52] Whether antibiotic treatment for *C. pneumoniae* will be effective in reducing risk after valve replacement remains to be tested in prospective trials. Prolonged treatment may be necessary, as infection in circulating monocytes is refractory to antibiotic treatment, although the organism can be more readily eliminated from endothelial cells[53] (Figure 8.7).

In patients with concomitant vascular disease, treatment with angiotensin-converting enzyme (ACE) inhibitors should be considered, as these drugs have been shown to significantly reduce the incidence of stroke in patients with coronary disease, cerebrovascular disease or peripheral vascular disease. In the HOPE study, there was a 32% reduction in relative risk of stroke and a 61% reduction in relative risk of fatal stroke with ramipril.[54] Hypercholesterolaemia should be treated with statins which have additional benefits in reducing the risk of stroke through antithrombotic, anti-inflammatory and antioxidant mechanisms.[55] Carotid endarterectomy should be considered in

---

Box 8.3 Risk factor modification to reduce thromboembolic risk

Modifiable risk factors	Action required
Systemic hypertension	Good blood pressure control
Diabetes	Good diabetic control
Chronic chlamydial infection	Antibiotic treatment
Factor VII 'resistance' to warfarin	Monitor factor VII level in addition to INR to optimise warfarin dose
	Reduce fat intake/statin therapy
Increased mean platelet volume	Investigate causes of increased platelet consumption (see text)
	Consider antiplatelet drug
Raised eosinophil count	Investigate and treat cause, e.g. allergic conditions, parasites, suspected malignant disease
Raised fibrinogen	Investigate and treat cause, e.g. chronic infection, chronic inflammation, dental disease
Raised reticulocyte count	Investigate cause of increased haemolysis and treat cause
Atrial fibrillation	Conversion to sinus rhythm pharmacologically or electrically
Cigarette smoking	Stop smoking
Poor left ventricular function/NYHA class IV/heart failure	Optimise drug treatment, including ACE inhibitors
Hypercholesterolaemia[a]	Statin therapy – anti-inflammatory and antithrombotic effects beneficial also
Obesity[a]	Reduce weight. Increase exercise
Pulmonary infection[a,b] (as an acute trigger factor)[63,64]	Treat pulmonary infections promptly and vigorously

ACE = angiotensin-converting enzyme, INR = international normalised ratio, NYHA = New York Health Association.
[a]Identified as risk factors for stroke in general, through prothrombotic and/or atherogenic mechanisms.
[b]Indirect evidence in prosthetic heart valve patients also.[22]

---

patients with carotid stenosis >70%, even if they are asymptomatic, as this has been shown to reduce stroke risk.[56]

Finally, an insufficiently reduced level of factor VII despite oral anticoagulation is a newly described risk factor for thromboembolism and deserves special mention. In the study mentioned above, this was the second strongest independent risk factor for thromboembolism after MVR on multivariate analysis[35] and confirms the view of other investigators that the degree of reduction in factor VII by oral anticoagulants may be equally as important as the degree of reduction in prothrombin (factor II).[57,58] At lower levels of INR, there is relatively less reduction of factor VII levels than prothrombin levels.[59] Acenocoumarol, because of its short half-life, allows greater fluctuation of factor VII levels than phenprocoumon,[57] and this may be an important consideration in choosing an oral anticoagulant drug, particularly for mitral patients (see below).

Factor VII levels normally fluctuate during the day. Factor VII has a short half-life and levels are increased by a fatty meal.[60] Levels also tend to rise with age and in obesity, pregnancy, hypercholesterolaemia, hypertriglyceridaemia and diabetes.[60] Raised levels of factor VII have been associated with increased coronary risk,[61] although this has not been confirmed in all studies and mechanisms have yet to be clarified, particularly with respect to the effect of poly-

morphisms in the factor VII gene.[62] Nevertheless, it is acknowledged that elevated factor VII coagulant activity is prothrombotic and this is consistent with the finding that relative 'resistance' of factor VII to oral anticoagulation, with lack of the anticipated reduction in levels, appears to act as a risk factor for thromboembolism in patients with prosthetic mitral valves. Such patients might benefit from factor VII monitoring to optimise their INR and should be advised to reduce their dietary fat intake. Statin therapy should also be considered, in view of the close relationship between lipid levels and factor VII.

Antithrombotic therapy according to type of surgery

Mechanical valves

It is generally agreed that all patients with mechanical prosthetic heart valves require anticoagulation for life, and there is no doubt that this is the safest approach under most circumstances.[1,2,65] Trials without anticoagulation and trials with antiplatelet therapy only have resulted in high rates of thromboembolism and/or valve thrombosis.[36] The details of how the intensity of anticoagulation should be adjusted according to the thrombogenicity of each type of mechanical valve are discussed in the section on Choosing the Optimum Intensity of Anticoagulation.

Bioprostheses, homografts and autografts

Bioprostheses in general are considered to be less thrombogenic than mechanical prostheses. However, they are still subject to thrombus deposition, both on the sewing ring and the leaflets, especially in the early postoperative months, and gross obstructive prosthesis thrombosis can occur, even in stentless bioprostheses. One randomised trial between mechanical valves on anticoagulation and porcine valves predominantly without anticoagulation showed no significant difference in the incidence of valve thrombosis at 15 years,[66] and valve thrombosis rates reported in the literature for mechanical valves and porcine valves in the mitral position are also very similar.[29] Bioprosthetic valve thrombosis, especially in the early postoperative period, is often related to low cardiac output.[67] Degenerating bioprostheses and homografts may also be subject to thrombus deposition which, through organisation and secondary calcification, may contribute to further stiffening of the leaflets.[67] Although warfarin has no effect on primary tissue calcification, one study has shown less secondary calcification in degenerating bioprostheses in patients treated with warfarin.[68] A retrospective study based on echocardiographic data suggests that statins may also delay the degenerative process,[69] perhaps through antithrombotic and anti-inflammatory mechanisms[56,70] and immunomodulation[71] in addition to reducing lipid infiltration. Prospective randomised trials are clearly required.

Whether patients with stented bioprostheses with no other indications for anticoagulation (e.g. atrial fibrillation) should receive anticoagulants during the first 3 months remains controversial, due to the absence of randomised trials. It is widely assumed that the thrombogenicity of a bioprosthesis will be less after 3 months, as by this time the sewing ring will be fully endothelialised. However, bioprosthetic sewing rings are sometimes incompletely covered by endothelium even years after implantation and it is doubtful whether the endothelium which is present actually functions normally in such an abnormal and hostile environment.[67] Thus, the 3-month period is somewhat arbitrary, although it has been shown that the risk of thromboembolism declines after this time period,[72,73] as it does with mechanical valves.

Some retrospective studies have found no difference in thromboembolism in the first 3 months between anticoagulated and non-anticoagulated patients,[72,74] whereas others have found fewer thromboembolic events in anticoagulated patients.[73,75] One randomised trial of two different intensities of anticoagulation (INR 2.0–2.25 vs. 2.5–4.0) found no difference in thromboembolism but a significantly higher incidence of bleeding with higher INRs.[30] Two retrospective comparisons of warfarin, aspirin and no treatment following hospital discharge from the pre-INR era in the USA[72,76] are therefore difficult to evaluate without knowledge of achieved INRs; both studies found that any possible benefit of warfarin was outweighed by a high incidence of bleeding, but anticoagulation intensity may have been too high, as in many American studies of that era.[77] A small European non-randomised study published in 2004 found no difference in either thromboembolism or bleeding events in the first 3 months between warfarin (INR 2.0–3.0) and aspirin (dose not stated) in patients following bioprosthetic aortic valve replacement who had no other risk factors for thromboembolism.[78] All bleeding events on aspirin therapy were gastrointestinal and all bleeding events on warfarin occurred with an INR >3.0.

A 2004 internet survey by CTSNet of 726 cardiac surgeons worldwide (45% from the USA, 33% from Europe) revealed that approximately 60% of respondents believed that antiplatelet therapy is an acceptable alternative to warfarin for the first 3 months after bioprosthetic aortic valve replacement in patients without co-morbidities. Almost 70% believed that warfarin for 3 months should no longer be the standard of care. This survey (available at www.CTSNet.org) highlights the current uncertainty about optimum antithrombotic management.

The largest and most recent study to date comparing early anticoagulation to no anticoagulation after bioprosthetic AVR was published in 2005.[79] The Mayo Clinic performed a retrospective analysis of 1151 patients operated between 1993 and 2000, of whom 624 received early anticoagulation and 527 did not, according to surgeon preference. The authors concluded that the use of warfarin did not appear to protect against neurological events during the first 3 months. There was no significant difference in the incidence of bleeding events. However, this retrospective study must be interpreted with great caution, as follow-up was only 87% complete and all follow-up data after discharge from hospital were collected by means of postal questionnaires, sent up to 10 years after surgery. It is well known that this method of data collection seriously underestimates event rates. Further caveats are that 78% of the no anticoagulation group received antiplatelet therapy and that the INRs of patients receiving warfarin were not recorded. The shortcomings of this study and others underline the need for prospective randomised trials in this area.

The current emphasis on earlier discharge from hospital should not be used as an argument in favour of no anticoagulation.[79] In the absence of firm guidance from randomised trials, recommendations can only be derived from basic principles and observational studies (see Box 8.4).

Box 8.4 Recommendations for bioprostheses

1. If there are no contraindications to anticoagulation, the use of low-intensity anticoagulation (target INR 2.5) is recommended for all patients for the first 3 months.
2. In patients with chronic atrial fibrillation and otherwise normal cardiac function, a target INR of 2.5 should be maintained indefinitely.
3. In patients with low cardiac output and heart failure due to impaired ventricular function, irrespective of whether they are in sinus rhythm or atrial fibrillation, a higher target INR of 3.0 should be used.
4. In patients with a high risk of bleeding on anticoagulation (Table 8.1), it is safer to avoid anticoagulation altogether, even in the first 3 months, if the patient is in sinus rhythm. In the presence of atrial fibrillation, low-intensity anticoagulation (INR 2.0) should be considered. Age per se is not a contraindication to anticoagulation.

Table 8.1 Risk factors for anticoagulation-related bleeding[145–149]

INR >4.0
- Poor anticoagulation control
- Drugs which potentiate the effect of oral anticoagulants

Underlying pathological conditions prone to bleeding:
- Peptic ulcer
- Angiodysplasia
- Diverticulitis
- Bladder papilloma
- Menorrhagia
- Cerebrovascular disease (history of stroke)
- Untreated hypertension
- Microvascular disease (diabetes)

Abnormal haemostasis:
- Coagulation disorders
- Anaemia
- Renal failure
- Concomitant antiplatelet therapy

Past history of major bleeding

Occupational or sports-related risk of trauma

Note: Many risk factors are additive, e.g. history of stroke, history of gastrointestinal bleeding, anaemia and renal failure.[149]

Controversy also surrounds the long-term antithrombotic management for bioprosthetic valve patients after the first 3 months. Current US guidelines recommend aspirin alone if the patient is in sinus rhythm,[1,2] but the evidence is weak, being derived from relatively small observational studies.[80–82] In one series of bioprosthetic AVR, the thromboembolism (TE) rate after 3 months was 1.3% per year on aspirin and 5.2% per year with no treatment ($p <0.02$), although concerns were raised in discussion about data collection methods and event definitions.[81] Other series have found no differences between aspirin therapy and no treatment.[72,83] In the absence of strong evidence, long-term antithrombotic management should be patient-specific, using aspirin for patients with established arterial disease and other stroke risk factors (diabetes, coronary disease, persistent smoking, etc.) and no contraindication to aspirin therapy (see section on Antiplatelet Therapy).

The evidence for aspirin following bioprosthetic MVR is even weaker. Nunez et al found an overall TE rate of 0.5% per year on high-dose aspirin (500 mg or 1 g) among 768 MVR and double valve replacement (DVR) patients in Spain, 76% of whom were in AF.[80] This surprisingly low TE rate may possibly be explained by the young age of the patients (mean age 44 years old), as the AFASAK and SPAF studies in patients with non-valvular AF found TE rates of 5.0% per year and 3.6% per year, respectively, in older patients on aspirin.[84,85] In the SPAF study, aspirin was also found to be much less effective in preventing cardioembolic stroke than non-cardioembolic stroke.[86] Thus, the study of Nunez et al cannot be used to support the recommendation of aspirin alone, particularly for patients in their 70s and 80s undergoing bioprosthetic MVR, if they are in atrial fibrillation. If the patient is in sinus rhythm, the recommendation for the use of aspirin is the same as for AVR (see above).

Regular follow-up of patients with bioprostheses is required not only to detect early signs of degeneration but also to detect the development of atrial fibrillation. The Edinburgh valve trial has shown that 33% of bioprosthetic AVR patients and 57% of MVR patients require anticoagulation by 15 years, mainly because of atrial fibrillation.[87] Risk factors for atrial fibrillation include older age, mitral valve disease, hypertension, diabetes, ischaemic heart disease and congestive heart failure.[88] Patients with these conditions will require extra vigilance. Patients with mitral bioprostheses who are not anticoagulated require particularly close follow-up as routine echocardiography reveals that a small percentage will develop thrombosis on the ventricular side of the bioprosthetic cusps, which may not always be symptomatic initially.[89] Patients who have had chordal preservation may be at higher risk.[90,91]

Homografts and autografts in the aortic position have no sewing ring and do not require anticoagulation if they are functioning normally, unless there are other indications.[92] However, degenerating homografts are subject to thrombus deposition[67,93,94] and antithrombotic treatment should be considered in this situation. Stentless aortic bioprostheses fall midway between homografts and stented bioprostheses in terms of potential thrombogenicity. They have no bulky sewing rings but do have artificial fabric exposed to the bloodstream at annular level and the cusps are susceptible, albeit rarely, to thrombosis,[95] usually associated with low cardiac output or technical factors leading to deformation of one or more cusps as the result of distortion at implantation or haematoma formation between the prosthesis and the aortic wall.[96,97] In the absence of trials, the same principles should be applied to stentless bioprostheses as apply to their stented counterparts.

Conservative valve surgery

There are no randomised trials on which to base firm recommendations about antithrombotic management. One of the purposes of conserving the patient's own valve is to avoid anticoagulation if possible. In the case of repair procedures on the aortic valve and in the case of mitral commissurotomy, no prosthetic material is used and there are therefore no artificial surfaces on which thrombus can form. Following these procedures anticoagulation is unnecessary if the patient is in sinus rhythm, providing that normal intracardiac flow conditions are restored. After mitral commissurotomy in particular, some degree of left atrial stasis may persist if relief of mitral stenosis is incomplete and the left atrium is significantly enlarged. Even in the presence of stable sinus rhythm, anticoagulation is advisable under these circumstances,[65] particularly if there is a history of previous embolism. The intensity of spontaneous echo contrast in the left atrium on echocardiography will provide a guide to the degree of stasis[98] and haematological evidence of coagulation activation may give further guidance for anticoagulation.[99]

Mitral valve repair for regurgitation nearly always involves the use of a prosthetic ring, closely resembling the sewing ring of a prosthetic valve, to support the repair and/or reduce the size of the annulus. As with prosthetic valves, this represents a thrombogenic surface until it becomes endothelialised and on general principles a strong case can be made for anticoagulation for the first 3 postoperative months.

If atrial fibrillation or congestive heart failure remain after mitral valve repair, long-term anticoagulation with a minimum INR of 2.0 will be necessary as antiplatelet therapy alone[100,101] or combined with ultra-low anticoagulation (INR <2.0)[102] provides insufficient protection against thromboembolism in atrial fibrillation. The recent Euro Heart Survey of current practice in 25 European countries revealed that approximately half of all patients following mitral valve repair are on chronic anticoagulation, mainly because of atrial fibrillation.[103,104] Increasing interest in the concomitant use of various ablation procedures[105,106] to restore sinus rhythm as an adjunct to mitral valve repair[107] may reduce the proportion of patients requiring anticoagulation in the future, although at present it remains uncertain whether restoration of electrical sinus rhythm corrects left atrial endothelial and contractile dysfunction and reduces thromboembolic risk,[108,109] or indeed whether correction of atrial fibrillation will remain stable in the long term.[110]

Anticoagulation in the early postoperative period

Immediately after any cardiac operation performed on cardiopulmonary bypass, the major concern is the prevention of excessive bleeding. Haemodilution, blood loss and platelet consumption caused by adherence to the bypass circuit result in moderate anaemia and a reduced platelet count. Platelet function is abnormal, fibrinogen levels are usually lower than normal and coagulation may be deranged in other ways also.[111,112] Consequently, the risk of bleeding from surgical sites is usually greater than the risk of thromboembolic complications at this time. Nevertheless, foreign surfaces exposed to the bloodstream will attract thrombus at a very early stage. Within seconds of exposure to blood, artificial surfaces are covered with a thin layer of plasma proteins, and platelet deposition follows rapidly.[113] In areas subject to conditions of low flow, macroscopic thrombus may develop. It is not unusual to see thrombus on the sewing ring of a prosthetic valve on TOE soon after implantation for example.[114] Similarly, thrombus may form in the left atrial appendage very soon after surgery in patients in atrial fibrillation, especially if the cardiac output is low, underlining the need for TOE monitoring in the early postoperative period if possible.[115]

The timing of anticoagulation in the early postoperative period is thus a matter of balancing the risks of bleeding and thromboembolism. After the first 24 hours, the risk of bleeding is usually very small, whereas the risk of thromboembolism progressively increases, as levels of fibrinogen and other coagulation proteins are restored, often exceeding preoperative levels as part of the physiological response to trauma,[116] and monocyte tissue factor expression increases.[117] Similarly, both platelet count and platelet aggregability may rise considerably above preoperative levels, an effect persisting for up to 3 weeks.[116]

As currently available oral anticoagulants work indirectly by suppressing the carboxylation of vitamin K-dependent coagulation proteins (prothrombin, factor VII, factor IX and factor X) by the liver, effective anticoagulation usually takes several days to establish.[59] In fact, in patients not taking oral anticoagulants preoperatively, a steady state in the level of prothrombin (factor II) in plasma may not be reached for 10–15 days, as a result of its long half-life (60–100 hours).[57] Relative resistance to oral anticoagulants, with the necessity for very large doses, can result from interaction with other drugs, impaired absorption, gross obesity, hypothyroidism, excessive vitamin K intake (unusual in a hospital setting) or genetic factors.[59] The latter is very rare. Asian patients, on average, require lower doses of oral anticoagulant drugs than patients of other ethnic origins.[59]

At least three protocols of anticoagulation initiation postoperatively are in widespread use, and no randomised comparison has yet been performed:

1. Intravenous heparin commenced as soon as postoperative bleeding from drainage tubes moderates and maintained until simultaneously or later commenced oral anticoagulation achieves a therapeutic level of INR.[65] This strategy has the potential to increase the risk of bleeding and tamponade. Therefore, strict activated partial thromboplastin time (aPTT) control is mandatory. It should not exceed twice the control value.
2. Oral anticoagulation commenced on the first postoperative day, and supplemented by intravenous heparin only if an effective INR is not achieved by the third postoperative day. If the patient is unable to take oral medication, or if there is doubt about absorption from the gastrointestinal tract (e.g. paralytic ileus, vomiting and diarrhoea), an intravenous preparation of warfarin can be substituted, although this is not available in all countries. This strategy has the potential to increase the risk of thromboembolism although in practice the risk is very small for the first 2 postoperative days. A study from Sweden in 534 patients using intravenous warfarin commenced the morning after surgery, and only supplemented by heparin if the INR was not therapeutic on the second postoperative day, reported no thromboembolic events in patients who followed the protocol.[118] However, this approach may not have wide applicability due to lack of availability of intravenous warfarin and, in any case, would need to be tested in other large series of patients, preferably randomised to other methods of initiating anticoagulation, before it could be recommended.
3. In recent years, subcutaneous low molecular weight heparin (LMWH) has been used increasingly as a bridge to therapeutic oral anticoagulation. This strategy is recommended as an alternative to intravenous unfractionated heparin (UFH) by the ACCP Guidelines.[2] Part of the motivation for using LMWH is to decrease length of stay in hospital and to reduce costs.[119] However, it must be emphasised that patient safety should be paramount, and at present there are no randomised studies to support the use of LMWH in this setting. If LMWH is used, factor Xa monitoring should ideally be employed to ensure optimum anticoagulation,[120] particularly in

patients with renal failure or obesity, in whom dosage may be difficult to determine,[121] and particularly immediately after surgery when the risk of bleeding will be higher at anti-Xa levels higher than 0.8 U/ml.[121]

Until randomised studies are available with echocardiographic control and adequate follow-up beyond the period of hospitalisation to detect thromboembolism after discharge, no particular method can be recommended, but regimen 1 (above) is likely to be associated with the greatest protection against thromboembolism. Whichever strategy is employed, it must be emphasised that inadequate anticoagulation beyond the second or third postoperative day in the presence of increasing prothrombotic conditions is potentially dangerous. The hazard function curve for thromboembolism shows the incidence to be highest during the first 30 days, only falling to a steady long-term level after 6 months.[116]

Initiation of oral anticoagulation after valve surgery requires care, particularly in elderly patients whose dosage requirement is usually less than younger patients due to decreased metabolic clearance of the unbound drug.[122] Variation from patient to patient in the warfarin dose required to achieve a specific INR is partly due to the effect of polymorphisms in factor II and factor VII genes.[123] No loading dose should be given.[124] Patients who have taken oral anticoagulants preoperatively can usually resume their previous dose, although drug interactions, low serum albumin or reduced dietary intake may necessitate a slightly lower dose initially.[125] More frequent INR measurements are necessary in the first few weeks until a steady state is reached.

Choosing the optimum intensity of anticoagulation

General principles and choice of drug

The new oral direct antithrombin drug ximelagatran has been shown to be equally as effective as vitamin K antagonists in the prevention of postoperative venous thromboembolism, stroke in atrial fibrillation and further events in acute coronary syndromes, with a slightly lower incidence of bleeding,[126] but has not yet been approved by the US Food and Drug Administration (FDA) due to concern about liver damage in long-term use in about 6% of patients. Until this issue is resolved and until trials are performed in patients with prosthetic valves, all patients will require anticoagulation using oral vitamin K antagonists. These drugs act indirectly by blocking the carboxylation of four coagulation proteins, factors II (prothrombin), VII,

IX and X, which confers their procoagulant activity. The carboxylation of these factors is not blocked to an equal extent and there is also considerable inter-individual variation in their plasma level at a given INR.[57–59] This biological variation, coupled with imprecision in measurement of the INR for technical reasons, results in some uncertainty as to the precise extent of anticoagulation achieved.[59,127] Further variation can occur between INR measurements due to fluctuation in dietary vitamin K, poor compliance, impaired absorption during gastrointestinal disturbance or drug interactions.[59] It is therefore important to appreciate that selection of a particular target INR level or a range of INR values is not an exact science, and that it is unrealistic to expect that a target INR will be maintained by all patients. INR variability is unfortunately very common, often due to poor compliance,[128] and is a major determinant of thromboembolic events[129] and reduced survival after valve replacement.[130] Furthermore, because of the many different pathogenetic mechanisms involved in thromboembolism after valve surgery,[6,35] anticoagulation at a particular INR may not prevent all events. In general, it is preferable to aim for a specific INR rather than a range when monitoring anticoagulation.

Warfarin is the most commonly used vitamin K antagonist worldwide, but two other drugs need to be mentioned, one shorter-acting and one longer-acting. The half-life of warfarin is 15–50 hours, that of acenocoumarol (widely used in France, Italy and Spain) about 10 hours and that of phenprocoumon (widely used in Germany and the Netherlands) 4–9 days.[59] Smoother control of the INR may be achieved with phenprocoumon in a steady state, but the disadvantages of this drug are the slower response to a dosage change, the necessity to stop the drug well in advance of any planned interruption in anticoagulation and its manufacture in tablets of only one dose. Two non-randomised studies have shown a higher incidence of bleeding complications with phenprocoumon than with acenocoumarol,[131,132] possibly because a high INR will take longer to return to the target range.[132] (See section on Management of the High INR.)

Given the increasing risk of bleeding with increasing anticoagulation intensity, the ideal INR for patients after valve surgery is the lowest which achieves effective reduction in the incidence of thromboembolic events, bearing in mind that the incidence cannot be lowered to zero in any large series of patients for the reasons discussed above. Evidence from several laboratory and clinical studies, both in patients with non-valvular atrial fibrillation[102,133,134] and in patients with prosthetic valves,[135,136] indicates that an INR in the range 2.0–2.5 is the *minimum* requirement for adequate prophylaxis against thrombosis occurring under conditions of relative stasis, but many patients will require a higher INR than this if adverse intracardiac conditions or a more thrombogenic prosthesis impose a greater risk of thrombosis (see below).

In a study of 1608 patients with a variety of different mechanical valves (3% caged ball/disc, 77% tilting disc, 20% bileaflet) followed for a mean of 4 years per patient in four anticoagulation clinics in the Netherlands, Cannegieter and colleagues found the lowest incidence of all events (thromboembolic and bleeding) occurred in the INR range 2.5–4.9.[137] However, this is a very broad range and almost certainly reflects not only the heterogeneity of the patient population in terms of age, risk factors, valve position (aortic or mitral) and valve type but also the inherent limitations of the study: the assumption that the change in INR from one measurement to the next (up to 8 weeks apart) would be linear, as this was the basis for calculating event rates for particular INR ranges.

A recent meta-analysis of heterogeneous observational series from the literature, comparing mean *target* INRs above and below 3.0, came to the conclusion that all patients, irrespective of individual risk factors, valve position and valve type, should have an INR between 3.0 and 4.5.[138] However, the methodology of the meta-analysis did not take into account differences among the series analysed in terms of data collection methods, selection bias, follow-up accuracy, patient risk factors or anticoagulation variability, all of which have been shown to influence thromboembolic rates.[139] In reaching their conclusion, the authors ignored evidence for a contrary view, including RCTs, current guidelines, the much higher mortality rate for anticoagulant-related intracerebral haemorrhage in comparison to ischaemic stroke and the finding that the risk of intracerebral haemorrhage rises steeply above an INR of 4.0. (See sections on Management of the High INR and Antiplatelet Therapy.) Nor did they take into account that many thromboembolic and bleeding events occur when the INR is outside the target range. Although having a uniform approach to anticoagulation intensity recommendations may have advantages for those managing the anticoagulation of large numbers of patients, this approach will not benefit individual patients who may be exposed to the risks of unnecessarily high anticoagulation intensity. In contrast, the trend in recent years has been towards lower-intensity anticoagulation, prosthesis- and patient-specific anticoagulation[116] and greater concentration on the management of patient risk factors, as discussed above.[6,35]

Patient-specific and prosthesis-specific anticoagulation

Unfortunately, currently available randomised trials of different INR ranges fail to provide widely applicable guidelines or to address the requirements of individual patients. All the randomised trials comparing different intensities of anticoagulation in patients with prosthetic heart valves suffer from limitations imposed by their selection criteria,

Table 8.2 Summary of randomised trials

Authors/trial name	Year	Country	Valve types	Target INR	Antiplatelet drugs also	% AVR	% SR	Mean age	Total no. of patients	FU years in each group
Turpie et al[30]	1988	Canada	Bioprostheses	2.0–2.25 vs 2.5–4.0	No	58%	76%	62	210	24[a] 24[a]
Saour et al[31]	1990	Saudi Arabia	B–S 23% S–C 22% S–E 21% Beall 19% SJM 14%	2.65 vs 9.0	DP after 1st TE	38%	83%	91% ≤40 71% ≤30	247	431 436
Altman et al[32]	1991	Argentina	Bicer (tilting disc)	2.0–3.0 vs 3.0–4.5	ASP + DP in all patients	67%	83%	52	99	52 41
AREVA[33]	1996	France	SJM 81% O/C 19%	2.0–3.0 vs 3.0–4.5	No	96%	100%	59	380	416[a] 416[a]
GELIA (AVR)[34]	2001	Germany	SJM 100%	2.0–3.5 vs 2.5–4.0 vs 3.0–4.5	No	100%	61%	60	2024	N/S
GELIA[140] (MVR + DVR)	2001	Germany	SJM 100%	2.0–3.5 vs 2.5–4.0 vs 3.0–4.5	No	0	N/S	N/S	711	N/S

AVR = aortic valve replacement, MVR = mitral valve replacement, DVR = double valve replacement, FU = follow-up, B–S = Bjork–Shiley, S–C = Smeloff–Cutter, S–E = Starr–Edwards, SJM = St. Jude Medical, O/C = Omnicarbon, DP = dipyridamole, TE = thromboembolism, ASP = aspirin, N/S = not stated.
[a] = approximate value. None of these trials showed any significant difference in thromboembolic rates between the different target INR ranges.

their patient population or their methodology (Table 8.2).[30–34,140] Almost all involve relatively small numbers of patients with short follow-up and, because of their fundamental differences and lack of uniformity of INR ranges, they are not suitable for meta-analysis. The AREVA trial, for example, although providing useful recommendations for selected low-risk patients with the St. Jude Medical valve in the aortic position, specifically excluded all patients with risk factors for thromboembolism, including atrial fibrillation, left atrial enlargement or thrombosis, and a previous history of thromboembolism.[33]

The most recently published randomised trial (German Experience with Low Intensity Anticoagulation – GELIA), a larger multicentre study based on patients with the St. Jude Medical prosthesis,[34,140] attempted to compare three overlapping INR ranges, 2.0–3.5, 2.5–4.0 and 3.0–4.5, for patients undergoing AVR, MVR or DVR, beginning 3 months after surgery. The relatively low event rates reported reflect the exclusion of the first 3 months, the period of highest risk. Unfortunately, the impact of the trial

was also severely blunted by the finding that many patients (57% in one subgroup) failed to maintain their INR within their allocated range. Each subgroup also contained a mixture of conventional anticoagulation management and patient self-managed anticoagulation. Not surprisingly perhaps, the trial failed to find any differences in either thromboembolic or bleeding rates between the three INR ranges. This trial amply illustrates the problem inherent in all trials of different *target* ranges of INR – that most events occur while the INR is outside the target range – emphasising the importance of good-quality INR control (see below).

Despite the lack of uniformity of INR ranges, patient characteristics and prostheses type in the various randomised trials, all trials share the same conclusions (in patients who were predominantly in sinus rhythm and who mostly had an aortic prosthesis): the lower range of INR tested did not increase the risk of embolism but did reduce the risk of bleeding. In the case of mechanical valve trials, the selected lower INR range equated with a mean INR of about 2.5 and this value has been accepted in recently

Table 8.3 Anticoagulation for valve replacement

		Without risk factors	With risk factors
Adjust target INR to: intracardiac conditions and prosthesis thrombogenicity		SR LA 0 MVgr 0 LV normal SEC 0 AVR	AF LA >50 mm MVgr + EF <35% SEC + MVR TVR PVR
Prosthesis thrombogenicity	Low	2.5	3.0
	Medium	3.0	3.5
	High	3.5	4.0

SR = sinus rhythm, AF = atrial fibrillation; LA = left atrium; MVgr = mitral valve gradient, EF = ejection fraction, SEC = spontaneous echo contrast, AVR = aortic valve replacement, MVR = mitral valve replacement, PVR = pulmonary valve replacement, TVR = tricuspid valve replacement.

Low = Medtronic Hall, St. Jude Medical (without Silzone), Carbomedics AVR.
Medium = Bileaflet valves with insufficient data, Björk–Shiley valves.
High = Lillehei Kaster, Omniscience, Starr–Edwards.

published guidelines as suitable for most patients with an aortic prosthesis in sinus rhythm.[1,2,65]

The randomised trials offer much less useful guidance on the ideal INR for patients with a mitral prosthesis (Table 8.2). The AREVA trial[33] largely excluded mitral patients, the trial from Saudi Arabia[31] was mainly in very young patients in sinus rhythm and the GELIA trial excluded from analysis the high-risk period of the first 3 months and had a high proportion of patients with INRs outside the target ranges.[34,140]

Following MVR, there are often additional prothrombotic conditions in the left atrium due to atrial fibrillation, left atrial enlargement, poor contractile performance of the appendage (even in sinus rhythm) or residual mitral valve gradient.[115] Hence, anticoagulation intensity must be sufficient to combat conditions of relative stasis in the left atrium in addition to preventing thrombus deposition on the prosthesis. Evidence from experimental laboratory studies,[7] and retrospective comparison of different mean INR levels following isolated MVR,[141] suggest that the lowest target INR for most MVR patients is 3.0, and this has also been recommended by recently published guidelines.[1,2,65] This additional anticoagulation intensity is probably sufficient to combat adverse left atrial conditions, as it has been shown to permit spontaneous regression of left atrial thrombus with return of elevated fibrinopeptide A levels to normal in previously un-anticoagulated

patients.[142] Patients with tricuspid or pulmonary prostheses will also be at higher risk and require a minimum INR of 3.0 (Table 8.3). In the case of some prostheses of higher thrombogenicity, an INR of 3.0 may not be high enough to prevent valve thrombosis, particularly in the presence of low-flow conditions or trigger factors for thrombosis such as dehydration or pulmonary infection. In some patients with prostheses of higher thrombogenicity or in newly introduced prostheses of uncertain thrombogenicity, it is probably safer to maintain a mean INR of 3.5 or 4.0. Thus, in selecting an appropriate INR for patients after valve replacement it is necessary to take into account both patient-related and prosthesis-related factors (Table 8.3).

It is not possible to define low-, medium- and high-thrombogenicity prostheses in exact scientific terms. Unstratified thromboembolic rates provide little guidance, as they can be influenced by so many non-prosthetic factors. On the other hand, prosthesis thrombosis rates are less influenced by extraneous factors, apart from the number of patients in the series who have had a period of anti-coagulation interruption. Relating prosthesis thrombosis rate to mean INR gives a better indication of prosthesis thrombogenicity, if sufficient large series exist in the literature for that prosthesis to provide points to construct a curve (Figure 8.8). For many prostheses on the market these data do not exist. In practical terms, from available data,[29,33,34,36,140,141,143] the Medtronic Hall tilting-disc valve, the St. Jude Medical bileaflet valve (without Silzone coating), the Carbomedics aortic prosthesis and all bioprostheses can be regarded as low-thrombogenicity prostheses.

However, in comparing the St. Jude Medical and Carbomedics valves there is a paradox and a caution. Average

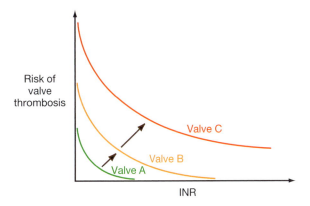

Figure 8.8
Diagrammatic representation of the risk of valve thrombosis according to INR level and prosthesis thrombogenicity. Valve A represents a prosthesis of low thrombogenicity which achieves a zero rate of valve thrombosis with a low level of INR. At the other end of the spectrum, Valve C is a very thrombogenic prosthesis, in which even high levels of INR do not abolish the risk of valve thrombosis altogether.

prosthesis thrombosis rates in the mitral position are higher with the Carbomedics valve, but in the aortic position the opposite is the case.[143] A possible explanation is that the raised pivot guard of the St. Jude valve projects into the left ventricle in the aortic position, where it can come into contact with periannular tissue, particularly if implanted in a supra-annular position. This makes the pivot guard more susceptible to tissue ingrowth, which was the explanation for a relatively high incidence of incomplete leaflet excursion among asymptomatic patients identified on cinefluoroscopy in one Japanese series.[144]

The Omniscience tilting disc valve has been shown to have a high susceptibility to valve thrombosis when exposed to low-intensity anticoagulation[67] and should be regarded as a high-thrombogenicity prosthesis in Table 8.3. It is no longer manufactured. Other tilting disc valves and other bileaflet valves not mentioned above probably occupy intermediate positions in terms of thrombogenicity and further data on *valve thrombosis* rates in relation to achieved INR are awaited in order to characterise them more accurately.

The ideal INR for patients following mitral valve repair using prosthetic ring annuloplasty depends primarily on left atrial conditions. On general principles, if the patient is in sinus rhythm, has no significant left atrial enlargement and good left ventricular function, an INR of 2.5 is probably sufficient, although there are no clinical data from trials to support this recommendation. On the other hand, if the patient is in atrial fibrillation, has moderate-to-severe left atrial enlargement or poor left ventricular function, a target INR of 3.0 is safer.

Management of the high INR

The risk of major bleeding begins to rise when the INR exceeds 4.5 and rises steeply and exponentially above an INR of 6.0.[145] Patients with risk factors for bleeding (Table 8.1)[145–149] are at higher risk. Among 23 patients experiencing fatal intracerebral haemorrhage in a recent large 20-year prosthetic valve series,[150] all had an INR >4.0, 74% had an INR >6.0, 39% were hypertensive and 39% were taking antiplatelet therapy in addition to warfarin. Other authors have also shown that the risk of intracerebral haemorrhage rises steeply above an INR of 4.0.[151] Intracerebral haemorrhage is associated with the highest mortality among bleeding complications, with mortality directly related to haematoma volume.[152] Pre-existing cerebrovascular disease is a risk factor.[146,149,151]

One of the commonest causes of an INR >6.0 is drug interaction with the oral anticoagulant.[59,153] Great care should be exercised when prescribing any of the drugs in the following list (see Box 8.5). The dose of the anticoagulant drug will almost certainly need to be reduced and more frequent INR measurements will need to be made

---

Box 8.5 Drugs which interact with oral anticoagulants to increase their effect[a]

Antibiotics
Almost all antibiotics (particularly cephalosporins) and sulphonamides potentiate the effect of oral anticoagulants, with the exception of *griseofulvin* and *rifampicin*, which have an antagonistic effect

Commonly used cardiovascular drugs
Amiodarone
Clofibrate
Diazoxide
Ethacrynic acid
Propafenone
Quinidine
Simvastatin

Analgesics
Paracetamol (acetaminophen) in prolonged use[b]
Azapropazone ⎫
Ketorolac ⎬ AVOID COMPLETELY
Diclofenac (given IV) ⎭ (danger of very high INR)

Endocrine drugs
Corticosteroids and anabolic steroids
Thyroid hormone

Gastrointestinal drugs
Cimetidine
Chlorpropamide
Metoclopramide

Central nervous system drugs
Chlorpromazine
Monoamine oxidase inhibitors
Tricylic antidepressants

Food
Cranberry juice – AVOID COMPLETELY

[a]*This is not a complete list.* Before prescribing any new or unfamiliar drug, check up-to-date drug information for interactions with oral anticoagulants.
[b]The commonest drug associated with an INR >6.0 in one study.[153]

---

until a steady state is achieved. Some drugs (as noted) should be avoided altogether. Medical conditions which can enhance the effect of oral anticoagulants include advanced malignant disease and recent diarrhoeal illness.[153]

An INR >6.0 is regarded as the threshold for reversal of anticoagulation, even in the absence of bleeding, either by discontinuation alone or by giving vitamin K in addition. However, the recommendation to give vitamin K is based upon analyses of this treatment in groups of patients with very varied indications for anticoagulation.[123,154,155] In some literature series, follow-up is limited to a few days only. No publications have addressed the issue specifically in patients with prosthetic heart valves, other than making risk calculations based on average valve thrombosis rates in non-anticoagulated patients.[155] No echocardiographic studies have been performed to identify early valve thrombosis in patients treated with vitamin K. *The commonest cause of valve thrombosis is anticoagulation interruption* (see Chapter 10). Valve thrombosis is associated with a high mortality, and prosthetic valve patients are therefore at higher risk than the average anticoagulated patient. Although, on average, the INR falls gradually to the therapeutic range with vitamin K,[154] the response in individual patients is unpredictable,[156] and herein lies the danger.

It is therefore recommended that a high INR (>6.0) without bleeding in prosthetic valve patients on warfarin or acenocoumarol should not be treated with intravenous vitamin K. In patients on phenprocoumon, it is permissible to use oral vitamin K, given in increments of 1 mg, as the long half-life of phenprocoumon allows the INR to fall more gradually following the administration of vitamin K. Because of the long half-life however, additional doses may be necessary as the INR often begins to rise again after the second day.[156] The response among individual patients is very variable.[156]

All patients with an INR >6.0 should be admitted to hospital for observation and their anticoagulation temporarily discontinued until the INR is <5.0. If the INR is >10.0, and the patient has risk factors for bleeding (Table 8.1) consideration should be given to the use of fresh frozen plasma at a dose of 15 ml/kg body weight, bearing in mind the very small risk of transmission of viruses[155] and variant Creutzfeldt–Jacob disease.[157] A pathogen inactivation process is now available for treating fresh frozen plasma without reducing its effectiveness.[158,159]

In patients who are bleeding with a high INR, a risk assessment must be made according to the severity, site and controllability of bleeding. If the risk to life from continued bleeding, inaccessible to local control, is greater than that of valve thrombosis (e.g. intracranial bleeding), cessation of anticoagulation should be accompanied by prothrombin complex concentrate. Intravenous vitamin K may also be necessary if bleeding continues, as the half-life of factor VII is only 6 hours. However, it should be recognised that both factor concentrates and vitamin K increase the risk of valve thrombosis.[155] Intracranial and, in particular, intracerebral haemorrhage, always necessitates reversal of anticoagulation.[160] The exact timing of the resumption of anticoagulation remains controversial but most agree that it should be resumed after 1 week[161,162] as the long-term risk of further intracranial bleeding is lower than that of valve thrombosis and thromboembolism.

Bleeding with a therapeutic INR is often related to an underlying pathological cause and it is important to identify and treat it. Anticoagulation often unmasks occult pathology, which is why 'anticoagulant-related' bleeding is commoner in the first few months.[146] Patients with intermittent major bleeding from the gastrointestinal tract sometimes represent a difficult problem. Peptic ulceration can usually be successfully treated but if intermittent bleeding is due to angiodysplasia not amenable to endoscopic ablation or surgery,[163] effective treatment is much more difficult. Bleeding in angiodysplasia has been linked to von Willebrand syndrome type 2A.[164] If local measures or hormone therapy with oestrogens[163] or octreotide[165] fail to control bleeding, lower-intensity anticoagulation or, in extreme cases with ongoing severe bleeding from widespread diffuse angiodysplasia, discontinuation of anticoagulation may be necessary. Fortunately, this is a very rare occurrence.

Self-management of oral anticoagulation

Traditional models of service provision for anticoagulation management vary in different countries, ranging from specialised anticoagulation clinics to general physicians managing anticoagulation in their individual patients. The introduction of the INR in 1983 represented a marked improvement in measurement of intensity of oral anticoagulation and in comparability of test results, but anticoagulation-related bleeding and thromboembolism remain the most common complications after heart valve replacement. Better anticoagulation control has been shown to improve survival after valve replacement, with anticoagulation variability being the strongest independent predictor of reduced survival.[130]

Anticoagulation control therefore is of prognostic importance, and poor control has significant healthcare costs. It has been calculated that lifetime management of cerebrovascular events caused by inadequate anticoagulation adds up to $85 000 in the USA.[166,167]

There is marked variation in the way that anticoagulation control is delivered, as shown in Europe by the Euro Heart Survey on Valvular Heart Disease.[103] The quality of these different anticoagulation control systems also varies considerably, with the percentage of INRs within the therapeutic range varying from 40% to 65%.[168,169]

The variability in quality of traditional anticoagulation control was the impetus for the introduction of patient self-management, as experience with self-management of blood sugar levels in diabetic patients had been successful for many years. In 1986, patient-managed control of anticoagulation began in Germany with the first patient performing a Quick-test.[170,171] Almost simultaneously, publications by Lucas et al[172] and White et al[173] in the USA described a novel capillary technique for measuring prothrombin time. This was the basis for home INR monitoring, and in 1994 the first anticoagulation monitors were introduced in Germany.

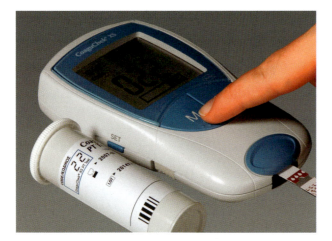

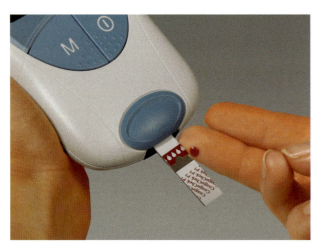

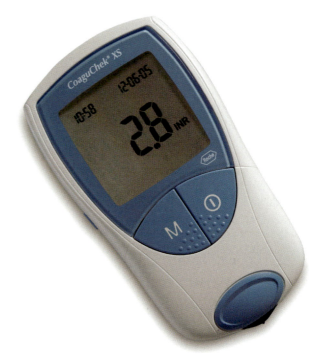

Figure 8.9
Procedure for INR self-assessment using the Coag-u-Chek device (Roche Diagnostics Ltd). The box containing the test strips also contains a calibration chip with a code number (in this case 022) which must be inserted into the device prior to use. A drop of capillary blood is then placed on the test strip. The INR is then read.

Patients can be trained to test a capillary sample for the INR using a portable monitor. Advice on dose can then be given by a physician, or alternatively the patient can be trained to adjust the anticoagulant dose. However, in the Euro Heart Survey on Valvular Heart Disease, self-assessment was used by less than 1% of the patients. Self-assessment is currently performed by about 3000 patients in Denmark and Sweden and about 60 000 patients in Germany (about 10% of all patients on anticoagulants).

The accuracy of the systems used for self-determination of the INR in comparison to conventional measurement has been assessed in several studies.[169,174–177] The R-value was found to be between 0.90 and 0.97.

Only patients on long-term anticoagulation who are able to follow a teaching course of 6–12 hours should be considered for self-management. They should have some manual skills to be able to puncture the finger, have no visual impairment and have sufficient understanding to recognise values outside the therapeutic range. The consent of their physician should be obtained.[169,178,179]

Teaching should include theoretical aspects, such as the effects of anticoagulation, how to monitor the blood, frequency of anticoagulation monitoring and resulting problems, interaction between anticoagulants and other drugs, the influence of nutrition, alcohol, intercurrent illnesses, travel, how to recognise and treat complications, overlapping heparin therapy and vaccinations. Practical teaching should include the operation of the coagulation monitor, practising the coagulation test, as well as an internal quality control, how to apply a correct fingerstick procedure, possible sources of error and recording of test results (Figure 8.9). Support for patients managing their own anticoagulation can be found on three helpful websites: www.ismaa-int.org and www.acfo-rum.org and www.anticoagulationeurope.org.

Effectiveness of self-management

In 9 randomised studies comparing conventional testing with self-testing, patients employing self-management were more frequently within the therapeutic range than with conventional testing, with 70–80% of INR values considered to be in range.[173,180–185] It has been shown that more frequent testing of the INR results in a higher percentage of INRs in the therapeutic range,[186] although for practical purposes a test interval of 8 days is considered sufficient.

Quality control of anticoagulation is an important determinant of prognosis,[130] and event-free survival in patients after valve replacement performing self-assessment has been shown to be significantly higher than in patients with conventional control.[185] Patients capable of performing self-assessment of anticoagulation are usually well educated and motivated and can be trained to be experts in anticoagulation. The frequency of testing (usually once per week in comparison to 4–13 weeks in physician-directed management) adds to improvement in control and also allows the flexibility to adjust testing intervals according to intercurrent events or diseases and changes in medication.

Nearly all studies have shown that most patients prefer self-management. Those who have been successfully trained consider their quality of life markedly improved. In one study, only 8.3% of those trained after valve surgery were unable to continue with self-management.[185]

Although the cost of the monitors, the test strips and the training course of the patient must be taken into account, these costs must be weighed against the high costs of treating the complications of conventionally managed anticoagulation, such as valve thrombosis, thromboembolism, stroke and bleeding complications. The cost-effectiveness of self-management has already been demonstrated in Germany.[177]

Antiplatelet therapy

The use of antiplatelet therapy either alone or in combination with anticoagulation remains controversial, particularly for patients with mechanical valves. There has been much less enthusiasm for combined therapy in Europe than in North America. One recent multicentre randomised trial, comparing two types of prosthesis, reported significant differences in antithrombotic management between the European and North American trial centres. Use of concomitant aspirin was zero in Europe, but 54.6% in the early postoperative period and 23.5% on discharge from hospital in North America.[187] Similarly, the recent Euro Heart Survey on Valvular Heart Disease in 25 European countries[103] found that only 9.2% of mechanical valve patients attending outpatient clinics were taking antiplatelet drugs in combination with anticoagulation.

In determining whether an antiplatelet agent should be added to anticoagulation in patients with prosthetic valves, it is important to distinguish between the possible benefits in cardiovascular disease in general and those specific to prosthetic valves, when computing the risk:benefit ratio.

Trials showing a benefit from antiplatelet drugs in vascular disease and trials showing apparent benefit in groups of patients with prosthetic valves *and vascular disease* should not be taken as evidence that patients with prosthetic valves and no vascular disease will also benefit.

It is also important to distinguish between the mechanisms of action of different antiplatelet drugs (Figure 8.10) rather than amalgamating them for the purposes of meta-analysis or extrapolating from the results of one drug when making recommendations about another. Aspirin, for example, does not significantly inhibit shear-induced platelet aggregation,[188] and experimental work in animals has shown that it does not prevent platelet adhesion to prosthetic surfaces, whereas dipyridamole does.[189]

Basic mechanisms

Antiplatelet agents are widely believed to be effective in preventing thrombotic events in the arterial, but much less in the venous circulation. However, this is not completely true, since deep vein thrombosis and pulmonary embolism were reduced by 36% by aspirin in the Pulmonary Embolism Prevention (PEP) trial in which almost half the patients also received heparin.[190] In atrial fibrillation (AF), a condition in which left atrial thrombi mostly occur because of blood stasis, aspirin alone has been shown to be effective in reducing the thromboembolic risk by 22% (95% confidence interval (CI) 0–38%, $p = 0.05$) in a combined analysis of 6 trials comparing aspirin with placebo. However, many of these patients also had arterial disease. In comparison, warfarin reduced the risk of thromboemboli in AF by 61% (95% CI 47–71%, $p < 0.001$).[191] Since the pathogenesis of thrombosis in patients with prosthetic valves also involves shear-induced platelet activation,[192] especially in the case of aortic valve replacement, the use of an appropriate antiplatelet agent in addition to oral anticoagulants seems to have a sound theoretical basis. However, this must be balanced against the additional risk of bleeding associated with the addition of antiplatelet agents to oral anticoagulant therapy.

Used alone, antiplatelet agents are known to provoke lower rates of intracranial haemorrhage than agents interfering with coagulation (anticoagulants and fibrinolytics).[193] Whereas the combination of the two is expected to result in more bleeding, some trials have addressed the hypothesis that a safe decrease in the intensity of anticoagulation might be possible, by adding an antiplatelet agent, while preserving optimal antithrombotic efficacy. In a direct comparison of high-INR warfarin (2.8–4.2) vs intermediate-INR warfarin (2.0–2.5) + aspirin 75 mg/day in patients after myocardial infarction (the Warfarin–Aspirin Reinfarction Study – II, WARIS II),[194] the combined therapy group had a slight trend to a better outcome (15.0%

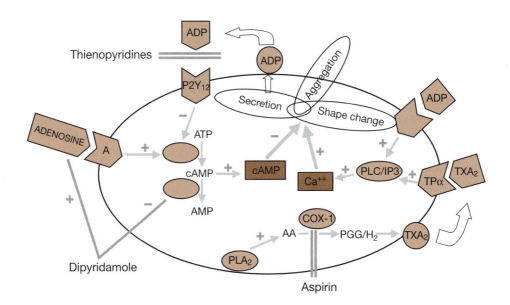

Figure 8.10
Mechanisms of action of the three antiplatelet drugs used in patients with prosthetic heart valves.

The antiplatelet effect of aspirin is due to the inhibition of the platelet cyclo-oxygenase-1 (COX 1)-dependent synthesis of thromboxane (TX) A_2, which is a powerful inducer of vasoconstriction and platelet aggregation deriving from arachidonic acid, a polyunsaturated fatty acid liberated from membrane phospholipids through the action of phospholipase (PL) A_2. The platelet receptor for TXA_2, TPα, stimulates, through G-protein activation, phospholipase (PL) C/inositol triphosphate (IP3)-dependent platelet activation and the release of intracellular calcium (Ca^{++}), which both contribute to platelet aggregation.

Thienopyridines (including ticlopidine and clopidogrel) block the platelet $P2Y_{12}$ ADP receptor, preventing ADP-induced platelet aggregation. $P2Y_{12}$ is one of the two main platelet ADP receptors, together with the $P2Y_1$ receptor. This latter, through G-protein activation, also stimulates PLC/IP3 activation and the increase in intracellular Ca^{++}, mediating shape change and transient aggregation. $P2Y_{12}$, the receptor blocked by thienopyridines, inhibits, through Gi-proteins, adenylate cyclase, and thus reduces intracellular concentrations of the anti-aggregatory cyclic adenosine monophosphate (cAMP), thus mediating sustained platelet aggregation and secretion.

The mechanism of action of dipyridamole as an antiplatelet agent has been the subject of controversy. Two main mechanisms of action have been suggested: the inhibition of cyclic nucleotide phosphodiesterase (PD) – the enzyme that degrades cAMP to AMP – resulting in the intraplatelet accumulation of cAMP; and the blockade of the uptake of adenosine, which acts through A_2 receptors stimulating platelet adenyl cyclase (AC) and thus increasing intracellular levels of cAMP.

COX-1-dependent synthesis of thromboxane TXA_2, ADP-receptor engagement, the inhibition of cyclic nucleotide phosphodiesterase or the blockade of the uptake of adenosine are only some of the possible targets for platelet inhibition. Other antiplatelet drugs, not used in the management of patients with prosthetic valves, include the glycoprotein (GP) IIb/IIIa inhibitors, affecting the surface activity of GP IIb/IIIa, a ligand for fibrinogen and the final common mediator of platelet aggregation; TX synthase inhibitors; and TX receptor antagonists. Apart from the GP IIb/IIIa inhibitors, all other antiplatelet agents affect single pathways of platelet activation, resulting in partial efficacy because of the multiple stimuli able to activate platelets (including ADP, TXA_2, thrombin, serotonin, epinephrine and collagen) and the important redundancy of intracellular controlling pathways.

Since platelets are also important for haemostatic competence, all such treatments entail an increased risk of bleeding as a result of interference with primary haemostasis.

rate of death, myocardial infarction and cerebrovascular accidents) than the warfarin arm (16.7%) in a 4-year follow-up, combined also with a trend towards less major bleeding (0.57% vs 0.68%),[194] although differences were small and non-significant.

A pooled analysis of all aspirin trials in cardiovascular disease concluded that the benefit from low-dose aspirin (75–150 mg/day) was not inferior to that with higher doses (160–325 mg/day), with no difference in the rate of bleeding,[195] but this analysis did not address the issue of com-

bined therapy with warfarin. Although gastrointestinal bleeding with aspirin has been shown to be dose-dependent,[196] this is not the case with intracerebral haemorrhage.[195–197] Meta-analysis of randomised controlled trials (RCTs) shows an 84% increase in the risk of intracerebral haemorrhage with aspirin (RR = 1.84, 95% CI 1.24–2.74, p <0.001).[198]

Apart from aspirin, dipyridamole is the only other agent which has been studied in clinical trials in combination with anticoagulation. The mechanism of action of dipyridamole is controversial,[199] but probably involves the inhibition of adenosine reuptake and potentiation of the effect of nitric oxide.[200] In contrast to all other available antiplatelet agents, dipyridamole is the only drug which does not prolong the bleeding time, an argument used by some to dispute its antiplatelet efficacy and by others to justify the limited, if not absent, excess bleeding risk reported in trials using this agent.[199] The inhibition of platelet adhesion to artificial surfaces by dipyridamole is of potential usefulness in patients with prosthetic heart valves.[189] Several studies have shown some therapeutic benefit with this drug in patients with prosthetic heart valves.[201] However most of these studies were carried out many years ago, mostly in patients with the Starr–Edwards caged-ball valve (which is unique in featuring high shear rates, causing ADP release, and areas of low shear at the apex of the cage), and with a formulation of dipyridamole now thought not to be very effective.[199] The renewed interest in dipyridamole after the publication of a large stroke prevention trial with a newer higher-dose and longer-acting formulation[202,203] should prompt new trials of this drug in the management of artificial heart valves. In a trial of 6602 patients, dipyridamole was equally as effective as aspirin but with half the risk of bleeding (no difference from placebo).[202,203] This absence of excess bleeding is in keeping with a meta-analysis of dipyridamole + warfarin trials[204] and the Mayo Clinic trial comparing warfarin alone, warfarin + dipyridamole and warfarin + aspirin after heart valve replacement.[205] A recent meta-analysis has also confirmed dipyridamole to be effective in reducing stroke recurrence in patients with previous cerebrovascular disease.[206]

Clopidogrel is a new thienopyridine, blocking the platelet $P2Y_{12}$ ADP receptor (Figure 8.10), with proven antithrombotic efficacy in a number of settings involving atherothrombosis. This drug has efficacy at least comparable to aspirin in patients with a previous myocardial infarction or a previous stroke/TIA, or with peripheral arterial disease.[207] Clopidogrel also has effects additive to those of aspirin in acute coronary syndromes and after coronary stenting, reducing the combination of death, myocardial infarction and stroke. Clopidogrel is now being investigated in combination with aspirin in comparison to warfarin in patients with AF at high risk of thromboembolic events (the ACTIVE trial, R De Caterina, pers comm).

Critique of previous recommendations

Recommendations for the use of antiplatelet therapy in patients with bioprostheses have already been discussed above. Recent US guidelines have broadened the indications for antithrombotic therapy with aspirin in the treat-

ment of patients with prosthetic heart valves in general and mechanical heart valves in particular.[1,2] However, the evidence for many of the recommendations is relatively weak, particularly as there was no stratification according to vascular disease in any of the trials cited.

In older trials, combining anticoagulation with aspirin tended to decrease the incidence and severity of embolic episodes, but caused increased, mainly gastrointestinal, bleeding.[205,208,209] This was particularly true when aspirin at doses greater than 500 mg/day was combined with high-intensity oral anticoagulation, as there is evidence that gastrointestinal symptoms and gastrointestinal bleeding associated with aspirin are dose-dependent, and that low doses of aspirin provide equal cardiovascular benefits.[195]

Turpie et al in 1993 reported on a comparison of aspirin 100 mg in association with oral anticoagulation (at INR 3.0–4.5) vs anticoagulation alone at the same INR range, with a 4-year follow-up.[210] In this small study with only about 300 follow-up years in each group, a high proportion of concomitant coronary artery surgery, and only 40% INRs in the target range, the authors showed that, in patients with mechanical heart valves and high-risk patients with prosthetic tissue valves, the addition of aspirin to warfarin therapy reduced mortality, particularly mortality from vascular causes, together with major systemic embolism, compared with oral anticoagulants alone (1.9% per year vs 8.5% per year, $p <0.001$). However, the effect of aspirin in patients without coronary disease was not analysed in this publication. Although the increase in the rate of major bleeding with aspirin was not statistically significant (8.5% per year vs 6.6% per year), the rate of bleeding in both groups was considerably higher than that reported in most recent prosthetic valve series in the literature (average 1.5–2.0% per year).[29] Of more concern, the rate of intracranial bleeding was doubled in the warfarin + aspirin group.[148,211]

After this study, a meta-analysis pooling data from six trials (including Turpie's trial) with either aspirin or dipyridamole as antiplatelet agents,[205,208–210,212,213] supported the contention that the rate of thromboembolism is further reduced with antiplatelet agents added to oral anticoagulants, by about two-thirds, in patients with mechanical prosthetic heart valves.[211] Major bleeding was, however, also increased. There was a 2.5-fold increase in major gastrointestinal haemorrhage from combination therapy. Analysing the risk:benefit ratio, it was at that time concluded that, for about every 1.6 patients in whom stroke was prevented by combination therapy, there was an excess of one major gastrointestinal bleeding. There was also a suggestion that aspirin plus oral anticoagulants resulted in some increase in intracranial bleeding, whereas this might not have occurred in studies using dipyridamole plus oral anticoagulants. These conclusions, although not supported by statistically significant differences,[211] are nevertheless in keeping with the meta-analysis of aspirin trials referred to above.[198]

In this context, it is important to emphasise that ischaemic stroke and intracerebral haemorrhage should not be considered as events of equivalent severity and prognosis. The 1-year survival after ischaemic stroke is about 80%, compared with about 20% after intracerebral haemorrhage.[214] Immediate (30-day) mortality from intracerebral haemorrhage ranges from 40% in the general population, through 60% in anticoagulated patients and 64% in patients with vascular disease on no treatment to 76% in patients on antiplatelet drugs for vascular disease.[148,195] In contrast, immediate mortality from ischaemic stroke is in the range 15–25%.[148,195]

The meta-analysis by Cappelleri et al in 1995[211] and the subsequent meta-analysis of Massel and Little published in 2001[215] illustrate the problems of attempting to apply meta-analysis to disparate trial settings. Meta-analysis was originally devised as a technique for amalgamating data from several RCTs *that had used the same methodology*. The trials utilised in both meta-analyses had numerous important differences between them:

1. Differences in definition of events.
2. Differences in patient selection and follow-up.
3. Differences in antiplatelet drug used. In the meta-analysis of Massel and Little, 6 of the 10 studies analysed had used dipyridamole.[215]
4. Differences in antiplatelet drug dose, particularly in the aspirin trials. Aspirin dose ranged from 100 mg/day to 1000 mg/day. As the gastrointestinal side-effects of aspirin are dose-related, rates of gastrointestinal bleeding are likely to be lower with low-dose aspirin (≤100 mg/day).
5. Differences in target anticoagulation intensity. In the Massel and Little meta-analysis, 8 of the 10 studies were from the pre-INR era (dating back to 1971), making exact anticoagulation intensity impossible to determine.[215]
6. Differences in prosthetic type, with a predominance of older design caged-ball valves.
7. The probability of differences in patient risk factors, particularly the prevalence of vascular disease, since the majority of trials did not provide this information.

There was also bias in the selection of the trials, most of which were small and of short duration. The meta-analysis of Cappelleri et al[211] utilised five trials performed between 1971 and 1993, including that of Chesebro et al reporting one of the largest trials from the Mayo Clinic, comparing warfarin alone, warfarin + aspirin and warfarin + dipyridamole.[205] Massel and Little[215] added only one more trial after 1993 (that of Meschengieser et al, see below), and five more from the 1970s and 1980s (including abstracts with limited information), but specifically excluded the Chesebro study which warned of the increased risk of major bleeding associated with the warfarin + aspirin (500 mg)

combination in comparison with warfarin alone (6.1% per year vs 1.8% per year, *p* <0.001), and showed no difference in bleeding risk between warfarin and warfarin + dipyridamole.[205] Despite the high dose of aspirin, the Chesebro study also found no reduction in thromboembolism from the combination of warfarin and aspirin.[205]

A separate meta-analysis of the dipyridamole trials only, supplemented by additional data submitted to the FDA by the trial centres,[204] confirmed the benefit of dipyridamole suggested by the Massel and Little meta-analysis (equivalent to aspirin)[215] but reached the different conclusion that there was no increased bleeding risk with dipyridamole, in keeping with the results of other trials.[202,203,205]

The most recent trial to address the issue of combined therapy (included in Massel and Little's meta-analysis) requires particular mention as it is widely quoted to support the safety of combined therapy with aspirin. Meschengieser et al compared the combination of 100 mg of aspirin in association with lower-intensity anticoagulation (INR 2.5–3.5) with higher-intensity anticoagulation alone (INR 3.5–4.5).[216] This study was performed in 503 patients receiving mostly AVR, and mostly with tilting-disc valves, and reported that the association of lower-intensity anticoagulation and low-dose aspirin therapy (100 mg/day) offered similar antithrombotic protection to higher-intensity anticoagulation alone, in terms of a composite rate of thromboembolism and valve thrombosis (1.3% per year vs 1.5% per year), without any increase in major bleeding (1.1% per year vs 2.3% per year). However, these results must be interpreted with caution for several reasons:

1. Patients were randomised at various different time intervals between operation and the start of the study, switching from a different therapy to one of the two arms of the study, thereby excluding the early peak in the hazard function curve for both anticoagulant-related bleeding and thromboembolism.
2. Patients with previous gastrointestinal bleeding (presumably while on a different therapy) or a *suspected haemorrhagic tendency* (undefined) were excluded.
3. Patients with previous thromboembolism were also excluded.

Thus, the study was not only blunted by the exclusion criteria but also biased in favour of the aspirin arm of the trial.

Combination therapy during pregnancy has been recommended by the ACC/AHA Guidelines for the Management of Patients with Valvular Heart Disease,[1] but this is not based on any trials and ignores the increased risk of fetal and neonatal intracranial haemorrhage with aspirin.[217,218] Furthermore, aspirin may cause premature closure of the ductus arteriosus.[219] Dipyridamole is not approved for use in pregnancy due to lack of data. In view of the lack of any data showing benefit and the potential risks to both mother and fetus, antiplatelet therapy should not be prescribed during pregnancy.

Despite the methodological concerns discussed above, the reduction in mortality and major systemic embolism observed in the Turpie et al trial and the lack of increased risk of bleeding observed in the Meschengieser et al trial, are the basis for the recommendation of the US guidelines (ACC/AHA) for the wider use of aspirin in combination with oral anticoagulants for patients with mechanical valves (ACC/AHA guidelines: *Addition of aspirin, 80–100 mg once daily if not on aspirin. Level of evidence IIa*).[1]

The latest ACCP Guidelines[2] restrict the use of aspirin in comparison to their previous recommendations, and now recommend anticoagulation with a target INR of 3.0 + aspirin 75–100 mg daily only in the following circumstances:

1. In patients who have mechanical valves and additional risk factors such as atrial fibrillation, myocardial infarction, left atrial enlargement, endocardial damage and low ejection fraction (grade 1C+).
2. In patients with caged-ball or caged-disc valves (grade 2A).
3. In patients with mechanical prosthetic heart valves who suffer systemic embolism despite a therapeutic INR (grade 1C+).

Neither the ACC/AHA nor the ACCP guidelines recommend the use of dipyridamole in combination with anticoagulants because of the lack of trials in patients with newer prosthetic valves and the lack of trials with the new dipyridamole formulation.

In our opinion, the above-mentioned trials and meta-analyses do not provide sufficient evidence to recommend aspirin in combination with oral anticoagulants for all patients with mechanical valves. Further evidence from RCTs in various subsets of patients – e.g. patients with no concomitant vascular disease, patients with atrial fibrillation, patients with concomitant coronary artery bypass grafting (CABG), etc. – is required to issue firm recommendations. At present, the scientific basis on which to recommend intermediate-intensity anticoagulation in combination with aspirin is extremely weak. The large comparisons available in the setting of coronary artery disease,[194] in which INR 2.8–4.2 and INR 2.0–2.5 + aspirin 75 mg/daily have proven roughly equivalent, cannot be extrapolated to the different setting of patients with a mechanical prosthetic valve, where thrombotic mechanisms are different. The use of aspirin in addition to the usual anticoagulation recommended for the type and position of the prosthetic valve should be restricted to patients with additional thrombotic risk factors that are *likely to be modified by aspirin*.

For each patient a balance must be struck between probable benefit and the increased risk of bleeding, particularly intracerebral haemorrhage, as the latter is such a lethal complication. All indications are thus *relative* rather than *absolute*. They represent situations in which antiplatelet

---

Box 8.6 Relative indications for antiplatelet therapy

1. Concomitant arterial disease, particularly coronary disease, aortic atheromatous plaques and carotid disease.
2. Following intracoronary stenting (although combining warfarin with both aspirin and clopidrogrel increases bleeding risk above that with warfarin and aspirin only. Preliminary data from a coronary stenting registry reveal a six-fold increase in the risk of bleeding with triple therapy versus dual therapy.[220]).
3. Recurrent embolism, but only after full investigation and treatment of risk factors, and optimisation of anticoagulation control with self-management (if appropriate) has failed to abolish the problem (see Chapter 9).
4. Increase in mean platelet volume, particularly if an embolic event has already occurred and there is no remediable cause for increased platelet consumption (see text).
5. In patients with caged ball valves in particular; dipyridamole should be considered rather than aspirin in view of its apparent efficacy in prostheses of this unique design in trials from the 1970s, with less risk of bleeding than aspirin.

Box 8.7 Relative contraindications for antiplatelet therapy

The following contraindications apply particularly to the use of aspirin:

1. Previous history of gastrointestinal bleeding, particularly from ulcer disease or angiodysplasia.
2. Hyper-responders to aspirin, with excessively prolonged bleeding time in response to aspirin.[221]
3. Poorly controlled hypertension, due to the increased risk of intracerebral haemorrhage[148] and the lack of efficacy of aspirin in preventing stroke in hypertension.[222–224]
4. Elderly patients, particularly women aged >75 years.[223]
5. Patients on multiple medications, patients who require frequent courses of antibiotics or patients whose anticoagulation control, despite all efforts, is extremely erratic. Frequent episodes of high INR due to drug interactions or poor compliance expose the patient to an increased risk if they are also taking aspirin.

therapy should be considered, rather than simply prescribed in all patients (see Boxes 8.6 and 8.7). In patients receiving combination therapy, antiplatelet therapy should, wherever possible, be combined with a target INR of 3.0 or less, and aspirin should only be used in low-dose formulations (≤100 mg/daily). There are some arguments for preferring dipyridamole to aspirin, as discussed above. For medical practitioners in the United Kingdom, it should be noted that only dipyridamole is recommended for combination therapy with anticoagulation by the British National Formulary (BNF published by the British Medical Association and the Royal Pharmaceutical Society of Great Britain), if an antiplatelet agent is considered necessary.[220]

It is important that further trials of dipyridamole combined with oral anticoagulation in various subsets of patients with and without vascular disease are undertaken, using the new higher-dose, slow-release formulation. Trials of combination therapy with statins and/or ACE inhibitors rather than antiplatelet agents would also be useful, particularly in patients with vascular disease.

Finally, it should not be forgotten that many drugs (other than conventional antiplatelet drugs) and some foods can have an adverse effect on platelet function and may prolong the bleeding time.[48] Caution should be advised in prescribing these drugs in anticoagulated patients, particularly if they are also taking an antiplatelet agent. Patients should also be advised of food items and supplements that may affect platelet function if consumed in large quantities (see Box 8.8).

Box 8.8 Drugs and foods which interfere with platelet function and prolong bleeding time (other than antiplatelet drugs)

Antibiotics
Penicillins
Cephalosporins
Tetracycline
Gentamicin
Nitrofurantoin

Non-steroidal anti-inflammatory drugs

Plasma expanders
Dextran
Hydroxyethyl starch

Alcohol (in high consumption)

Foods and supplements
N-3 fatty acids
Garlic and onion
Ginger
Cloves, cumin and turmeric
Chinese black tree fungus
Vitamins C and E

References

1. ACC/AHA Task Force on Practice Guidelines. ACC/AHA guidelines for the management of patients with valvular heart disease. J Am Coll Cardiol 1998; 32:1486–588.

2. Salem DN, Stein PD, Al-Ahmad A, et al. Antithrombotic therapy in valvular heart disease – native and prosthetic. Chest 2004; 126(Suppl):457S-82S.

3. Oxford Community Stroke Project. Incidence of stroke in Oxfordshire: first year's experience of community stroke register. BMJ 1983; 287:713–17.

4. Murray CJ, Lopez AD. Cerebrovascular disease. Global health statistics. Geneva. World Health Organisation, 1996: 655–7.

5. Gibbs RGJ, Newson R, Lawrenson R, Greenhalgh RM, Davies AH. Diagnosis and initial management of stroke and transient ischaemic attack across UK health regions from 1992 to 1996. Stroke 2001; 32:1085–90.

6. Butchart EG, Moreno de la Santa P, Rooney SJ, Lewis PA. Arterial risk factors and cerebrovascular events following aortic valve replacement. J Heart Valve Dis 1995; 4:1–8.

7. Inauen W, Bombeli T, Baumgartner HR, Haeberli A, Straub PW. Effects of the oral anticoagulant phenprocoumon on blood coagulation and thrombogenesis induced by rabbit aorta subendothelium exposed to flowing human blood: role of dose and shear rate. J Lab Clin Med 1991; 118:280–8.

8. Wolf PA, Abbott RD, Kannel WB. Atrial fibrillation as an independent risk factor for stroke: the Framingham Study. Stroke 1991; 22:983–8.

9. Jones EF, Kalman JM, Calafiore P, Tonkin AM, Donnan GA. Proximal aortic atheroma – an independent risk factor for cerebral ischaemia. Stroke 1995; 26:218–24.

10. Wolf PA, Kannel WB, Cupples LA, D'Agostino RB. Risk factor interaction in cardiovascular and cerebrovascular disease. In: Furlan AJ, ed. The heart and stroke. London: Springer-Verlag, 1987: 331–55.

11. MacMahon S, Peto R, Cutler J, et al. Blood pressure, stroke and coronary heart disease; part 1, prolonged differences in blood pressure: prospective observational studies corrected for the regression dilution bias. Lancet 1990; 335:765–74.

12. Bowler JV, Hachinski V. Epidemiology of cerebral infarction. In: Gorelick PB, ed. Atlas of cerebrovascular disease. Philadelphia: Current Medicine 1996: 1.2–1.22.

13. Manolio TA, Kronmal RA, Burke GL, O'Leary DH, Price TR. Short-term predictors of incident stroke in older adults. Stroke 1996; 27:1479–86.

14. Shinton R, Beevers G. Meta-analysis of relation between cigarette smoking and stroke. BMJ 1989; 298:789–94.

15. Butchart EG, Lewis PA, Bethel JA, Breckenridge IM. Adjusting anticoagulation to prosthesis thrombogenicity and patient risk factors: recommendations for the Medtronic Hall valve. Circulation 1991; 84(5 Suppl):III61–9.

16. Harrison DG, Minor RL, Guerra R, Wuillen JE, Sellke FW. Endothelial dysfunction in atherosclerosis. In: Rubanyi GM, ed. Cardiovascular significance of endothelium-derived vasoactive factors. Mount Kisco, NY: Futura, 1991: 263–80.

17. Burrig KF. The endothelium of advanced arteriosclerotic plaques in humans. Arteriosclerosis Thromb 1991; 11:1678–89.

18. Packham MA, Kinlough-Rathbone RL. Mechanisms of atherogenesis and thrombosis. In: Bloom AL, Forbes CD, Thomas DP, Tuddenham EGD, eds. Haemostasis and thrombosis, 3rd edn. Edinburgh: Churchill Livingstone, 1994: 1107–38.

19. Yoganathan AP, Wick TM, Reul H. The influence of flow characteristics of prosthetic valves on thrombus formation. In: Butchart EG, Bodnar E, eds. Current issues in heart valve disease: thrombosis, embolism and bleeding. London: ICR Publishers, 1992: 123–48.

20. Jones M, Eidbo EE. Doppler color flow evaluation of prosthetic

mitral valves: experimental epicardial studies. J Am Coll Cardiol 1989; 13:234–40.

21. Yasaka M, Beppu S. Hypercoagulability in the left atrium. Part II: coagulation factors. J Heart Valve Dis 1993; 2:25–34.

22. Butchart EG. Fibrinogen and leukocyte activation – the keys to understanding prosthetic valve thrombosis? J Heart Valve Dis 1997; 6:9–16.

23. Ruggeri ZM. Mechanisms of shear-induced platelet adhesion and aggregation. Thromb Haemost 1993; 70:119–23.

24. Alkhamis TM, Beissinger RL, Chediak J. Artificial surface effect on red blood cells and platelets in laminar shear flow. Blood 1990; 75:1568–75.

25. Kroll MH, Hellums JD, McIntyre LV, Schaefer AI, Moake JL. Platelets and shear stress. Blood 1996; 88:1525–41.

26. Okazaki Y, Wika KE, Matsuyoshi T, et al. Platelets are deposited early post-operatively on the leaflet of a mechanical valve in sheep without post-operative anticoagulants or antiplatelet agents. A scanning electron microscopic observation of the pyrolitic carbon surface in a mechanical heart valve. ASAIO J 1996; 42:M750–4.

27. Janicek MJ, Van den Abbeele AD, DeSisto WC, et al. Embolization of platelets after endothelial injury to the aorta in rabbits. Assessment with ¹¹¹indium-labelled platelets and angiography. Invest Radiol 1991; 26:655–9.

28. Butchart EG, Moreno de la Santa P, Rooney SJ, Lewis PA. The role of risk factors and trigger factors in cerebrovascular events after mitral valve replacement: implications for antithrombotic management. J Card Surg 1994; 9(Suppl):228–36.

29. Grunkemeier GL, Li HH, Naftel DC, Starr A, Rahimtoola SH. Long-term performance of heart valve prostheses. Curr Probl Cardiol 2000; 25:73–156.

30. Turpie AGG, Gunstensen J, Hirsh J, Nelson H, Gent M. Randomised comparison of two intensities of oral anticoagulant therapy after tissue heart valve replacement. Lancet 1988; 1:1242–5.

31. Saour JN, Sieck JO, Mamo LAR, Gallus AS. Trial of different intensities of anticoagulation in patients with prosthetic heart valves. N Engl J Med 1990; 322:428–32.

32. Altman R, Rouvier G, Gurfinkel E, et al. Comparison of two levels of anticoagulant therapy in patients with substitute heart valves. J Thorac Cardiovasc Surg 1991; 101:427–31.

33. Acar J, Iung B, Boissel JP, et al. AREVA: multicenter randomized comparison of low-dose versus standard-dose anticoagulation in patients with mechanical prosthetic heart valves. Circulation 1996; 94:2107–12.

34. Huth C, Friedl A, Rost A. Intensity of oral anticoagulation after implantation of St. Jude Medical aortic prosthesis: analysis of GELIA database. Eur Heart J Suppl 2001; 3(Suppl Q):Q33–8.

35. Butchart EG, Ionescu A, Payne N, et al. A new scoring system to determine thromboembolic risk after heart valve replacement. Circulation 2003; 108(SupplII):68–74.

36. Butchart EG. Thrombogenesis and its management. In: Acar J, Bodnar E, eds. Textbook of acquired heart valve disease. London: ICR Publishers, 1995: 1048–120.

37. Blood Pressure Lowering Treatment Trialists' Collaboration. Effects of different blood-pressure-lowering regimens on major cardiovascular events: results of prospectively-designed overviews of randomised trials. Lancet 2003; 362:1527–35.

38. Ambrose JA, Barua RS. The pathophysiology of cigarette smoking and cardiovascular disease: an update. J Am Coll Cardiol 2004; 43:1731–7.

39. Kuusisto J, Mykkanen L, Pyorala K, Laakso M. Non-insulin-dependent diabetes and its metabolic control are important predictors of stroke in elderly subjects. Stroke 1994; 25:1157–64.

40. Sacco RL. Reducing the risk of stroke in diabetes: what have we learned that is new? Diabetes Obes Metab 2002; 4(Suppl 1):S27–34.

41. Stroke Prevention in Atrial Fibrillation Investigators. Prediction of thromboembolism in atrial fibrillation. II Echocardiographic features of patients at risk. Ann Intern Med 1992; 116:6–12.

42. Rosito GA, D'Agostino RB, Massaro J, et al. Association between obesity and a prothrombotic state: the Framingham Offspring Study. Thromb Haemost 2004; 91:683–9.

43. Kurth T, Gaziano M, Berger K, et al. Body mass index and the risk of stroke in men. Arch Intern Med 2002; 162:2557–62.

44. Jood K, Jern C, Wilhelmsen L, Rosengren A. Body mass index in mid-life is associated with a first stroke in men. Stroke 2004; 35:2764–9.

45. Rexrode KM, Hennekens CH, Willett WC, et al. A prospective study of body mass index, weight change and risk of stroke in women. JAMA 1997; 277:1539–45.

46. Bath P, Algert C, Chapman N, et al. Association of mean platelet volume with risk of stroke among 3134 individuals with history of cerebrovascular disease. Stroke 2004; 35:622–6.

47. Sharpe PC, Trinick T. Mean platelet volume in diabetes mellitus. Q J Med 1993; 86:739–42.

48. Warkentin TE, Kelton JG. Acquired platelet disorders. In: Bloom AL, Forbes CD, Thomas DP, Tuddenham EGD, eds. Haemostasis and thrombosis. Edinburgh: Churchill Livingstone, 1994: 767–818.

49. Martin JF, Trowbridge EA, Salmon G, et al. The biological significance of platelet volume: its relationship to bleeding time, platelet thromboxane B_2 production and megakaryocyte nuclear DNA concentration. Thromb Res 1983; 32:443–60.

50. Ernst E, Resch KL. Therapeutic interventions to lower plasma fibrinogen concentration. Eur Heart J 1995; 16(Suppl A):47–53.

51. Cook PJ, Honeybourne D, Lip GYH, et al. Chlamydia pneumoniae antibody titres are significantly associated with acute stroke and transient cerebral ischaemia. Stroke 1998; 29:404–10.

52. Elkind MSV, Lin IF, Grayston JT, et al. Chlamydia pneumoniae and the risk of first ischaemic stroke. Stroke 2000; 31:1521–5.

53. Gieffers J, Fullgraf H, Jahn J, et al. Chlamydia pneumoniae infection in circulating human monocytes is refractory to antibiotic treatment. Circulation 2001; 103:351–6.

54. Bosch J, Yusuf S, Pogue J, et al. Use of ramipril in preventing stroke: double blind randomised trial. BMJ 2002; 324:699–702.

55. Di Napoli P, Taccardi AA, Oliver M, DeCaterina R. Statins and stroke: evidence for cholesterol-independent effects. Eur Heart J 2002; 23:1908–21.

56. MRC Asymptomatic Carotid Surgery Trial Collaborative Group. Prevention of disabling and fatal strokes by successful carotid endarterectomy in patients without recent neurological symptoms: randomised controlled trial. Lancet 2004; 363:1491–502.

57. Thijssen HHW, Hamulyak K, Willigers H. 4–hydroxycoumarin oral anticoagulants: pharmacokinetics–response relationship. Thromb Haemost 1988; 60:35–8.

58. Weinstock DM, Chang P, Aronson DL, et al. Comparison of plasma prothrombin and factor VII and urine prothrombin F1 concentrations in patients on long-term warfarin therapy and those in the initial phase. Am J Hematol 1998; 57:193–9.

59. van den Besselaar AMHP. Oral anticoagulant therapy. In: Bloom AL, Forbes CD, Thomas DP, Tuddenham EGD, eds. Haemostasis and thrombosis. Edinburgh: Churchill Livingstone 1994: 1439–58.

60. Miller GJ, Meade TW. Hypercoagulability. In: Butchart EG, Bodnar E, eds. Current issues in heart valve disease: thrombosis, embolism and bleeding. London: ICR Publishers, 1992: 81–92.

61. Meade TW, Mellows S, Brozovic M, et al. Haemostatic function and ischaemic heart disease: principal results of the Northwick Park Heart Study. Lancet 1986; 2:533–7.

62. Eriksson-Berg M, Deguchi H, Hawe E, et al. Influence of factor VII gene polymorphisms and environmental factors on plasma coagulation factor VII concentrations in middle-aged women with and without manifest coronary heart disease. Thromb Haemost 2005; 93:351–8.

63. Syrjanen J, Valtonen VV, Ivanainen M, et al. Preceding infection as an important risk factor for ischaemic brain infarction in young and middle-aged patients. BMJ 1988; 296:1156–60.

64. Grau AJ, Buggle F, Heindl S, et al. Recent infection as a risk factor for cerebrovascular ischaemia. Stroke 1995; 26:373–9.

65. Gohlke-Bärwolf C, Acar J, Oakley C, et al. Guidelines for the prevention of thromboembolic events in valvular heart disease. Eur Heart J 1995; 16:1320–30.

66. Hammermeister K, Sethi GK, Henderson WG, et al. Outcomes 15 years after valve replacement with a mechanical valve versus a bioprosthetic valve: final report of the Veterans Affairs randomized trial. J Am Coll Cardiol 2000; 36:1152–8.

67. Butchart EG. Thrombogenicity, thrombosis and embolism. In: Butchart EG, Bodnar E, eds. Current issues in heart valve disease: thrombosis, embolism and bleeding. London: ICR Publishers, 1992: 172–205.

68. Stein PD, Riddle JM, Kemp SR, et al. Effect of warfarin on calcification of spontaneously degenerated porcine bioprosthetic valves. J Thorac Cardiovasc Surg 1985; 90:119–25.

69. Antonini-Canterin F, Zuppiroli A, Popescu BA, et al. Effect of statins on the progression of bioprosthetic aortic valve degeneration. Am J Cardiol 2003; 92:1479–82.

70. Undas A, Brummel KE, Musial J, Mann KG, Szczeklik A. Simvastatin depresses blood clotting by inhibiting activation of prothrombin, factor V and factor XIII and by enhancing factor Va inactivation. Circulation 2001; 103:2248–53.

71. Palinski W. Immunomodulation: a new role for statins? Nature Med 2000; 6:1311–12.

72. Blair KL, Hatton AC, White WD, et al. Comparison of anticoagulation regimens after Carpentier–Edwards aortic or mitral valve replacement. Circulation 1994; 90(Suppl II): 214-19.

73. Heras M, Chesebro JH, Fuster V, et al. High risk of thromboemboli early after bioprosthetic cardiac valve replacement. J Am Coll Cardiol 1995; 25:1111–19.

74. Moinuddeen K, Quin J, Shaw R, et al. Anticoagulation is unnecessary after biological aortic valve replacement. Circulation 1998; 98(Suppl II):95–9.

75. Silverton NP, Abdulali SA, Yakirevich VS, Tandon AP, Ionescu MI. Embolism, thrombosis and anticoagulant haemorrhage in mitral valve disease. A prospective study of patients having valve replacement with the pericardial xenograft. Eur Heart J 1984; 5(Suppl D):19–25.

76. Hill JD, LaFollette L, Szarnicki RJ, et al. Risk-benefit analysis of warfarin therapy in Hancock mitral valve replacement. J Thorac Cardiovasc Surg 1982; 83:718–23.

77. Hirsh J, Levine M. Confusion over the therapeutic range for monitoring oral anticoagulation therapy in North America. Thromb Haemost 1988; 59:129–32.

78. Gherli T, Colli A, Fragnito C, et al. Comparing warfarin with aspirin after biological aortic valve replacement: a prospective study. Circulation 2004; 110:496–500.

79. Sundt TM, Zehr KJ, Dearani JA, et al. Is early anticoagulation with warfarin necessary after bioprosthetic aortic valve replacement? J Thorac Cardiovasc Surg 2005; 129:1024–31.

80. Nunez L, Aguado ML, Larrea JL, Celemin D, Oliver J. Prevention of thromboembolism using aspirin after mitral valve replacement with porcine bioprostheses. Ann Thorac Surg 1984; 37:84–7.

81. David TE, Ho WIC, Christakis GT. Thromboembolism in patients with aortic porcine bioprostheses. Ann Thorac Surg 1985; 40:229–33.

82. Goldsmith I, Lip GYH, Mukundan S, Rosin MD. Experience with lose-dose aspirin as thromboprophylaxis for the Tissuemed porcine aortic bioprosthesis: a survey of five years' experience. J Heart Valve Dis 1998; 7:574–9.

83. Jamieson WRE, Lemieux MD, Sullivan JR, et al. Comparing warfarin with aspirin after biological aortic valve replacement. Ann Thorac Surg 1985; 40:232–3.

84. Petersen P, Boysen G, Godtfredsen J, Andersen ED, Andersen B. Placebo-controlled, randomised trial of warfarin and aspirin for prevention of thromboembolic complications in chronic atrial fibrillation. Lancet 1989; 1:175–9.

85. SPAF Study Group Investigators. Preliminary report of the stroke prevention in atrial fibrillation study. N Engl J Med 1990; 322:863–8.

86. Miller VT, Rothrick JF, Pearce LA, et al. Ischaemic stroke in patients with atrial fibrillation: effect of aspirin according to stroke mechanism. Neurology 1993; 43:32–6.

87. Oxenham H, Bloomfield P, Wheatley DJ, et al. Twenty year comparison of a Bjork–Shiley mechanical heart valve with porcine prostheses. Heart 2003; 89:715–21.

88. Kannel WB, Wolf PA, Benjamin EJ, Levy D. Prevalence, incidence, prognosis and predisposing conditions for atrial fibrillation: population-based estimates. Am J Cardiol 1998; 82:2–9N.

89. Oliver JM, Gallego P, Gonzalez A, et al. Bioprosthetic mitral valve thrombosis: clinical profile, transesophageal echocardiographic features and follow-up after anticoagulant therapy. J Am Soc Echocardiogr 1996; 9:691–9.

90. Fasol R, Lakew F. Early failure of bioprosthesis by preserved mitral leaflets. Ann Thorac Surg 2000; 70:653–4.

91. Korkolis DP, Passik CS, Marshalko SJ, Koullias GJ. Early bioprosthetic mitral valve 'pseudostenosis' after complete preservation of the native mitral apparatus. Ann Thorac Surg 2002; 74:1689–91.

92. Unger P, Plein D, Pradier O, LeClerc JL. Thrombosis of aortic valve homograft associated with lupus anticoagulant antibodies. Ann Thorac Surg 2004; 77:312–14.

93. Davies M, Missen GAK, Blandford G, et al. Homograft replacement of the aortic valve. A clinical and pathological study. Am J Cardiol 1968; 22:195–217.

94. Doty DB. Aortic valve replacement with homograft and autograft. Semin Thorac Cardiovasc Surg 1996; 8:249–58.

95. Medtronic Inc. Freestyle aortic root bioprosthesis. Clinical compendium. Data on file at Medtronic.

96. van Nooten G, Ozaki S, Herijgers P, et al. Distortion of the stentless porcine valve induces accelerated leaflet fibrosis and calcification in juvenile sheep. J Heart Valve Dis 1999; 8:34–41.

97. Bach DS. Echocardiographic assessment of stentless aortic bioprosthetic valves. J Am Soc Echocardiogr 2000; 13:941–8.

98. Fraser AG. Ultrasonic detection of increased embolic risk. In: Butchart EG, Bodnar E, eds. Current issues in heart valve disease: thrombosis, embolism and bleeding. London: ICR Publishers, 1992: 223–44.

99. Adams JE, Jaffe AS. Scintigraphic and haematological detection of thrombosis and increased embolic risk. In: Butchart EG, Bodnar E, eds. Current issues in heart valve disease: thrombosis, embolism and bleeding. London: ICR Publishers, 1992: 206–22.

100. Yamamoto K, Ikeda U, Fukazawa H, Shimada K. Effects of aspirin on status of thrombin generation in atrial fibrillation. Am J Cardiol 1996; 77:528–30.

101. Kamath S, Blann AD, Chin BSP, Lip GYH. A prospective randomized trial of aspirin-clopidogrel combination therapy and dose-adjusted warfarin on indices of thrombogenesis and platelet activation in atrial fibrillation. J Am Coll Cardiol 2002; 40:484–90.

102. SPAF Investigators. Adjusted-dose warfarin versus low-intensity, fixed dose warfarin plus aspirin for high risk patients with atrial fibrillation: Stroke Prevention in Atrial Fibrillation III randomised clinical trial. Lancet 1996; 348:633–8.

103. Iung B, Baron G, Butchart EG, et al. A prospective survey of patients with valvular heart disease in Europe: The Euro Heart Survey on Valvular Heart Disease. Eur Heart J 2003; 24:1231–43.

104. Gohlke-Bärwolf C, Iung B, Butchart EG, et al. Unexpected findings in anticoagulation management in patients with valvular heart disease after valve surgery. Eur Heart J 2003; 24(Suppl):abstract No. 2278.

105. Ng FS, Camm AJ. Catheter ablation of atrial fibrillation. Clin Cardiol 2002; 25:384–94.

106. Viola N, Williams MR, Oz MC, Ad N. The technology in use for surgical ablation of atrial fibrillation. Semin Thorac Cardiovasc Surg 2002; 14:198–205.

107. Ad N, Cox JW. The significance of atrial fibrillation ablation in patients undergoing mitral valve surgery. Semin Thorac Cardiovasc Surg 2002; 14:193–7.

108. Lip GY. The prothrombotic state in atrial fibrillation: the atrium, the endothelium... . And tissue factor? Thromb Res 2003; 111:133–5.

109. Marin F, Roldan V, Climent V, et al. Is thrombogenesis in atrial fibrillation related to matrix metalloproteinase-1 and its inhibitor, TIMP-1? Stroke 2003; 34:1181–6.

110. Pacifico A, Henry PD. Ablation for atrial fibrillation: are cures really achieved? J Am Coll Cardiol 2004; 43:1940–2.

111. Woodman RC, Harker LA. Bleeding complications associated with cardiopulmonary bypass. Blood 1990; 76:1680–97.

112. Kouchoukos NT, Blackstone EH, Doty DB, Hanley FL, Karp RB. Hypothermia, circulatory arrest and cardiopulmonary bypass. In: Kirklin JW, Barratt-Boyes B, eds. Cardiac surgery, 3rd edn. Philadelphia: Churchill Livingstone, 2003: 66–130.

113. Anderson JM, Schoen FH. Interactions of blood with artificial surfaces. In: Butchart EG, Bodnar E, eds. Current issues in heart valve disease: thrombosis, embolism and bleeding. London: ICR Publishers, 1992: 160–71.

114. Laplace G, Lafitte S, Labèque JN, et al. Clinical significance of early thrombosis after prosthetic mitral valve replacement. J Am Coll Cardiol 2004; 43:1283–90.

115. Beppu S. Hypercoagulability in the left atrium: part I: echocardiography. J Heart Valve Dis 1993; 2:18–24.

116. Butchart EG. Prosthesis-specific and patient-specific anticoagulation. In: Butchart EG, Bodnar E, eds. Current issues in heart valve disease: thrombosis, embolism and bleeding. London: ICR Publishers, 1992: 293–317.

117. Ernofsson M, Thelin S, Siegbahn A. Monocyte tissue factor expression, cell activation and thrombin formation during cardiopulmonary bypass: a clinical study. J Thorac Cardiovasc Surg 1997; 113:576–84.

118. Thulin LI, Olin CL. Initiation and long-term anticoagulation after heart valve replacements. Arq Bras Cardiol 1987; 49:265–8.

119. Fanikos J, Tsilimingras K, Kucher N, et al. Comparison of efficacy, safety and cost of low-molecular-weight heparin with continuous infusion unfractionated heparin for initiation of anticoagulation after mechanical prosthetic valve implantation. Am J Cardiol 2004; 93:247–50.

120. Montalescot G, Polle V, Collet JP, et al. Low molecular weight heparin after mechanical heart valve replacement. Circulation 2000; 101:1083–6.

121. Hirsh J, Warkentin TE, Shaughnessy SG, et al. Heparin and low-molecular-weight heparin. Mechanisms of action, pharmacokinetics, dosing, monitoring, efficacy and safety. Chest 2001; 119(Suppl):64S–94S.

122. Russman S, Gohlke-Bärwolf C, Jähnchen E, Trenk D, Roskamm H. Age-dependent differences in the anticoagulant effect of phenprocoumon in patients after heart valve surgery. Eur J Clin Pharmacol 1997; 52:31–5.

123. D'Ambrosio RL, D'Andrea G, Cappucci F, et al. Polymorphisms in factor II and factor VII genes modulate oral anticoagulation with warfarin. Haematologica 2004; 89:1510–16.

124. Ansell J, Hirsh J, Dalen J, et al. Managing oral anticoagulant therapy. Chest 2001; 119(Suppl):22–38S.

125. Ageno W, Turpie AGG. Exaggerated initial response to warfarin following heart valve replacement. Am J Cardiol 1999; 84:905–8.

126. Gurewich V. Ximelagatran – promises and concerns. JAMA 2005; 293:736–9.

127. McKernan A, Thomson JM, Poller L. The reliability of international normalised ratios during short-term oral anticoagulant treatment. Clin Lab Haematol 1988; 10:63–71.

128. Arnsten JH, Gelfand JM, Singer DE. Determinants of compliance with anticoagulation: a case-control study. Am J Med 1977; 103:11–17.

129. Huber KC, Gersh BJ, Bailey KR, et al. Variability in anticoagulation control predicts thromboembolism after mechanical cardiac valve replacement: a 23 year population-based study. Mayo Clin Proc 1997; 72:1103–10.

130. Butchart EG, Payne N, Li HH, et al. Better anticoagulation control improves survival after valve replacement. J Thorac Cardiovasc Surg 2002; 123:715–23.

131. Sixty Plus Reinfarction Study Research Group. Risks of long-term oral anticoagulant therapy in elderly patients after myocardial infarction: second report of the Sixty Plus Reinfarction Study Research Group. Lancet 1982; 1:64–8.

132. van der Meer FJM, Rosendaal FR, Vandenbroucke JP, Briet E. Bleeding complications in oral anticoagulant therapy. Arch Intern Med 1993; 153:1557–62.

133. Feinberg WM, Cornell ES, Nightingale SD, et al. Relationship between prothrombin activation fragment F1.2 and international normalized ratio in patients with atrial fibrillation. Stroke Prevention in Atrial Fibrillation Investigators. Stroke 1997; 28:1101–6.

134. Koefoed BG, Fedddersen C, Gullov AL, Petersen P. Effect of minidose warfarin, conventional dose warfarin and aspirin on INR and prothrombin fragment 1 + 2 in patients with atrial fibrillation. Thomb Haemost 1997; 77:845–8.

135. van Wersch JWJ, van Mourik-Alderliesten CH, Coremans A. Determination of markers of coagulation activation and reactive fibrinolysis in patients with mechanical heart valve prosthesis at different intensities of oral anticoagulation. Blood Coag Fibrinol 1992; 3:183–6.

136. Tientadakul P, Opartkiattikul N, Sangtawesin W, et al. Effect of different oral anticoagulant intensities on prothrombin fragment 1 + 2 in Thai patients with mechanical heart valve prostheses. J Med Assoc Thai 1997; 80:81–6.

137. Cannegieter SC, Rosendaal FR, Wintzen AR, et al. Optimal oral anticoagulant therapy in patients with mechanical heart valves. N Engl J Med 1995; 333:11–17.

138. Vink R, Kraaijenhagen RA, Hutten BA, et al. The optimal intensity of vitamin K antagonists in patients with mechanical heart valves. A meta-analysis. J Am Coll Cardiol 2003; 42:2042–8.

139. Butchart EG, Gohlke-Bärwolf C. Anticoagulation management of patients with prosthetic heart valves. J Am Coll Cardiol 2004; 44:1143–4.

140. Pruefer D, Dahm M, Dohmen G, et al. Intensity of oral anticoagulation after implantation of St. Jude Medical mitral or multiple valve replacement: lessons learned from GELIA. Eur Heart J Suppl 2001; 3(Suppl Q):Q39–43.

141. Butchart EG, Lewis PA, Bethel JA, Breckenridge IM. Adjusting anticoagulation to prosthesis thrombogenicity and patient risk factors. Recommendations for the Medtronic Hall valve. Circulation 1991; 84(Suppl III):61–9.

142. Yasaka M, Yamaguchi T, Miyashita T, Tsuchiya T. Regression of intracardiac thrombus after embolic stroke. Stroke 1990; 21:1540–4.

143. Grunkemeier GL, Wu YX. Our complication rates are lower than theirs: statistical critique of heart valve comparisons. J Thorac Cardiovasc Surg 2003; 125:290–300.

144. Aoyagi S, Nishimi M, Kawano H, et al. Obstruction of St. Jude Medical valves in the aortic position: significance of a combination of cineradiography and echocardiography. J Thorac Cardiovasc Surg 2000; 120:142–7.

145. Palareti G, Leali N, Manotti C, et al. Bleeding complications of oral anticoagulant treatment: an inception-cohort, prospective collaborative study (ISCOAT). Lancet 1996; 348:423–8.

146. Landefeld CS, Goldman L. Major bleeding in outpatients treated with warfarin: incidence and prediction by factors known at the start of outpatient therapy. Am J Med 1989; 87:144–52.

147. Launbjerg J, Egeblad H, Heaf J, et al. Bleeding complications to oral anticoagulant therapy: multivariate analysis of 1010 treatment years in 551 outpatients. J Intern Med 1991; 229:351–5.

148. Hart RG, Boop BS, Anderson DC. Oral anticoagulants and intracranial haemorrhage: facts and hypotheses. Stroke 1995; 26:1471–7.

149. Beyth RJ, Quinn LM, Landefeld S. Prospective evaluation of an index for predicting the risk of major bleeding in outpatients treated with warfarin. Am J Med 1998; 105: 91–9.

150. Butchart EG, Li HH, Payne N, Buchan K, Grunkemeier GL. Twenty years' experience with the Medtronic Hall valve. J Thorac Cardiovasc Surg 2001; 121:1090–100.

151. Hylek EM, Singer DE. Risk factors for intracranial hemorrhage in outpatients taking warfarin. Ann Intern Med 1994; 120:897–902.

152. Radberg JA, Olsson JE, Radberg CT. Prognostic parameters in spontaneous intracerebral hematomas with special reference to anticoagulant treatment. Stroke 1991; 22:571–6.

153. Hylek EM, Heiman H, Skates SJ, et al. Acetaminophen and other risk factors for excessive warfarin anticoagulation. JAMA 1998; 279:657–62.

154. Crowther MA, Julian J, McCarty D, et al. Treatment of warfarin-associated coagulopathy with oral vitamin K: a randomised controlled trial. Lancet 2000; 356:1551–3.

155. Makris M, Watson HG. The management of coumarin-induced over-anticoagulation. Br J Haematol 2001; 114:271–80.

156. Penning-van Beest FJA, Rosendaal FR, Grobbee DE, van Meegan E, Stricker BHC. Course of the International Normalized Radio in response to oral vitamin K_1 in patients overanticoagulated with phenprocoumon. Br Haematol 1999; 104:241–5.

157. Llewellyn CA, Hewitt PE, Knight RS, et al. Possible transmission of variant Creutzfeldt–Jakob disease by blood transfusion. Lancet 2004; 363:417–21.

158. Wollowitz S. Fundamentals of the psoralen-based Helinx technology for inactivation of infectious pathogens and leukocytes in platelets and plasma. Semin Hematol 2001; 38(Suppl 11):4–11.

159. Hambleton J, Wages D, Radu-Radulescu L, et al. Pharmacokinetic study of FFP photochemically treated with amotosalen (S-59) and UV light compared to FFP in healthy volunteers anticoagulated with warfarin. Transfusion 2002; 42:1302–7.

160. Butler AC, Tait RC. Management of oral anticoagulant-induced intracranial haemorrhage. Blood Rev 1998; 12:35–44.

161. Butler AC, Tait RC. Restarting anticoagulation in prosthetic heart valve patients after intracranial haemorrhage: a 2–year follow-up. Br J Haematol 1998; 103:1064–6.

162. Wijdicks EFM, Schievink WI, Brown RD, Mullany CJ. The dilemma of discontinuation of anticoagulation therapy for patients with intracranial hemorrhage and mechanical heart valves. Neurosurgery 1998; 42:769–73.

163. Sharma R, Gorbien MJ. Angiodysplasia and lower gastrointestinal tract bleeding in elderly patients. Arch Intern Med 1995; 155:807–12.

164. Warkentin TE, Moore JC, Anand SS, Lonn EM, Morgan DG. Gastrointestinal bleeding, angiodysplasia, cardiovascular disease and acquired von Willebrand syndrome. Transfus Med Rev 2003; 17:272–86.

165. Blich M, Fruchter O, Edelstein S, Edoute Y. Somatostatin therapy ameliorates chronic and refractory gastrointestinal bleeding caused by diffuse angiodysplasia in a patient on anticoagulation therapy. Scand J Gastroenterol 2003; 38:801–3.

166. Lafata JE, Martin SA, Kaatz S, Ward RE. The cost-effectiveness of different management strategies for patients on chronic warfarin therapy. J Gen Intern Med 2000; 15:31–7.

167. Rosengart TK. Anticoagulation self-testing after heart valve replacement. J Heart Valve Dis 2001; 11(Suppl 1)S61–5.

168. Rose P. Audit of anticoagulant therapy. J Clin Pathol 1996; 40:5–9.

169. Fitzmaurice DA, Machin SJ, on behalf of the British Society of Haematology Task Force for Haemostasis and Thrombosis. Recommendations for patients undertaking self management of oral anticoagulation. BMJ 2001; 323:985–9.

170. Halhuber C. Quick test self-determination by patients. Adequate long-term anticoagulation can often only be performed with great difficulty. Fortschr Med 1988; 106:615–17.

171. Bernardo A, Halhuber C, Horstkotte D. Home prothrombin time estimation. In: Butchart EG, Bodnar E, eds. Current issues in heart valve disease: thrombosis, embolism and bleeding. London: ICR Publishers, 1992: 325–30.

172. Lucas FV, Duncan A, Jay R, et al. A novel whole blood capillary technique for measuring the prothrombin time. Am J Clin Pathol 1987; 88:442–6.

173. White R, McCurdy SY, von Marensdorff H, Woodruff DE, Leftgoff PA. Home prothrombin time monitoring after the initiation of warfarin therapy. Ann Intern Med 1989; 111:730–6.

174. Ansell JE, Holden A, Knapic N. Patient self-management of oral anticoagulation guided by capillary (fingerstick) whole-blood prothrombin times. Arch Intern Med 1989; 149:2509–11.

175. White RH, McKittrick T, Hutchinson R, Twitchell J. Temporary discontinuation of warfarin therapy: changes in the international normalized ratio. Ann Intern Med 1995; 122:40–2.

176. Jacobson AK. Patient self-management of oral anticoagulant therapy: an international update. J Thromb Thrombolys 1998; 5:S25–8.

177. Taborski VWE, Wittstamm FJ, Bernado A. Cost-effectiveness of self-management anticoagulant therapy in Germany. Semin Thromb Haemost 1999; 25:103–7.

178. Körtke H, Gohlke-Bärwolf C, Heik SCW, Horstkotte D. Empfehlungen zum INR – Selbstmanagement bei oraler Antikoagulation. Z Kardiol 1998; 87:983–5.

179. Bernardo A, Völler H. Leitlinien 'Gerinnungsselbstmanagement'. Medizinische Wochenzeitschrift 2001; 126:346–51.

180. Ansell JE, Hughes R. Evolving models of warfarin management: anticoagulation clinics, patient self-monitoring, and patient self-management. Am Heart J 1996; 132:1095–1100.

181. Hasenkam JM, Knudsen L, Kimose HH, et al. Practicability of patient self-testing of oral anticoagulant therapy by the International Normalized Ratio (INR) using a portable whole blood monitor. A pilot investigation. Thromb Res 1997; 85:77–82.

182. Beyth RJ, Quinn L, Landefeld CS. A multicomponent intervention to prevent major bleeding complications in older patients receiving warfarin. A randomised controlled trial. Ann Intern Med 2000; 133:687–95.

183. Sawicki PT. A structured teaching and self-management program for patients receiving oral anticoagulation: a randomised controlled trial. JAMA 1999; 281:145–50.

184. Gadisseur AP, Breuking-Engbers WG, van der Meer FJ, et al. Comparison of the quality of oral anticoagulant therapy through patient self-management of oral anticoagulation. Arch Intern Med 2003; 163:2639–46.

185. Körtke H, Körfer R. International normalized ratio self-management after mechanical heart valve replacement: is an early start advantageous? Ann Thorac Surg 2001; 72:44–8.

186. Horstkotte D, Piper C, Wiemer M. Optimal frequency of patient monitoring and intensity of oral anticoagulation therapy in valvular heart disease. J Thromb Thrombolys 1998; 5:19–24.

187. Engelberger L, Carrel T, Schaff HV, Kennard ED, Holubkov R. Differences in heart valve procedures between North American and European centres: a report from the Artificial Valve Endocarditis Reduction Trial (AVERT). J Heart Valve Dis 2001; 10:562–71.

188. Moake JL, Turner NA, Stathopoulos NA, Nolasko L, Hellums JD. Shear-induced platelet aggregation can be mediated by vWF released from platelets, as well as by exogenous large or unusually large vWF multimers, requires adenosine diphosphate, and is resistant to aspirin. Blood 1988; 71:1366–74.

189. Harker LA, Hanson SR, Kirkman TR. Experimental arterial thromboembolism in baboons: mechanisms, quantitation and pharmacologic prevention. J Clin Invest 1979; 64:559–69.

190. The PEP Trial Investigators. Prevention of pulmonary embolism

and deep vein thrombosis with low dose aspirin: Pulmonary Embolism Prevention (PEP) trial. Lancet 2000; 355:1295–302.

191. Hart RG, Benavente O, McBride R, Pearce LA. Antithrombotic therapy to prevent stroke in patients with atrial fibrillation: A meta-analysis. Ann Intern Med 1999; 131:492–501.

192. Butchart EG. Rationalising antithrombotic management for patients with prosthetic heart valves. J Heart Valve Dis 1995; 4:106–13.

193. Da Silva MS, Sobel M. Anticoagulants: to bleed or not to bleed, that is the question. Semin Vasc Surg 2002; 15:256–67.

194. Hurlen M, Abdelnoor M, Smith P, Erikssen J, Arnesen H. Warfarin, aspirin, or both after myocardial infarction. N Engl J Med 2002; 347 969–74.

195. Antithrombotic Trialists' Collaboration. Collaborative meta-analysis of randomised trials of antiplatelet therapy for prevention of death, myocardial infarction, and stroke in high risk patients. BMJ 2002; 324:71–86.

196. Kelly JP, Kaufman DW, Jurgelon JM, et al. Risk of aspirin-associated major upper-gastrointestinal bleeding with enteric-coated or buffered product. Lancet 1996; 348:1413–16.

197. Hart RG, Pearce LA. In vivo antithrombotic effect of aspirin: dose versus nongastrointestinal bleeding. Stroke 1993; 24:138–9.

198. He J, Whelton PK, Vu B, Klag MJ. Aspirin and risk of hemorrhagic stroke: a meta-analysis of randomised controlled trials. JAMA 1998; 238:1930–5.

199. FitzGerald GA. Dipyridamole. N Engl J Med 1987; 316:1247–57.

200. Bult H, Fret HR, Jordaens FH, Herman AG. Dipyridamole potentiates platelet inhibition by nitric oxide. Thromb Haemost 1991; 66:343–49.

201. Fuster V, Israel DH. Platelet inhibitor drugs after prosthetic heart valve replacement. In: Butchart EG, Bodnar E, eds. Current issues in heart valve disease: thrombosis, embolism and bleeding. London: ICR Publishers, 1992: 247–62.

202. European Stroke Prevention Study 2. Efficacy and safety data. J Neurol Sci 1997; 151(Suppl):S1–77.

203. Forbes CD. Secondary stroke prevention with low-dose aspirin, sustained release dipyridamole alone and in combination. ESPS Investigators. European Stroke Prevention Study. Thromb Res 1998; 92:S1–6.

204. Pouleur H, Buyse M. Effects of dipyridamole in combination with anticoagulant therapy on survival and thromboembolic events in patients with prosthetic heart valves. A meta-analysis of the randomized trials. J Thorac Cardiovasc Surg 1995; 110:463–72.

205. Chesebro J, Fuster V, Elveback LR. Trial of combined warfarin plus dipyridamole or aspirin therapy in prosthetic heart valve replacement: danger of aspirin compared with dipyridamole. Am J Cardiol 1983; 51:1537–41.

206. Leonardi-Bee J, Bath PMW, Bousser MG, et al. Dipyridamole for preventing recurrent ischemic stroke and other vascular events. Stroke 2005; 36:162–8.

207. CAPRIE Steering Committee. A randomised, blinded, trial of clopidogrel versus aspirin in patients at risk of ischaemic events (CAPRIE). Lancet 1996; 348:1329–39.

208. Altman R, Boullon F, Rouvier J, de la Fuente L, Favaloro R. Aspirin

and prophylaxis of thromboembolic complications in patients with substitute heart valves. J Thorac Cardiovasc Surg 1976; 72:127–9.

209. Dale J, Myhre E, Storstein O, Stormorken H, Efskind L. Prevention of arterial thromboembolism with acetylsalicylic acid. A controlled clinical study in patients with aortic ball valves. Am Heart J 1977; 94:101–11.

210. Turpie AG, Gent M, Laupacis A, et al. A comparison of aspirin with placebo in patients treated with warfarin after heart valve replacement. N Engl J Med 1993; 329:524–9.

211. Cappelleri JC, Fiore LD, Brophy MT, Deykin D, Lau J. Efficacy and safety of combined anticoagulant and antiplatelet therapy versus anticoagulant monotherapy after mechanical heart valve replacement: a meta-analysis. Am Heart J 1995; 130:547–52.

212. Sullivan JM, Harken DE, Gorlin R. Pharmacologic control of thromboembolic complications of cardiac valve replacement. N Engl J Med 1971; 284:1391–4.

213. Dale J, Myhre E, Loew D. Bleeding during acetylsalicylic acid and anticoagulant therapy in patients with reduced platelet reactivity after aortic valve replacement. Am Heart J 1980; 99:746–52.

214. Taylor TN, Davis PH, Torner JC, et al. Lifetime cost of stroke in the United States. Stroke 1996; 27:1459–66.

215. Massel D, Little SH. Risks and benefits of adding anti-platelet therapy to warfarin among patients with prosthetic heart valves: a meta-analysis. J Am Coll Cardiol 2001; 37:569–78.

216. Meschengieser S, Fondevila C, Frontroth J, et al. Low-intensity oral anticoagulation plus low-dose aspirin versus high-intensity oral anticoagulation alone: a randomized trial in patients with mechanical prosthetic heart valves. J Thorac Cardiovasc Surg 1997; 113:910–16.

217. Rumack CM, Guggenheim MA, Rumack BH, et al. Neonatal intracranial hemorrhage and maternal use of aspirin. Obstet Gynecol 1981; 58:52–6S.

218. Stuart MJ, Gross SJ, Elrad H, Graeber JE. Effects of acetylsalicylic acid ingestion on maternal and neonatal hemostasis. N Engl J Med 1982; 307:909–12.

219. Chesebro JH, Fuster V. Valvular heart disease and prosthetic valves. In: Verstraete M, Fuster V, Topol EJ, eds. Cardiovascular thrombosis. Philadelphia: Lippincott-Raven, 1998: 365–94.

220. Sambola A, Tomos P, Angel J, et al. Therapeutic strategies after stent placement in chronic anticoagulated patients: effectiveness and safety in daily clinical practice. Eur Heart J 2005; 26(Suppl):A2233.

221. Fiore LD, Brophy MT, Lopez A, et al. The bleeding time response to aspirin; identifying the hyperresponder. Am J Clin Pathol 1990; 94:292–6.

222. Hansson L, Zanchetti A, Carruthers SG, et al. Effects of intensive blood-pressure lowering and low-dose aspirin in patients with hypertension: principal results of the Hypertension Optimal Treatment (HOT) randomised trial. Lancet 1998; 351:1755–62.

223. Hart RG, Pearce LA, McBride R, Rothbart RM, Asinger RW. Factors associated with ischemic stroke during aspirin therapy in atrial fibrillation. Analysis of 2012 participants in the SPAF I-III clinical trials. Stroke 1999; 30:1223–9.

224. Meade TW, Brennan PJ. Determination of who may derive most benefit from aspirin in primary prevention: subgroup results from a randomised controlled trial. BMJ 2000; 321:13–17.

9

Investigation and management of recurrent embolism

Alec Vahanian, Olivier Nallet and Eric G Butchart

Introduction

Embolism remains one of the most important causes of morbidity and mortality in patients who have undergone prosthetic valve replacement. Cerebral or peripheral emboli, which may present during the early or late follow-up period, may also have important prognostic implications.

More specifically, we shall deal here with the predictors and management of patients who present embolic complications after prosthetic valve replacement.

Definitions and mechanisms

Embolism, as defined by the American Association for Thoracic Surgery and the Society of Thoracic Surgeons, comprises all embolic events that occur after the postoperative period, in the absence of ongoing infection.[1] Most cases of embolic events after prosthetic valve replacement are prosthesis-related. However, embolism may also be due to other cardiac causes, such as those originating from the left atrium, in particular the left atrial appendage, or the left ventricle, as well as extracardiac causes.[2] Most embolic complications are cerebral in location and it is important to remember that in the general population ischaemic strokes are of non-cardiac origin in around 75–80% of cases. After prosthetic valve replacement, this proportion naturally decreases; however, this does not mean that all the other potential mechanisms of ischaemic stroke, such as atheroma of the aorta, the supra-aortic vessels and even the small intracranial vessels, do not still also play a role.[3] The relative proportion of ischaemic stroke of arterial origin is variable and increases with the presence of cerebral vascular risk factors, as is the case in elderly patients with aortic stenosis, who represent a large proportion of the patient population currently undergoing valve replacement.[4]

Incidence and predictors

The incidence of the embolic complications, in particular cerebral vascular events, recorded after valve replacement depends greatly on the population studied as regards the prevalence of stroke risk factors and the type of prosthesis used, in addition to the regimen of antithrombotic management.[5] Furthermore, the methodology used is of crucial importance as regards the length of follow-up, the quality of data collection, which can be prospective or retrospective, as well as more or less detailed: i.e. if a simple questionnaire is used, the incidence will be lower than with clinical examination at the outpatient clinic, which will in turn be lower than with cerebral imaging. Cerebral embolism may well be asymptomatic in patients with valve prosthesis,[6] as shown by the AREVA study, where computed tomography (CT) showed an incidence of asymptomatic cerebral events as high as 46% when systematically performed postoperatively and 1 year after aortic valve replacement.[7] These factors explain why reported thromboembolic rates may vary from 0 to 7.5% per year.

The occurrence of thromboembolism after prosthetic valve replacement is multifactorial, being related to the prosthesis, the patient and the quality of anticoagulation.[3,8]

Prosthesis-related factors

Embolism is more frequent after mitral than after aortic valve replacement.[9–15] The difference in incidence between aortic combined with mitral valve replacement and mitral valve replacement alone is not significant. As would be expected, embolic complications occur less frequently with contemporary valves, such as bileaflet or disc prosthesis, than with first-generation mechanical prosthesis (ball valves).[9] Furthermore, bioprostheses and homografts are less thrombogenic than mechanical prostheses.[16–19]

Patient-related factors

The most important predictor of recurring embolism is a previous history of embolism. Atrial fibrillation and congestive heart failure also significantly increase the risk of embolism, regardless of the prosthesis. Cardiovascular risk factors, such as older age primarily, but also diabetes, hypertension and smoking, increase the risk of cerebral events. Beyond clinical examination, the widespread use of echocardiography provides important data for the stratification of embolic risk. Dilatation of left atrium[20] and left ventricular systolic dysfunction, as well as the presence of dense spontaneous echo contrast in the left atrium,[21–23] are all strong predictors of embolic risk.[24–26] More recently, the prognostic value of small strands on the prosthesis has been emphasised.[24,25] Finally, the embolic risk is higher within 3 months of valve replacement, which justifies the use of anticoagulation for biological valves during this period. For mechanical prostheses, the time of increased risk extends to the end of the first postoperative year.[8,9]

Anticoagulation-related factors

The quality of anticoagulation has a strong bearing on the incidence of embolism.[9,12–14,27] In a given patient, embolic complications are more frequent when variations in the level of anticoagulation occur, such as during a postoperative period.[9,24] They are also more frequent in patients in whom the level of anticoagulation is highly variable for a long period of time.[8,27]

Diagnostic strategy

Clinical evaluation and echocardiography are the cornerstones of diagnostic strategy.[28]

Clinical evaluation

Clinical evaluation is always the first step in diagnosis; it relies upon medical history, physical elimination, electrocardiography (ECG), X-ray and conventional blood testing. Medical history provides the information required to evaluate the quality of anticoagulation in the months leading up to the embolism as well as at the time of its occurrence. This is usually done by looking for recent changes in the level of anticoagulation due to possible drug interactions or changes in diet. Further research into the patient's history may also reveal cardiovascular risk factors. Physical examination looks for changes in the auscultatory signs of the prosthesis or the appearance of a regurgitant murmur as well as signs of heart failure. The disappearance of the click characteristic of mechanical valves upon cardiac auscultation is the fastest diagnostic clue to acute and massive valve thrombosis.[28] In conjunction, physical examination can reveal other clinical signs that may point towards another aetiology for stroke such as a cervical murmur. Finally, the presence of bacterial endocarditis will be systematically excluded on the basis of clinical findings, blood cultures and echocardiographic findings.

Echocardiography

Echocardiography should be systematically performed as soon as possible after an embolic event. Transthoracic echocardiography is the first step and it evaluates the size of the left atrium and the left ventricular function. The presence of obstructive prosthetic thrombosis can be detected through abnormalities in the movement of the mobile elements of the prosthetic valve, an increase in transprosthetic gradient as compared to reported values in the literature for this type of prosthesis and, more importantly, to the patient's previously reported values. In practice, however, if it is not occlusive, prosthetic thrombosis is seldom diagnosed by transthoracic echocardiography. On the other hand, this method is the best way to detect left ventricular thrombosis.

Transoesophageal echocardiography is the reference method in echocardiography. It should always be performed, except in cases where emergency surgery is required due to occlusive thrombosis diagnosed through transthoracic echocardiography and poor haemodynamic condition.[24,29,30] It should be clearly established whether or not the thrombosis is obstructive; in addition, its length

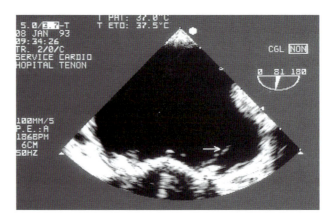

Figure 9.1
Strands on a mitral prosthesis. Transoesophageal view of a bileaflet mitral prosthesis (bileaflet). Small strands can be seen in the left atrial aspect of the prosthesis annulus.

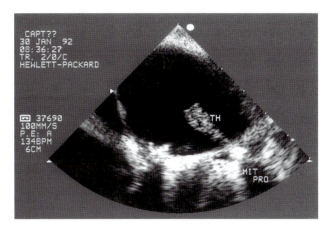

Figure 9.2
Non-occlusive thrombosis of a mitral prosthesis. Transoesophageal view of a mechanical (bileaflet) mitral prosthesis (MIT PRO). The cusps are in open position and a large non-obstructive thrombus can be seen (TH).

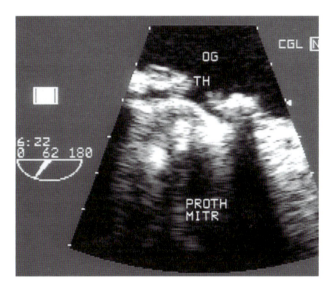

Figure 9.3
Occlusive thrombosis of a mitral prosthesis. Transoesophageal view of a mechanical mitral prosthesis. An occlusive thrombosis (TH) can be seen on both aspects of the valve: left atrium (OG) and ventricle (PROTH MITR).

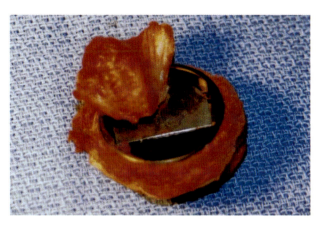

Figure 9.4
Occlusive thrombosis of a mitral prosthesis. A large thrombus impeding the movement of the leaflets of a mitral prosthesis can be seen.

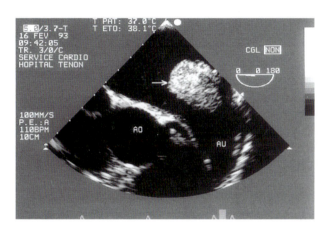

Figure 9.5
Thrombosis of the left atrial appendage. Transoesophageal view. A large thrombus is located in the left atrial appendage (arrow). AO = aorta, AU = left atrial appendage.

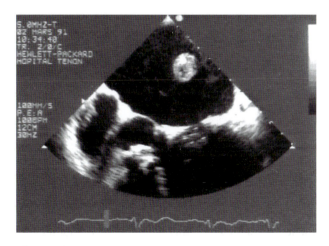

Figure 9.6
Thrombosis of the left atrium. Transoesophageal view. A ball thrombus can be seen floating in the atrial cavity.

and mobility should be precisely defined.[31] Valve thrombosis should be differentiated from a pannus, which is denser. This distinction is often difficult in practice, even more so because pannus and thrombosis can often be found in the same patient.[32] Non-obstructive prosthetic thrombosis should also be differentiated from strands or vegetations (Figures 9.1–9.4). On top of the presence of thrombosis, transoesophageal echocardiographic examination should also evaluate the movement of the leaflets or of the disc and look for abnormal regurgitation, the presence of thrombosis in the left atrium or the left atrial appendage (Figures 9.5

and 9.6), as well as the presence of spontaneous echo contrast in the left atrium.[33,34] Finally, transoesophageal examination should also search for non-cardiac causes of embolism such as atheroma of the aorta or patent foramen ovale with aneurysm of the interatrial septum.

Other evaluations

Fluoroscopy is a useful adjunct to echocardiography when occlusive fibrinolysis is suspected. It is a simple examination that is non-invasive; however, interpretation is subject to error and to inter-observer variability. The angle of opening and closing of the disc or leaflets will be measured and compared with normal values and previous recordings in the same patient. The negative and positive predictive values of fluoroscopic examination are superior to that of transthoracic echocardiography. When both examinations are concurrent with the diagnosis of occlusive prosthetic thrombosis, this hypothesis is consistently confirmed by transoesophageal examination.[28,35]

Specific organ-orientated examinations may be necessary according to the location of the embolic complication. Cerebral imaging using CT, or magnetic resonance imaging (MRI), should be performed in the case of a cerebral vascular accident in order to exclude intracerebral haemorrhage and to evaluate the size of the cerebral infarction. Doppler examination of the carotid arteries should also be performed in elderly patients and/or in the presence of a cervical murmur. Coronary or peripheral angiography is indicated in cases with myocardial infarction or embolism in the limbs. Finally, blood tests for prothrombotic factors should also be performed as part of a thrombophilia screen.[8]

Treatment strategy

The treatment strategy chosen will depend on whether or not prosthetic valve thrombosis, and more specifically obstructive thrombosis, is present.

Patients with obstructive thrombosis

In cases of suspected acute left-sided valve thrombosis, the patient should be transferred as soon as possible to a tertiary heart centre after intravenous injection of a bolus of heparin followed by continuous perfusion.

The two major therapeutic options available are surgery (valve replacement) or medical treatment with heparin and/or thrombolytics. The treatment strategy needs to be individualised according to several parameters: cause of valve thrombosis, clinical status, bleeding risk and presence of co-morbidity.[36] The choice of the best treatment is still controversial.[37]

Urgent valve replacement[38] should be considered in critically ill patients with valve thrombosis, without serious co-morbidities, and with easy access to surgery.[12–14,39] The type of valve substitute to be used for reoperation is dependent on the circumstances. Patients who have a mechanical prosthesis could receive another mechanical prosthesis if the long-term quality of anticoagulation was adequate. However, a bioprosthetic valve replacement could be recommended in patients who receive a highly variable level of anticoagulation or in those with contraindications for anticoagulation, such as cerebral complications.

Fibrinolysis could be performed in critically ill patients (pulmonary oedema, hypotension) with serious co-morbidities or if surgery is not urgently available and the patient cannot be transferred.[40–43] In such cases, if no contraindications are present, these patients should be treated with intravenous rtPA (recombinant tissue plasminogen activator) or SK (streptokinase). If neither of these are available, urokinase can be used. Oral anticoagulation should be resumed as soon as clinical status is stable and heparin continued until the INR (international normalised ratio) is within the therapeutic range for a mechanical valve, which is between 3.0 and 3.5 in the mitral position and between 2.5 and 3.0 in the aortic position.[9,12–14,39] Aspirin 100 mg should be added.[12,13]

Serial echocardiographic studies should be performed, and repeated infusions of thrombolytic therapy could be administered if complete resolution of prosthetic valve thrombus is not achieved.

Patients in whom acute discontinuation of oral anticoagulation or recent inadequate anticoagulation is considered the most likely cause for valve thrombosis represent a special subset. In the absence of haemodynamic compromise, a short treatment course of unfractionated heparin can be initiated under close echocardiographic monitoring. In patients with good initial results as demonstrated by clinical improvement, as well as a decrease in gradient on echocardiography, treatment should be continued until resolution of obstruction. If this strategy is not successful within 12–24 hours, an operation should be carried out, whereas fibrinolysis can be given to patients with contraindication for surgery.

Patients without obstructive valve thrombosis

When non-obstructive thrombosis is present, or even if thrombosis cannot be demonstrated, the diagnosis of prosthesis-related complications is highly probable if no other cause of thrombosis, such as intracardiac embolism or carotid stenosis, can be found.

The treatment armamentarium comprises antithrombotic agents, surgery and treatment of the cardiovascular risk factors.

The antithrombotic treatment will vary according to whether or not anticoagulation is adequate at the time of the embolic complications.

If the anticoagulation is not sufficient, intravenous unfractionated heparin should be given while the dose of oral anticoagulation is increased until the target INR level is achieved. If the patient did not receive aspirin in addition to anticoagulation, a dose of aspirin of 80–100 mg/day should be given. Clopidogrel could be used as an alternative or an additional treatment; however, this cannot be recommended without further evaluation.

If the anticoagulation is adequate, it should be continued and aspirin should be added if not previously given. It should be noted that the recommendation to add aspirin is based on the extrapolation of data showing a favourable effect on embolism, firstly, in the general population, then in patients with valve prostheses and no embolic events who were given aspirin 100 mg/day or sometimes a higher dose.[44–49] However , it should be acknowledged that even if these recommendations do not rely on strong evidence-based data, it is common practice to use aspirin as adjunctive therapy in patients who have had embolic complications; thus, the performance of a randomised trial to further prove its efficacy is unlikely.

The superiority of aspirin over other antiplatelet agents in such situations has not been proven. Dypiridamole may be preferred because of equivalent efficacy with a lower rate of bleeding.[50–53] However, despite these findings, dypiridamole is seldom used in practice in this indication, mostly due to poor digestive tolerance.

Finally, it is recommended that patients with bioprosthetic valves who have a history of systemic embolism should be treated with long-term oral anticoagulation. The INR intensity and duration are undetermined. The general consensus is to treat with oral anticoagulation between 3 and 12 months, with dose sufficient to prolong the INR at 2.5. These recommendations, however, are not based on published series.[9,12–14,39]

Surgery is indicated in cases of recurrent embolic episodes despite adequate anticoagulation and control of stroke risk factors. It could also be considered in the case of a large non-obstructive thrombus (>1 cm) that fails to regress with optimal anticoagulation. The indication for surgery should be discussed on an individual basis after the careful assessment of the risk-to-benefit ratio.[9,12–14,39] In addition, specific surgical treatment, such as embolectomy in the limbs, may be necessary according to the clinical situation.

After a cerebral event, there is no consensus on the indication or the timing of surgery. In cases with obstructive thrombosis, the haemodynamic condition is the leading factor in the decision to operate early, whereas in other cases the consensus is to wait a few weeks whenever possible.

Finally, in the rare cases of patients presenting early with acute myocardial infarction, percutaneous coronary intervention is preferable to fibrinolysis.

Particular situations of patients who have presented with a stroke

What treatment strategy to use with patients who present with a stroke still remains controversial and should take into account the balance between the risk of recurrence of embolism on the one hand, and the risk of cerebral haemorrhage on the other: the risk of occurrence is higher during the first 2 weeks, at around 1% per day, whereas the risk of haemorrhage ranges from 0 to 24%.[54–57]

In patients with mechanical valve prostheses, anticoagulation can be restarted immediately when the initial CT scan – which is performed within 24–48 hours of stroke – does not indicate haemorrhage and shows that the embolic stroke is of small to moderate size. On the other hand, anticoagulation is contraindicated in cases of haemorrhage, or large cerebral infarction, also indicated by the level of the clinical deficit, disturbances of consciousness, or finally by the presence of uncontrolled systemic hypertension. In these latter cases, anticoagulation is usually postponed for at least 5 days. This delay allows time to perform another CT scan to exclude haemorrhagic transformation. During this period, heparin therapy is usually recommended at a therapeutic range of 1.5–2 times the control. Here again, the recommendations are not evidence-based but result from expert consensus.[58–60]

After the acute phase

Patients who have a thromboembolic complication after valve replacement are at high risk of recurrence; therefore, all necessary measures should be taken to minimise the thromboembolic and haemorrhagic risk.

Clinical follow-up should be performed together with systematic transoesophageal echocardiography, usually repeated 1 week after the initial episode. Thereafter, in the absence of complications, regular follow-up transthoracic echocardiographic examinations are recommended twice a year.

Anticoagulation should be optimised. The most appropriate monitoring technique must be chosen according to local facilities, e.g. general physician, cardiologist, or anticoagulation clinic. When the necessary facilities are available, self-assessment methods improve the event-free survival and are cost-effective.[61] The recommended level of anticoagulation should be adapted to the individual risk of the patient.[12–14,39,61,62] Better control is, in the first instance, preferable to increasing the target INR. Antiplatelet agents are usually recommended after weighing up the individual risk-to-benefit ratio.[8,12–14,39,44] This combined antithrombotic treatment is of particular interest for patients with concomitant arterial disease.

Control of modifiable risk factors for embolism is mandatory and should be systematically performed. In cases of recent atrial fibrillation, electric counter shock should be considered in the absence of prosthetic or cardiac thrombosis. Hypertension, diabetes and dislipidaemia should be treated. It is of the utmost importance that the patient stops smoking.[63–66]

As well as these important measures, a very thorough education of the patient is paramount in preventing further embolism. This should include education on the choice of the most adequate target INR, measures for adaptation of dose, regular monitoring, and also possible drug or alimentary interactions. This education should concern both the patient and his physician.

Conclusion

The management of patients with valve prosthesis who present with embolic complications is often difficult and requires a close interdisciplinary collaboration. In the future, improvement will result from the performance of trials assessing the efficacy of the combination of antiplatelet agents and oral anticoagulant, as well as the evaluation of new antithrombotic agents such as direct antithrombins[67] or new antiplatelet agents. However, above all, the key factor in decreasing embolism remains to better educate the patient.

References

1. Edmunds LH Jr, Clark RE, Cohn LH, et al. Guidelines for reporting morbidity and mortality after cardiac valvular operations. The American Association for Thoracic Surgery. Committee for Standardizing Definitions of Prosthetic Heart Valve Morbidity. Ann Thorac Surg 1996; 62(3):932–5.
2. Cerebral Embolism Task Force. Cardiogenic brain embolism. Arch Neurol 1986; 43(1):71–84.
3. Butchart EG, Moreno de la Santa P, Rooney SJ, Lewis PA. Arterial risk factors and ischemic cerebrovascular events after aortic valve replacement. J Heart Valve Dis 1995; 4(1):1–8.
4. Iung B, Baron G, Butchart EG, et al. A prospective survey of patients with valvular heart disease in Europe: the Euro Heart Survey on Valvular Heart Disease. Eur Heart J 2003; 24(13):1231–43.
5. Grunkemeier GL, Starr A, Rahimtoola SH. Prosthetic heart valve performance: long-term follow-up. Curr Probl Cardiol 1992; 17(6):329–406.
6. Kempster PA, Gerraty RP, Gates PC. Asymptomatic cerebral infarction in patients with chronic atrial fibrillation. Stroke 1988; 19(8):955–7.
7. Acar J, Iung B, Boissel JP, et al. AREVA: multicenter randomized comparison of low-dose versus standard-dose anticoagulation in patients with mechanical prosthetic heart valves. Circulation 1996; 94(9):2107–12.
8. Butchart EG, Ionescu A, Payne N, et al. A new scoring system to determine thromboembolic risk after heart valve replacement. Circulation 2003; 108(Suppl 1):II68–74.
9. Butchart EG. Prosthetic heart valves. In: Verstraete M, Fuster V, Topol EJ, eds. Cardiovascular thrombosis, 2nd edn. Philadelphia: Lippincott-Raven, 1998: 399–418.
10. Cannegieter SC, Rosendaal FR, Wintzen AR, et al. Optimal oral anticoagulant therapy in patients with mechanical heart valves. N Engl J Med 1995; 333(1):11–17.
11. Baudet EM, Puel V, McBride JT, et al. Long-term results of valve replacement with the St. Jude Medical prosthesis. J Thorac Cardiovasc Surg 1995; 109(5):858–70.
12. ACC/AHA guidelines for the management of patients with valvular heart disease. A report of the American College of Cardiology/American Heart Association. Task Force on Practice Guidelines (Committee on Management of Patients with Valvular Heart Disease). J Am Coll Cardiol 1998; 32(5):1486–588.
13. Gohlke-Bärwolf C, Acar J, Oakley C, et al. Guidelines for the prevention of thromboembolic events in valvular heart disease. Eur Heart J 1995; 16(10):1320–30.
14. Stein PD, Alpert JS, Bussey HI, Dalen JE, Turpie AG. Antithrombotic therapy in patients with mechanical and biological heart valves. Chest 2001; 119(1 Suppl):220S-7S.
15. Casselman FP, Bots ML, Van Lommel W, et al. Repeated thromboembolic and bleeding events after mechanical aortic valve replacement. Ann Thorac Surg 2001; 71(4):1172–80.
16. Puvimanasinghe JP, Steyerberg EW, Takkenberg JJ, et al. Prognosis after aortic valve replacement with a bioprosthesis: predictions based on meta-analysis and microsimulation. Circulation 2001; 103(11):1535–41.
17. Khan SS, Trento A, DeRobertis M, et al. Twenty-year comparison of tissue and mechanical valve replacement. J Thorac Cardiovasc Surg 2001; 122(2):257–69.
18. Hammermeister K, Sethi GK, Henderson WG, et al. Outcomes 15 years after valve replacement with a mechanical versus a bioprosthetic valve: final report of the Veterans Affairs randomized trial. J Am Coll Cardiol 2000; 36(4):1152–8.
19. Grunkemeier GL, Li HH, Naftel DC, Starr A, Rahimtoola SH. Long-term performance of heart valve prostheses. Curr Probl Cardiol 2000; 25(2):73–156.
20. Burchfiel CM, Hammermeister KE, Krause-Steinrauf H, et al. Left atrial dimension and risk of systemic embolism in patients with a prosthetic heart valve. Department of Veterans Affairs Cooperative Study on Valvular Heart Disease. J Am Coll Cardiol 1990; 15(1):32–41.
21. Leung DY, Black IW, Cranney GB, Hopkins AP, Walsh WF. Prognostic implications of left atrial spontaneous echo contrast in nonvalvular atrial fibrillation. J Am Coll Cardiol 1994; 24(3):755–62.
22. Ozkan M, Kaymaz C, Kirma C, et al. Predictors of left atrial thrombus and spontaneous echo contrast in rheumatic valve disease before and after mitral valve replacement. Am J Cardiol 1998; 82(9):1066–70.
23. Agmon Y, Khandheria BK, Gentile F, Seward JB. Echocardiographic assessment of the left atrial appendage. J Am Coll Cardiol 1999; 34(7):1867–77.
24. Iung B, Cormier B, Dadez E, et al. Small abnormal echos after mitral valve replacement with bileaflet mechanical prostheses: predisposing factors and effect on thromboembolism. J Heart Valve Dis 1993; 2(3):259–66.

25. Freedberg RS, Goodkin GM, Perez JL, Tunick PA, Kronzon I. Valve strands are strongly associated with systemic embolization: a transesophageal echocardiographic study. J Am Coll Cardiol 1995; 26(7):1709–12.

26. Orsinelli DA, Pearson AC. Detection of prosthetic valve strands by transesophageal echocardiography: clinical significance in patients with suspected cardiac source of embolism. J Am Coll Cardiol 1995; 26(7):1713–18.

27. Butchart EG, Payne N, Li HH, et al. Better anticoagulation control improves survival after valve replacement. J Thorac Cardiovasc Surg 2002; 123(4):715–23.

28. Ledain LD, Ohayon JP, Colle JP, et al. Acute thrombotic obstruction with disc valve prostheses: diagnostic considerations and fibrinolytic treatment. J Am Coll Cardiol 1986; 7(4):743–51.

29. Malergue MC, Temkine J, Slama M, et al. [Value of early systematic postoperative transesophageal echocardiography in mitral valve replacements. A prospective study of 50 patients]. Arch Mal Coeur Vaiss 1992; 85(9):1299–304 [in French].

30. Shiran A, Weissman NJ, Merdler A, et al. Transesophageal echocardiographic findings in patients with nonobstructed prosthetic valves and suspected cardiac source of embolism. Am J Cardiol 2001; 88(12):1441–4, A8–9.

31. Gueret P, Vignon P, Fournier P, et al. Transesophageal echocardiography for the diagnosis and management of nonobstructive fibrinolysis of mechanical mitral valve prosthesis. Circulation 1995; 91(1):103–10.

32. Barbetseas J, Nagueh SF, Pitsavos C, et al. Differentiating thrombus from pannus formation in obstructed mechanical prosthetic valves: an evaluation of clinical, transthoracic and transesophageal echocardiographic parameters. J Am Coll Cardiol 1998; 32(5):1410–17.

33. Barbetseas J, Pitsavos C, Aggeli C, et al. Comparison of frequency of left atrial thrombus in patients with mechanical prosthetic cardiac valves and stroke versus transient ischemic attacks. Am J Cardiol 1997; 80(4):526–8.

34. Alton ME, Pasierski TJ, Orsinelli DA, Eaton GM, Pearson AC. Comparison of transthoracic and transesophageal echocardiography in evaluation of 47 Starr-Edwards prosthetic valves. J Am Coll Cardiol 1992; 20(7):1503–11.

35. Montorsi P, De Bernardi F, Muratori M, Cavoretto D, Pepi M. Role of cine-fluoroscopy, transthoracic, and transesophageal echocardiography in patients with suspected prosthetic heart valve fibrinolysis. Am J Cardiol 2000; 85(1):58–64.

36. Hering D, Piper C, Horstkotte D. Management of prosthetic valve fibrinolysis. Eur Heart J 2001; Suppl 3:Q22–6.

37. Lengyel M, Fuster V, Keltai M, et al. Guidelines for management of left-sided prosthetic valve thrombosis: a role for thrombolytic therapy. Consensus Conference on Prosthetic Valve Thrombosis. J Am Coll Cardiol 1997; 30(6):1521–6.

38. Martinell J, Jimenez A, Rabago G, et al. Mechanical cardiac valve thrombosis. Is thrombectomy justified? Circulation 1991; 84(5 Suppl):III70–5.

39. Salem DN, Stein PD, Al-Ahmad A, et al. Antithrombotic therapy in valvular heart disease – native and prosthetic: the Seventh ACCP Conference on Antithrombotic and Thrombolytic Therapy. Chest 2004; 126(3 Suppl):457S-82S.

40. Roudaut R, Lafitte S, Roudaut MF, et al. Fibrinolysis of mechanical prosthetic valve thrombosis: a single-center study of 127 cases. J Am Coll Cardiol 2003; 41(4):653–8.

41. Lengyel M, Vandor L. The role of thrombolysis in the management of left-sided prosthetic valve thrombosis: a study of 85 cases diagnosed by transesophageal echocardiography. J Heart Valve Dis 2001; 10(5):636–49.

42. Gupta D, Kothari SS, Bahl VK, et al. Thrombolytic therapy for prosthetic valve thrombosis: short- and long-term results. Am Heart J 2000; 140(6):906–16.

43. Jost CM, Yancy CW Jr, Ring WS. Combined thrombolytic therapy for prosthetic mitral valve thrombosis. Ann Thorac Surg 1993; 55(1):159–61.

44. Massel D, Little SH. Risks and benefits of adding anti-platelet therapy to warfarin among patients with prosthetic heart valves: a meta-analysis. J Am Coll Cardiol 2001; 37(2):569–78.

45. Altman R, Boullon F, Rouvier J, et al. Aspirin and prophylaxis of thromboembolic complications in patients with substitute heart valves. J Thorac Cardiovasc Surg 1976; 72(1):127–9.

46. Turpie AG, Gent M, Laupacis A, et al. A comparison of aspirin with placebo in patients treated with warfarin after heart-valve replacement. N Engl J Med 1993; 329(8):524–9.

47. Dale J, Myhre E, Storstein O, Stormorken H, Efskind L. Prevention of arterial thromboembolism with acetylsalicylic acid. A controlled clinical study in patients with aortic ball valves. Am Heart J 1977; 94(1):101–11.

48. Dale J, Myhre E, Loew D. Bleeding during acetylsalicylic acid and anticoagulant therapy in patients with reduced platelet reactivity after aortic valve replacement. Am Heart J 1980; 99(6):746–52.

49. Laffort P, Roudaut R, Roques X, et al. Early and long-term (one-year) effects of the association of aspirin and oral anticoagulant on thrombi and morbidity after replacement of the mitral valve with the St. Jude medical prosthesis: a clinical and transesophageal echocardiographic study. J Am Coll Cardiol 2000; 35(3):739–46.

50. Forbes CD. Secondary stroke prevention with low-dose aspirin, sustained release dipyridamole alone and in combination. ESPS Investigators. European Stroke Prevention Study. Thromb Res 1998; 92(1 Suppl 1):S1–6.

51. Pouleur H, Buyse M. Effects of dipyridamole in combination with anticoagulant therapy on survival and thromboembolic events in patients with prosthetic heart valves. A meta-analysis of the randomized trials. J Thorac Cardiovasc Surg 1995; 110(2):463–72.

52. Chesebro JH, Fuster V, Elveback LR, et al. Trial of combined warfarin plus dipyridamole or aspirin therapy in prosthetic heart valve replacement: danger of aspirin compared with dipyridamole. Am J Cardiol 1983; 51(9):1537–41.

53. British National Formulary (BNF) 47. London: British Medical Association and the Royal Pharmaceutical Society of Great Britain, 2004.

54. Sacco RL, Foulkes MA, Mohr JP, et al. Determinants of early recurrence of cerebral infarction. The Stroke Data Bank. Stroke 1989; 20(8):983–9.

55. Yasaka M, Yamaguchi T, Oita J, et al. Clinical features of recurrent embolization in acute cardioembolic stroke. Stroke 1993; 24(11):1681–5.

56. Hart RG, Putnam C. Hemorrhagic transformation of cardioembolic stroke. Stroke 1989; 20(8):1117.

57. Rothrock JF, Dittrich HC, McAllen S, Taft BJ, Lyden PD. Acute anticoagulation following cardioembolic stroke. Stroke 1989; 20(6):730–4.

58. Immediate anticoagulation of embolic stroke: a randomized trial. Cerebral Embolism Study Group. Stroke 1983; 14(5):668–76.

59. Cerebral Embolism Study Group. Immediate anticoagulation of embolic stroke: brain hemorrhage and management options. Stroke 1984; 15(5):779–89.

60. Albers GW, Amarenco P, Easton JD, Sacco RL, Teal P. Antithrombotic and thrombolytic therapy for ischemic stroke. Chest 2001; 119(1 Suppl):300S-20S.

61. Taborski U, Wittstamm FJ, Bernardo A. Cost-effectiveness of self-managed anticoagulant therapy in Germany. Semin Thromb Hemost 1999; 25(1):103–7.

62. Vink R, Kraaijenhagen RA, Hutten BA, et al. The optimal intensity of vitamin K antagonists in patients with mechanical heart valves: a meta-analysis. J Am Coll Cardiol 2003; 42(12):2042–8.

63. Ambrose JA, Barua RS. The pathophysiology of cigarette smoking and cardiovascular disease: an update. J Am Coll Cardiol 2004; 43(10):1731–7.

64. Sacco RL. Reducing the risk of stroke in diabetes: what have we learned that is new? Diabetes Obes Metab 2002; 4(Suppl 1):S27–34.

65. Lowe GD. Dental disease, coronary heart disease and stroke, and inflammatory markers: what are the associations, and what do they mean? Circulation 2004; 109(9):1076–8.

66. European Stroke Prevention Study 2. Efficacy and safety data. J Neurol Sci 1997; 151 (Suppl):S1–77.

67. Sinnaeve PR, Van de Werf FJ. Will oral antithrombin agents replace warfarin? Heart 2004; 90(8):827–8.

10

Management of valve thrombosis

Christa Gohlke-Bärwolf, Alec Vahanian and Eric G Butchart

Thrombosis of a mechanical heart valve (Figure 10.1A,B) is an infrequent, yet potentially life-threatening complication, requiring immediate diagnosis and treatment. It occurs more frequently in patients who are non-compliant with anticoagulation therapy, but may occur in the presence of adequate anticoagulation. The clinical presentation may vary from insidious dyspnoea, to pulmonary oedema and cardiogenic shock. Cerebral or peripheral emboli, or acute myocardial infarction due to a coronary emboli (Figure 10.2A,B) may be the initial signs of valve thrombosis,[1–5] but the most frequent clinical finding is congestive heart failure, in about half of the patients.[6]

Definition and incidence

Valve thrombosis can occur acutely or chronically and can be obstructive or non-obstructive. Obstructive thrombosis is defined as a thrombotic occlusion of the prosthetic valve, leading to severe haemodynamic compromise.[7] It may begin as non-obstructive thrombosis, which is defined as a thrombus located usually at the sewing ring of the prosthesis without significantly increased gradient across the prosthesis or interference with movement of the occluder. Peripheral or cerebral emboli are usually the only symptoms of this type of valve thrombosis, but many instances of

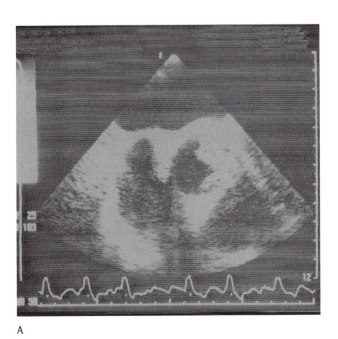

A

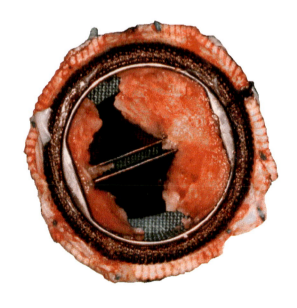

B

Figure 10.1
(A) Large thrombus on an aortic bileaflet prosthesis on transoesophageal echocardiography. (B) The surgically removed prosthesis from the same patient.

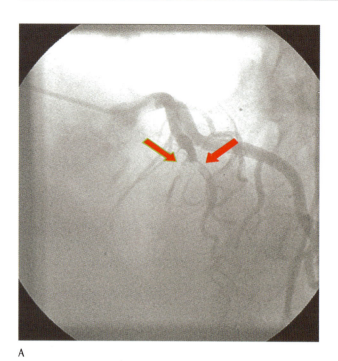

A

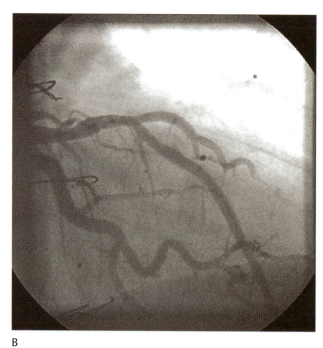

B

Figure 10.2

Coronary embolus in a 65-year-old patient 5 days after discontinuation of oral anticoagulation and treatment with LMWH (low molecular weight heparin) once daily. (A) Coronary angiography showing a saddle embolus (arrows) in the left anterior descending artery and diagonal branch. (B) Both arteries are patent after intracoronary fibrinolysis and glycoprotein IIb/IIIa antagonist (abciximab). The gradient across the aortic valve was moderately increased, but no thrombus was detected on transoesophageal echocardiography (TOE).

non-obstructive thrombosis are chronic and silent, and are only discovered on routine transoesophageal echocardiography (TOE). In one series, the pathological substrate of obstruction was pannus ingrowth in 11% of patients and a combination of pannus and thrombus in 12%.[5] Yet, in a recent study pannus was present in 63%.[8] Pannus can occur as early as 1 month after the initial surgery, but more often occurs late after operation (later than 30 days in 80%[6]).

Valve thrombosis is often associated with subtherapeutic or interrupted anticoagulation,[2,9] although other patient- and prosthesis-related factors may also play a role. The most frequent reasons for deliberate interruption of the anticoagulation leading to valve thrombosis are elective non-cardiac surgery or severe bleeding events,[2,5] underlining the importance of careful anticoagulation management in these situations. The risk is determined by the inherent thrombogenicity and haemodynamic performance of the prosthesis, patient-related risk factors and other trigger factors such as infection, as well as by the quality of anticoagulation management,[10–13] and the time interval from the operation. Other risk factors for valve thrombosis are prior stroke, atrial fibrillation and impaired left ventricular function (see Chapter 8).

With improvements in valve design and materials, the incidence of valve thrombosis has decreased over the last 20 years, but it has not been eliminated. The true incidence of the different types of valve thrombosis is not known, as many cases are not diagnosed or are only diagnosed post-mortem. In one study,[5] up to two-thirds of cases were fatal and most were diagnosed only after death. Diagnosis depends on the type of investigations performed, particularly if TOE has been included in the work-up.

Among anticoagulated patients with mechanical valves, the incidence varies from zero to 0.5% per year in the aortic position and from zero to 3% per year in the mitral position.[14] The incidence of valve thrombosis in the tricuspid position is markedly higher.[15] Thrombosis of a bileaflet prosthetic valve often leads more rapidly to severe haemodynamic impairment than thrombosis of a tilting disc valve, because even quite small amounts of thrombus at the hinge points can immobilise both leaflets.[16] Also, initial immobilisation of only one leaflet may go unnoticed until the clot impairs the movement of the other leaflet.

Bioprostheses and homografts are less thrombogenic than mechanical prostheses, but bioprosthetic valve thrombosis may occur in the absence of anticoagulation.[16–19] Predisposing factors include low cardiac output, chordal preservation in mitral valve replacement and structural valve deterioration.[16,20,21] Porcine valves appear to be more thrombogenic than pericardial valves,[14] with

Table 10.1 Diagnostic procedures for valve thrombosis

History
- High index of suspicion in any patient with inadequate or interrupted anticoagulation, sudden onset or insidious occurrence of dyspnoea
- Cerebral or peripheral embolism

Auscultation (Figure 10.3)
- Loss of or muffled valve clicks
- New stenotic or insufficiency murmur

Echocardiography
- Transthoracic: increased valve gradient
- Transoesophageal: thrombus, location, size, mobility

Cinefluoroscopy
- Mobility of valve leaflets

rates of thrombosis without anticoagulation similar to those of mechanical valves with anticoagulation.[14,22] Thrombosis of an aortic valve homograft has been reported in association with lupus anticoagulant antibodies.[23]

Diagnosis

Acute obstructive valve thrombosis requires urgent diagnosis (Table 10.1, Figure 10.3). It should be considered as a strong probability after valve replacement in all patients who present in pulmonary oedema or shock, particularly if there is loss of or muffled mechanical valve clicks on auscultation or new stenosis or regurgitant murmurs.

In a recent study, the delay between first symptoms to hospitalisation ranged from 1 to 45 days.[24] The diagnosis is confirmed by transthoracic and/or transoesophageal Doppler echocardiography.[25,26] Transthoracic Doppler echocardiography is useful in the assessment of gradients across the valve, detection of regurgitation and occasionally demonstration of thrombus, whereas TOE is important for delineation of size, structure and location of thrombi. TOE is also helpful in assessing the risk of thrombolytic therapy. A thrombus area <0.8 cm^2 identifies patients at lower risk for complications from thrombolysis.[27] Non-obstructive valve thrombosis is usually discovered only on TOE, often during investigation of an embolic event (see below).

Cinefluoroscopy permits rapid assessment of leaflet motion of valves with radio-opaque occluders[28,29] and is complementary to echocardiography. In bileaflet valves it is possible to determine if one or both leaflets are involved and to what degree. Finally, multidetector-row computed tomography (CT) is helpful in the detection of pannus formation.[30]

Therapy

Basically, two therapeutic options are available:

- valve surgery
- medical therapy with heparin or thrombolysis.

Which treatment strategy is preferred depends on several factors: the presence or absence of obstruction; the location of the prosthesis; the acuteness of the thrombosis; the severity of clinical symptoms; the patient's age; and the co-morbidities. In addition, the degree of organisation of the

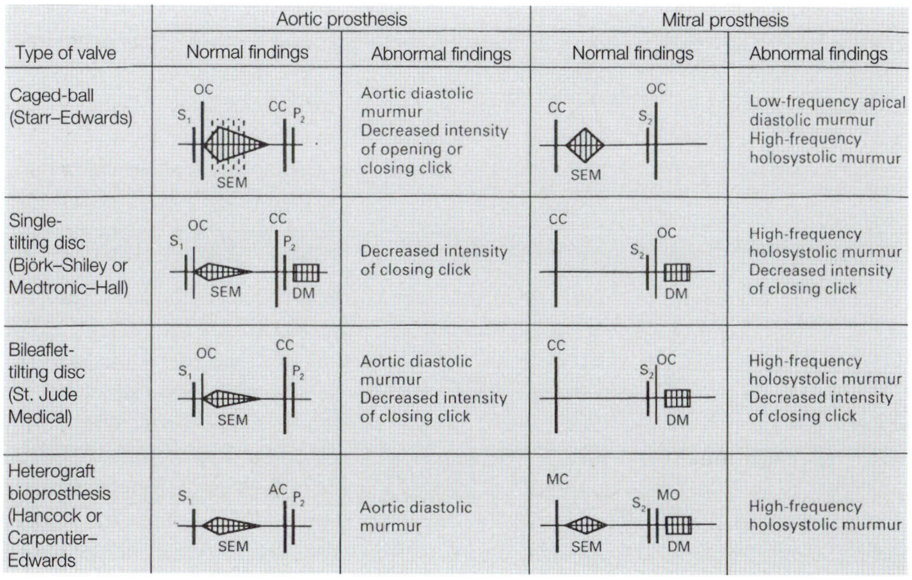

Figure 10.3
Auscultatory findings in normally and abnormally functioning prosthetic valves. OC = opening click, CC = closing click, SEM = systolic ejection murmur, DM = diastolic murmur, AC = aortic closure, MC = mitral valve closure, MO = mitral opening, S1 = first heart sound, S2 = second heart sound, P2 = pulmonic component of the second heart sound. Reproduced from Vongpatanasin W, Hillis LD, Lang RA. Prosthetic heart valves. New Engl J Med 1996; 335:407–16, with permission.

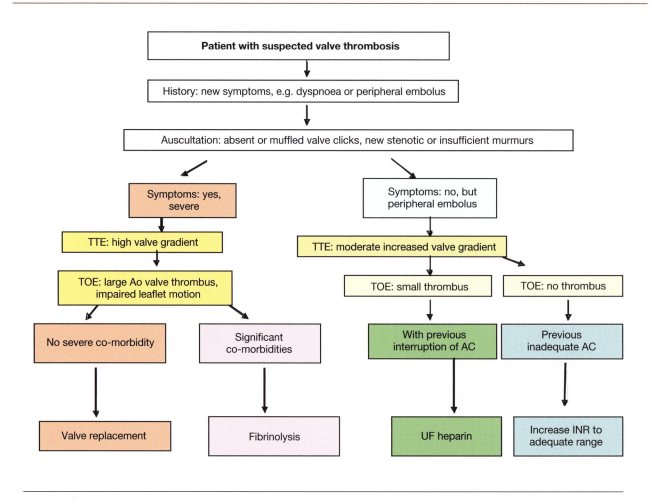

Figure 10.4
Management of valve thrombosis. INR = international normalised ratio, TOE = transoesophageal echocardiography, TTE = transthoracic echocardiography, UF = unfractionated, Ao = ascending aorta, AC = anticoagulation.

thrombus and the presence of pannus influence treatment. It is generally agreed that valve thrombosis in the right heart is best treated with fibrinolysis, because of the high success rate and low incidence of embolism.[31,32] The following recommendations therefore apply primarily to aortic and mitral valve thrombosis.

Patients with mitral valve thrombosis have a higher complication rate with thrombolysis than patients with aortic valve thrombosis.[27]

Management of obstructive valve thrombosis

If valve thrombosis is suspected, the patient should be transferred as soon as possible to a tertiary care heart cen-

tre after intravenous injection of a bolus of heparin (5000 units) followed by continuous heparin infusion. Thereafter, the choice of treatment strategy (Figure 10.4) depends on the factors mentioned above:

1. Urgent or emergency *valve replacement* should be considered in critically ill and symptomatic patients without serious co-morbidities, a large thrombus (area >1 cm^2), history of stroke or other emboli and readily available surgical treatment. Surgical thrombectomy is not often performed now because of high recurrence rates, as success of this procedure depends on good access to both sides of the prosthesis and secondly on the underlying cause of the valve thrombosis and whether it can be subsequently eliminated.[1] Video-assisted thrombectomy was used by Dürrleman et al[6] in 47% of patients treated surgically, particularly in cases of early postoperative valve thrombosis. Overall operative mortality was 9%, which is markedly higher in the video-assisted thrombectomy group. Surgical mortality depends on the clinical status of the patients and varies between 4.7% and 40%.[5,8] Ten-year actuarial survival after prosthetic valve thrombosis was 46% ± 10%.[6]

Patients with a mechanical prosthesis should receive another mechanical prosthesis, preferably of lower thrombogenicity, providing that the long-term quality of anticoagulation can be assured. Bioprosthetic valve replacement should be considered in patients with high variability of anticoagulation level or in those with contraindications to anticoagulation, for example due to recent intracranial haemorrhage.

2. *Fibrinolysis* is the treatment of choice in patients with tricuspid and pulmonary valve thrombosis.[31] It should also be performed in critically ill patients with serious co-morbidities (e.g. cancer or renal failure), small thrombi (thrombus area <0.6 cm²) or if surgery is not immediately available and the patient is haemodynamically compromised and cannot be transferred. Providing that there are no contraindications to fibrinolysis (e.g. recent major surgery, recent intracranial bleeding, large thrombi), these patients should be treated with intravenous recombinant tissue plasminogen activator (rtPA) (in total 100 mg should be administered; 10 mg immediate intravenous bolus followed by 90 mg infused over 90 minutes) or *streptokinase* (500 000 IU over 20 minutes, followed by 1.5 million IU infused over 10 hours). If both are unavailable, *urokinase* can be used in high dose (4500 IU/kg/h for 12 hours) without heparin, or low dose (2000 IU/kg/h) given with heparin for 24 hours. All suggested doses might need adjustment according to individual patient characteristics. Serial TOE studies should be performed, with repeated infusions of thrombolytic therapy if complete resolution of prosthetic valve thrombus is not achieved.

The overall initial success rate of fibrinolysis is 70–80%.[4,33–35] Fibrinolysis is less likely to be successful in chronic thrombosis or in the presence of pannus, and is associated with a risk of systemic embolism and recurrent thrombosis (both about 14–20%) and of death in about 5% of patients.[27] There is also a 5% risk of major bleeding. Success is less likely in mitral prostheses in comparison to aortic prostheses.[4,27] In multivariate analysis, two variables were independent predictors of complications with fibrinolysis: thrombus area by TOE (odds ratio (OR) of 2.41 per 1 cm² increment (confidence interval (CI) 1.12–5.19)) and prior history of stroke (OR = 4.55, CI 1.35–15.38).[27] A thrombus area of <0.8 cm² identifies patients at lower risk for complications from thrombolysis, irrespective of New York Heart Association (NYHA) functional class. Symptoms are also important predictors of outcome. Patients in NYHA classes III and IV had a death rate of 8.2 and 10.5% with thrombolysis versus 0% in patients in NYHA classes I and II.[27]

3. In haemodynamically stable patients with mild obstruction, in whom recent acute discontinuation of oral anticoagulation or inadequate anticoagulation is considered the most likely cause for valve thrombosis, a short treatment course of *intravenous unfractionated heparin*, as a bolus, followed by infusion, should be applied first, closely monitored by echocardiography and/or cinefluoroscopy.[28,31] In patients with a good initial response, treatment should be continued until full resolution of the obstruction. If heparin (with an activated partial thromboplastin time (aPTT) twice control value) is not successful within 12–24 hours, thrombolysis should be started. When fibrinogen level is above 0.5 g/L, unfractionated heparin infusion should be recommenced to obtain an aPTT 1.5–2 times the control value. In patients with no co-morbidities, unsuccessful treatment with heparin should be followed by valve surgery rather than fibrinolysis.

Oral anticoagulation should be resumed as soon as clinical status is stable and heparin continued until the international normalised ratio (INR) is within the therapeutic range for the mechanical valve and position (mitral valve 3.0–3.5, aortic valve 2.5–3.0).

Management of non-obstructive valve thrombosis

Initial treatment comprises optimisation of oral anticoagulation, if this was previously poorly controlled or subtherapeutic, together with intravenous heparin. Thereafter, treatment should be directed at underlying contributory factors, e.g. prothrombotic intracardiac conditions such as atrial fibrillation, dehydration and pulmonary infection. Factors related to the prosthesis itself, e.g. pannus or silver coating of the sewing ring in the case of the St. Jude Silzone valve,[36] may also be important contributors and necessitate reoperation.

In the case of a large non-obstructive thrombus (>1 cm) that fails to regress with heparin and optimum oral anticoagulation, consideration should be given to reoperation or thrombolysis in patients with co-morbidities at high risk for surgery.

When the thrombus regresses with conservative treatment and correction of contributory factors, future management must be carefully considered. If the anticoagulation was previously adequate, it should be continued with a higher target INR. However, an INR of more than 4.0 has not been shown to be of benefit, and considerably increases the risk of bleeding.

On the basis of one randomised study in patients without non-obstructive valve thrombosis, some have recommended aspirin in this setting in addition to oral anticoagulants at a therapeutic INR of about 3.5.[31,37,38] However, the risk of bleeding is further increased with the combination of oral anticoagulants and aspirin. There may be theoretical advantages to the use of dipyridamole, which inhibits platelet deposition on artificial surfaces, and is less likely to increase bleeding risk, but as yet there are no studies available in patients with non-obstructive valve thrombosis to recommend this combination (see Chapter 8).

It is also important to treat other risk factors which may increase thrombogenicity, such as smoking, hypercholesterolaemia, hypertension, diabetes and other acquired forms of hypercoagulability.

Summary and recommendations

- The most frequent cause of prosthetic valve thrombosis is inadequate or interrupted oral anticoagulation. Overall mortality and morbidity with prosthetic valve thrombosis is still high, irrespective of form of treatment.
- Maintaining therapeutic levels of anticoagulation adjusted to the patient's individual risk factor profile is essential and requires intensive patient and physician education about anticoagulation, risk factors for thromboembolism and their treatment as well as signs of impending valve thrombosis.
- Patients and physicians should be instructed about the possibility of valve thrombosis in any patient with a prosthetic valve, whether mechanical or bioprosthesis.
- Valve thrombosis should be suspected in any patient who presents with a recent increase in shortness of breath or fatigue, systemic or cerebral emboli.
- If valve thrombosis is suspected because of absent or muffled valve sounds on auscultation, the diagnosis should be confirmed by transthoracic and transoesophageal echocardiography. Cinefluoroscopy is of additional value.
- Patients with suspected or proven valve thrombosis should be immediately transferred to a cardiac centre with cardiac surgical facilities after being given 5000 units of heparin intravenously, followed by continuous infusion of heparin.
- Urgent or emergency valve replacement is the treatment of choice for obstructive thrombosis of aortic or mitral prostheses in critically ill patients without serious co-morbidities.
- Thrombolysis should be preferred in critically ill patients with obstructive thrombosis of aortic or mitral prostheses unlikely to survive surgery because of serious co-morbidities and impaired general health status prior to developing valve thrombosis.
- Thrombolysis is the treatment of choice in patients with thrombosis of the tricuspid or pulmonary valve prosthesis.
- Thrombolysis is less likely to be successful in patients with obstructive thrombosis of mitral prostheses, in chronic thrombosis or in the presence of pannus.
- In haemodynamically stable patients with mild or no obstruction, in whom acute discontinuation or recent subtherapeutic anticoagulation is considered the most likely cause for valve thrombosis, a short course of intravenous heparin should be used first, closely monitored by echocardiography and/or cinefluoroscopy.

References

1. Martinell J, Jimenez A, Rabago G, et al. Mechanical cardiac valve fibrinolysis: is thrombectomy justified? Circulation 1991; 84(Suppl III):70–5.
2. Silber H, Khan SS, Matloff JM, et al. The St. Jude valve. Thrombolysis as the first line of therapy for cardiac valve thrombosis. Circulation 1993; 87:30–7.
3. Bollag L, Attenhofer Jost CH, Vogt PR, et al. Symptomatic mechanical heart valve thrombosis: high morbidity and mortality despite successful treatment options. Swiss Med Wkly 2001; 131:109–16.
4. Roudaut R, Lafitte S, Roudaut MF, et al. Fibrinolysis of mechanical prosthetic valve thrombosis: a single-center study of 127 cases. J Am Coll Cardiol 2003; 41:653–8.
5. Deviri E, Sareli P, Wisenbaugh T, Cronje SL. Obstruction of mechanical heart valve prostheses: clinical aspects and surgical management. J Am Coll Cardiol 1991; 17:646–50.
6. Dürrleman N, Pellerin M, Bouchard D, et al. Prosthetic valve thrombosis: twenty-year experience at the Montreal Heart Institute. J Thorac Cardiovasc Surg 2004; 127:1388–92
7. Edmunds LH Jr, Clark RE, Cohn LH, et al. Guidelines for reporting morbidity and mortality after cardiac valvular operations. Ad Hoc Liaison Committee for Standardizing Definitions of Prosthetic Heart Valve Morbidity of The American Association for Thoracic Surgery and The Society of Thoracic Surgeons. J Thorac Cardiovasc Surg 1996; 112:708–11.
8. Renzulli A, Onorati F, De Feo M, et al. Mechanical valve thrombosis: a tailored approach for a multiplex disease. J Heart Valve Dis 2004; 13(Suppl 1):S37–42.
9. Lengyel M, Fuster V, Keltai M, et al. Guidelines for management of left-sided prosthetic valve thrombosis: a role for thrombolytic therapy. Consensus Conference on Prosthetic Valve Thrombosis. J Am Coll Cardiol 1997; 30:1521–6.
10. Butchart EG, Ionescu A, Payne N, et al. A new scoring system to determine thromboembolic risk after heart valve replacement. Circulation 2003; 108(Suppl II):68–74.
11. Butchart EG, Payne N, Li HH, et al. Better anticoagulation control improves survival after valve replacement. J Thorac Cardiovasc Surg 2002; 123:715–23.
12. Butchart EG, Moreno de la Santa P, Rooney SJ, Lewis PA. The role of risk factors and trigger factors in cerebrovascular events after mitral valve replacement: implications for antithrombotic management. J Card Surg 1994; 9(Suppl):228–36.
13. Butchart EG. Fibrinogen and leukocyte activation – the keys to understanding prosthetic valve thrombosis? J Heart Valve Dis 1997; 6:9–16.
14. Grunkemeier GL, Li HH, Naftel DC, Starr A, Rahimtoola SH. Long-term performance of heart valve prostheses. Curr Probl Cardiol 2000; 25:73–156.
15. Edmunds LH Jr. Thromboembolic complications of current cardiac valvular prostheses. Ann Thorac Surg 1982; 34:96–106.

16. Butchart EG. Thrombogenicity, thrombosis and embolism. In: Butchart EG, Bodnar E, eds. Current issues in heart valve disease: thrombosis, embolism and bleeding. London: ICR Publishers, 1992: 172–205.

17. Edmond JJ, Greaves SC, French JK, et al. Thrombotic risk in patients with aortic bioprothesis. J Heart Valve Dis 2004; 13:525–8.

18. Oliver JM, Gallego P, Gonzalez A, et al. Bioprosthetic mitral valve thrombosis: clinical profile, transesophageal echocardiographic features, and follow-up after anticoagulant therapy. J Am Soc Echocardiogr 1996; 9:691–9.

19. Renzulli A, De Luca L, Caruso A, et al. Acute thrombosis of prosthetic valves: a multivariate analysis of the risk factors for a life-threatening event. Eur J Cardiothorac Surg 1992; 6:412–42.

20. Fasol R, Lakew F. Early failure of bioprosthesis by preserved mitral leaflets. Ann Thorac Surg 2000; 70:653–4.

21. Korkolis DP, Passik CS, Marshalko SJ, Koullias GJ. Early bioprosthetic mitral valve 'pseudostenosis' after complete preservation of the native mitral apparatus. Ann Thorac Surg 2002; 74: 1689–91.

22. Hammermeister K, Sethi GK, Henderson WG, et al. Outcomes 15 years after valve replacement with a mechanical valve versus a bioprosthetic valve: final report of the Veterans Affairs randomized trial. J Am Coll Cardiol 2000; 36:1152–8.

23. Unger P, Plein D, Pradier O, et al. Thrombosis of aortic valve homograft associated with lupus anticoagulant antibodies. Ann Thorac Surg 2004; 77:312–14.

24. Buttard P, Bonnefoy E, Chevalier P, et al. Mechanical cardiac valve thrombosis in patients in critical hemodynamic compromise. Eur J Cardiothorac Surg 1997; 11:710–13.

25. Barbetseas J, Nagueh SF, Pitsavos C, et al. Differentiating thrombus from pannus formation in obstructed mechanical prosthetic valves: an evaluation of clinical, transthoracic and transesophageal echocardiographic parameters. J Am Coll Cardiol 1998; 32:1410–17.

26. Shiran A, Weissman NJ, Merdler A, et al. Transesophageal echocardiographic findings in patients with nonobstructed prosthetic valves and suspected cardiac source of embolism. Am J Cardiol 2001; 88:1441–4.

27. Tong AT, Roudaut R, Özkan M, et al. Transesophageal echocardiography improves risk assessment of thrombolysis of prosthetic valve thrombosis: results of the international PRO-TEE registry. J Am Coll Cardiol 2004; 43:77–84.

28. Montorsi P, De Bernardi F, Muratori M, et al. Role of cinefluoroscopy, transthoracic, and transesophageal echocardiography in patients with suspected prosthetic heart valve fibrinolysis. Am J Cardiol 2000; 85:58–64.

29. Shapira Y, Herz I, Sagie A. Fluoroscopy of prosthetic heart valves: does it have a place in the echocardiography era? J Heart Valve Dis 2000; 9:594–9.

30. Teshima H, Hayashida N, Fukunaga S, et al. Usefulness of computed tomography scanner for detecting pannus formation. Ann Thorac Surg 2004; 77: 523–6.

31. Bonow RO, Carabello B, de Leon AC, et al. ACC/AHA Guidelines for the Management of Patients with Valvular Heart Disease. Executive Summary. A report of the American College of Cardiology/American Heart Association Task Force on Practice Guidelines (Committee on Management of Patients with Valvular Heart Disease). J Am Coll Cardiol 1998; 32:1486–588.

32. Peterffy A, Henze A, Savidge GF, Landon C, Björk VO. Late thrombosis of the Björk–Shiley tilting disc valve in the tricuspid position. Scand J Thorac Cardiovasc Surg 1980; 14:33–41.

33. Roudaut R, Labbé T, Lorient-Roudaut MF, et al. Mechanical cardiac valve thrombosis. Is fibrinolysis justified? Circulation 1992; 86(Suppl):II8–15.

34. Lengyel M, Vandor L. The role of thrombolysis in the management of left-sided prosthetic valve thrombosis: a study of 85 cases diagnosed by transesophageal echocardiography. J Heart Valve Dis 2001; 10:636–49.

35. Lengyel M. Management of prosthetic valve thrombosis. J Heart Valve Dis 2004; 13:329–34.

36. Ionescu A, Payne N, Fraser AG, et al. Incidence of embolism and paravalvular leak after St. Jude Silzone valve implantation. Heart 2003; 89:1055–61.

37. Turpie AG, Gent M, Laupacis A, et al. A comparison of aspirin with placebo in patients treated with warfarin after heart valve replacement. N Engl J Med 1993; 329:524–9.

38. Gohlke-Bärwolf C, Acar J, Oakley C, et al. Guidelines for the prevention of thromboembolic events in valvular heart disease. Eur Heart J 1995; 16:1320–30.

11

Haemolysis after valve surgery

Raffaele De Caterina and Manola Soccio

Although haemolysis is a relatively frequent complication of prosthetic valve implantation, only rarely does it become severe enough to cause anaemia, which may determine a choice of reintervention. The recognition and estimation of severity of haemolysis after valve implantation are important steps in the patient follow-up and the premise for a rational treatment.

Incidence

Because of the improvement in the haemodynamic profile and, to a lesser extent, because of the improvement in surgical techniques, the incidence of haemolysis after valve surgery in general has notably decreased throughout the years: estimated to be at 15% in 1975, it was reported to be 7% in 1983 and has probably further decreased more recently.[1] However, the frequency of haemolysis may depend on the accuracy by which it is searched for and on accurate investigation, and it may occur in up to one-half of patients with commonly used mechanical prostheses.[2] Haemolytic anaemia (or haemolysis severe enough to cause anaemia) is a rare consequence of haemolysis, being reported in less than 4% of cases presenting detectable haemolysis.[3]

Haemolysis has been shown to occur with variable incidence in the various valve models used. Biological prostheses usually feature a low degree of haemolysis: albeit modest, this may become clinically relevant in the presence of valve lesions, structural alterations of the haemodynamic profile, paraprosthetic leaks and calcifications.[4] The capacity of inducing haemolysis in bioprostheses seems mostly due to the presence of the sewing ring; indeed, the only prostheses in which no haemolysis has been demonstrated are stentless valves.[5] Recently, the presence of haemolysis has been demonstrated also after mitral repair and the use of rings for annuloplasty. Free tendinous chordae and loss of suture stitches are possible causes.[6] The haemolytic potential of bioprostheses is attributable to alterations of the valve haemodynamic profile induced by

structural changes, with the subsequent increase in turbulence.[1] Experiments on bioprostheses have shown that these structures are capable of generating modest flow turbulences, sufficient to cause haemolysis but not, usually, haemolytic anaemia if not accompanied by paraprosthetic leaks and valve dysfunctions. The absence of haemolysis only with stentless valves is probably attributable to a better haemodynamic profile of natural, non-artificially manipulated valves.

In mechanical prostheses, conversely, turbulences are common also in the presence of a normally functioning valve. This condition leads by itself to an increased risk of thrombosis on the one hand, and to haemolysis on the other. For these reasons, a modest degree of intravascular haemolysis is common among patients with even perfectly functioning valvular prostheses, being found in 40–85% of patients with such characteristics.[2,7–9]

The highest degree of haemolysis has been demonstrated for ball-and-cage Starr–Edwards valves, especially cloth-covered ones.[10,11] Bileaflet mechanical prostheses apparently cause a slightly higher degree of haemolysis than single-disc valves in a comparison of the St. Jude with the Medtronic Hall valve in a black population[2] and in a series of multiple valve types.[12] This is to some extent unexpected, considering the usually better haemodynamic profile of bileaflet valves. A possible explanation is the presence of a double hinge, which determines a higher reflow volume (from 4 to 15% of the antegrade flow, depending on the size of the valve, transvalvular gradient, cardiac rhythm and heart rate).[12,13] Considering the small magnitude of reported differences and the substantial uncertainty in these comparisons, it is doubtful that they should substantially influence practical use. The incidence and severity of haemolysis are higher in cases of double or multiple substitution.[2,5] Recently, the reported incidence has been 46% vs 24% on average for double- vs single-valve replacement.[5] In older reports, and for most prostheses, the aortic site entails the greater risk of haemolysis,[14–16] but this has not been confirmed in newer ones,[2,5] underscoring the relative importance of factors other than the central transvalvular shear stress – obviously higher in the passage through the aortic than the mitral orifice – imposed on red blood cells. Besides the number, site and type of valves, surgical factors are relevant in producing haemolysis. A paraprosthetic leak, defined as an abnormal reflow around the circumference of valve implantation,[17] is the most common cause of severe haemolysis in a patient with a valve prosthesis, independent of the type of valve and of the site of implantation. Infections are a frequent cause of leaks, and are responsible for 67% of substitutions in the aortic position and for 79% of substitutions in the mitral position.[18] Patients with Marfan's syndrome are more prone to develop leaks, probably because of the disarray of elastic fibres in the tissue around the implantation site.[19] It has also been reported that calcifications, because of the difficulty in sewing and the less stable support for the suture, are a frequent cause of leaks,[20] emphasising the importance of a proper decalcification of the annulus before proceeding to the implant. Leaks have also been associated with other technical factors, such as the use of single-filament and continuous sutures, as well as lesions produced by the suture thread at the sites of anchoring of the prosthesis.[21] Small paraprosthetic leaks usually cause haemolysis, but are less associated with infection than larger ones.[21]

Pathophysiology

The development of a chronic severe haemolytic anaemia in the first carriers of mechanical valves since 1964 led to an effort to shed light on the nature of the potentially severe disease associated with valve implantation.[22] Haemolysis is a condition of premature destruction of red blood cells (i.e. less than the average survival of about 120 days) that may occur either because intrinsically defective red blood cells are produced, or because causes of damage are present in the intravascular environment. Studies of erythrocyte survival using [51]chromium-labelled red blood cells confirmed that not only autologous red blood cells but also red blood cells from possibile donors had a reduced half-life in carriers of a prosthetic valve, indicating the presence of a cause extrinsic to the red blood cell itself.[23]

The mechanical trauma of red blood cells is the first cause of haemolysis in carriers of prosthetic valves. The main mechanism involved is flow turbulence produced by the passage of blood through the prosthesis, which causes excess shear stress on the cells themselves. All factors that increase turbulence increase the likelihood of haemolysis. The passage of part of the blood jet between the occluding leaflet and the hinge during the closure phase of a mechanical valve is a relevant and inevitable site of damage.[24] Conditions favouring red blood cell damage and predisposing the patient to the risk of a clinically relevant haemolysis are blood pressure variations, high transvalvular gradients, undersized prostheses, intrinsic red blood cell anomalies,

interactions with other foreign surfaces and unfavourable flow within the valve caused by specific features of the valve itself. Also a patient–prosthesis mismatch, i.e. an inappropriate dimensional choice of the valve, generating substantial transvalvular pressure gradients, can be a cause of intravascular haemolysis.[1,25]

The characteristic disc-like shape and the capability of modifying their shape are peculiar aspects of red blood cells that confer on them the possibility of repeated passage in the microvasculature, enabling them to perform their function of oxygen transport.[26] Red blood cell deformability is determined by three main components: cytoplasmic viscosity, membrane deformability and the surface/volume ratio.[27] This last factor accounts for the fact that globular red blood cells are more susceptible to haemolysis than normal disc-like cells. As a result of these properties, the red blood cell is capable of resisting low-intensity and short-duration stresses, ultimately returning to the original shape.[26] An irreversible cell damage occurs when cell tolerance limits are exceeded. It has been calculated that laminar shear stress induces haemolysis for intensities >1500–2500 dynes/cm^2. However, the concomitance of other conditions and the interaction of blood with abnormal foreign surfaces may make red blood cells more susceptible to shear stresses. Indeed, only 500 dynes/cm^2 are necessary to induce red blood cell damage in the case of turbulent flow, and even lower values are necessary in the case of a foreign body.[28,29] It should be noted that turbulent shear stresses in excess of 1200 dynes/cm^2 have been measured 11 mm downstream of the St. Jude Medical bileaflet valve in the aortic position,[28] and that similar values have also been reported in more modern valves such as the CarboMedics bileaflet valve, designed specifically to improve upon the design of the St. Jude Medical valve.[24,30]

The duration of exposure of red blood cells to increased shear stress is also important. It is likely that moderately increased shear stresses mostly cause the haemolysis of older red blood cells, which become more fragile compared with younger ones. It is conceivable that younger and younger red blood cells are haemolysed with a progressive increase in shear stress intensity and in the exposure time, without the existence of a real threshold.

As a consequence of membrane damage, a reduced mean red blood cell survival occurs.[26] One of the first biochemically demonstrable changes is the loss of asymmetry in the arrangement of cell membrane phospholipids. Normally, phosphatidylcholine is located in the outer membrane layer, whereas phosphatidylserine and phosphatidylethanolamine are in the inner layer; this asymmetry is ensured by the presence of specific membrane enzymes. The exposure of phosphatidylserine allows the recognition of red blood cells by macrophages and cells of the reticuloendothelial system, and is an important mechanism of cell removal in the extravascular spaces, mostly in the spleen and the liver.[31–33] The appearance of

Table 11.1 Laboratory criteria for the diagnosis of haemolytic anaemia

Test	Result	Conclusion
Haemoglobin	<13.8 g/dl in men; <12.4 g/dl in women	Criterion for the diagnosis of anaemia
Reticulocytes (%)	>2%	Sign of increased bone marrow production
Schistocytes	Present	Sign of red blood cell membrane lesion
Haptoglobin	Reduced	Due to haemoglobinuria, and indicates a rapid intravascular haemolysis
Plasma iron (transferrin)	Possibly reduced	Expression of increased turnover
LDH	Increased	Expression of red blood cell destruction

LDH = lactate dehydrogenase.

phosphatidylserine on the outer layer is also associated with numerous pathological phenomena in cells other than erythrocytes. For example, the asymmetrical distribution of the above-mentioned phospholipids is lost in activated platelets, with phosphatidylserine rendered available on the cell surface. This phenomenon has a role in the regulation of haemostatic events, such as the activation of the prothrombin complex. In red blood cells, the exposure of phosphatidylserine has a similar biological effect on haemostasis.[26] In peripheral blood smears the appearance of schistocytes, i.e. fragmented or deformed red blood cells, indicates an increased red blood cell fragility.

Haptoglobin is a glycoprotein synthesised by the liver that is able to bind haemoglobin after haemolysis, thus preventing – up to the saturation of its binding capacity – the appearance of haemoglobinuria. Haptoglobin has a half-life of about 4 days, but, when bound to haemoglobin, the resulting complex is removed from plasma within a few minutes. Hepatic reticuloendothelial cells catabolise both components of the complex. When haptoglobin catabolism exceeds its rate of synthesis, plasma levels decrease down to non-measurable levels. If the amount of haemoglobin in plasma exceeds haptoglobin-binding capacity, haemoglobin appears in the glomerular filtrate as dimers. Dimers are easily reabsorbed from cells in the proximal tubule that incorporate haem iron in ferritin and haemosiderin. When the load of filtered dimer exceeds the absorbing capacity of the proximal tubule, haemoglobin appears in the urine.

The presence of haemolysis does not necessarily result in anaemia, which only occurs when the rate of red blood cell destruction exceeds bone marrow regenerative capacity. Therefore, the appearance of anaemia in the presence of haemolysis usually indicates a severe degree of haemolysis and/or the concomitance of conditions (deficiency of iron, vitamin B_{12}, folates) that limit the bone marrow production reserve. In contrast to subclinical haemolysis, severe clinical haemolytic anaemia, diagnosed by haemoglobin levels <10 g/L and/or by transfusion requirements, is a quite rare phenomenon in carriers of prosthetic valves.

Diagnostic approach

The first approach to a patient with haemolysis and a valve prosthesis is an anamnestic evaluation that allows the identification of the type of valve implanted and the time since implantation (biological prostheses have a more limited duration than mechanical prostheses). History and laboratory investigations should rule out the possibility that haemolysis pre-dated valve surgery as a result of haemoglobinopathies or other causes intrinsic or extrinsic to red blood cells.[34,35] An echocardiogram will allow the recognition of a dysfunction of the prosthesis and the presence of significant paraprosthetic leaks. Laboratory data allow one to establish the possible presence of anaemia, to determine its severity and to evaluate the possible contribution of associated factors such as iron or folate deficiency as a result of increased loss or increased consumption. To diagnose and assess the severity of a haemolytic anaemia, the following laboratory tests need to be performed: haemoglobin levels; reticulocyte count; the demonstration of schistocytes on a smear; serum levels of lactic dehydrogenase (LDH), haptoglobin and iron (Table 11.1).

Criteria to diagnose intravascular haemolysis are serum LDH levels >460 U/L and at least two of the following four criteria:

- levels of haemoglobin <13.8 g/dl in men and <12.4 g/dl in women
- levels of haptoglobin <0.5 g/L
- reticulocyte count >2%
- presence of schistocytes in a peripheral blood smear.[2]

The need of multiple criteria in addition to LDH elevation is due to the relative non-specificity of LDH elevation as an indication of haemolysis.

The decrease in plasma levels of haptoglobin – despite being influenced by conditions of hepatic insufficiency – is an index of intravascular haemolysis, and sometimes reaches undetectable levels by common biochemical

Table 11.2 A classification of the intensity of haemolysis based on laboratory parameters

	Mild	Moderate	Severe
LDH	<500 U/L	>500 U/L	≥500 U/L
Haptoglobin	<0.5 g/L	absent	absent
Reticulocytes	<5%	>5%	≥5%
Schistocytes	<1%	>1%	≥1%

LDH = lactate dehydrogenase.

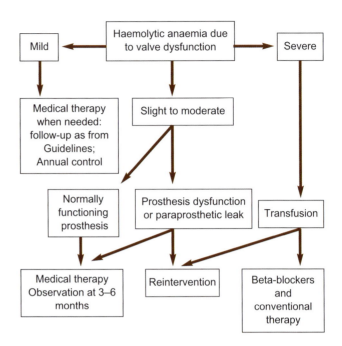

Figure 11.1
Therapeutic algorithm in carriers of cardiac valve prostheses with haemolytic anaemia.

methods. Reticulocytes are non-nucleated cells; they are direct precursors of mature red blood cells and their count is an index of the bone marrow haematopoietic activity.

The severity of haemolysis has been evaluated as mild for LDH values <500 U/L, with reduced haptoglobin, reticulocyte count <5% and <1% schistocytes; it is moderate or severe for values higher or much higher than those used to diagnose mild haemolysis, respectively (Table 11.2).[5] Again, one needs to remember that the absence of anaemia does not exclude the presence of a relevant haemolysis, as anaemia (to a certain degree) is compensated by an adequate erythropoiesis.[1]

Treatment

Treatment of haemolysis appears to be necessary only when it is severe enough to cause anaemia. Medical treatment is effective in most patients with haemolytic disease induced by cardiac valve prostheses. Treatment includes supplementation with iron in all those patients in whom a significant iron loss is evident, also in the absence of anaemia. Transfusions are necessary only in cases of severe anaemia that are refractory to treatment. In the presence of haemolytic anaemia not responsive to treatment with iron, the possibility of a concomitant folate deficiency has to be contemplated and, in this case, folate supplementation is also required.[1]

The use of beta-blockers appears to decrease the severity of haemolysis, probably because of the bradycardia and the negative inotropic effects, which together decrease transvalvular flow velocities and the associated shear stresses.[25] The use of beta-blockers needs therefore to be contemplated in patients with prosthetic valve-related haemolytic anaemia. For the same reasons, patients should be instructed to avoid strenuous exercise, which increases transvalvular shear stresses, although such a recommendation is based on common sense and not from properly conducted prospective trials.

Since 1989, when human recombinant erythropoietin was introduced for the treatment of anaemia in cases of terminal renal insufficiency, the use of this hormone in haemolytic anaemias induced by cardiac valve prostheses has also been contemplated.[36] Erythropoietin is a hormone that promotes the maturation of the erythroid series. It has been demonstrated that chronic administration of human recombinant erythropoietin causes an increased concentration of all progenitors of haematopoietic cells.[37,38] Some cases of erythropoietin treatment of haemolytic anaemias caused cardiac valve prostheses have been described, with favourable outcome.[36,39] The reduction in transfusion requirements in some treated patients has stimulated the use of erythropoietin, but its widespread use in this indication is today only justified in cases where endogenous erythropoietin production is inadequate.[36] Today, its use should probably be restricted to patients with severe haemolytic anaemia in whom repair surgery is contraindicated, or when transfusions need to be avoided or postponed.[36] However, it should be remarked that the risk of reoperation is most probably increased when endogenous red cell production is insufficient, and that a short-term trial with erythropoietin is probably warranted when insufficient bone marrow compensation is suspected, through the easy monitoring of reticulocyte count possible upon the administration of the recombinant hormone.

When haemolytic anaemia is severe and medical therapy is ineffective, a reintervention has to be considered:[40] this consists of the substitution of the prosthesis or in the correction of the paraprosthetic leak.

Although the operative risk of valve surgery is, in general, slowly but steadily declining, a reintervention for the substitution of a cardiac valve prosthesis is a serious clinical event. Early mortality for this operation is around 17.4 and 11% for substitutions of mechanical and biological prostheses, respectively.[41] A patient in stable clinical condition and without endocarditis can undergo a reoperation when necessary, after adequate clinical and instrumental evaluation, assuming that the increased operative risk compared with the first operation is acceptable. The indication for a reintervention has to be formulated also on the basis of symptoms, the state of left ventricular function and the type of prosthesis, considering the shorter duration of biological vs mechanical valves. In some cases, a paraprosthetic leak, an important cause of haemolysis, may be repaired without changing the valve. If haemolytic anaemia occurs in a patient with a Starr–Edwards valve, a replacement with a more modern valve type is warranted. When valve repair or substitution is not possible, the use of beta-blockers and other supportive measures are indicated (Figure 11.1).[25]

Conclusions

Haemolytic anaemia, albeit rare, needs to be kept in mind as one of the complications in patients with valve prostheses, exposing the patient to a considerable risk and most often underscoring a suboptimal condition of the prosthetic valve.

Although a subclinical intravascular haemolysis, as highlighted by the increase in LDH, reticulocytosis and the reduction of haptoglobin, can be demonstrated in most patients with normally functioning valve prostheses, severe cases of haemolytic anaemia are not common and, when present, suggest the presence of a paraprosthetic leak due to partial suture failure.[11] Carriers of a ball-and-cage prosthesis, or of multiple prostheses, have a higher incidence and a more severe haemolytic anaemia than patients with valves of more recent introduction and undergoing single-valve substitution.

Carriers of prosthetic valves and with haemolytic anaemia should be treated with iron and folates or with transfusions; those with a severe para-prosthetic leak or with intractable anaemia should be reoperated. In the presence of contraindications to a reintervention, beta-blockers, which may reduce the intensity of haemolysis, in association with iron and folate, should be considered. The possibility of adding erythropoietin is being evaluated. Experimental studies with erythropoietin have shown that its administration may decrease the severity of anaemia, thus reducing the need for reinterventions or transfusion requirements, but its use has still to be considered experimental.

References

1. Maraj R, Jacobs L, Ioli A, Kotler M. Evaluation of hemolysis in patients with prosthetic heart valves. Clin Cardiol 1998; 21: 387–92.
2. Skoularigis J, Essop R, Skudicky D, Middlemost S, Sareli P. Frequency and severity of intravascular hemolysis after left-sided cardiac valve replacement with Medtronic Hall and St. Jude medical prostheses, and influence of prosthetic type, position, size and number. Am J Cardiol 1993; 71:587–91.
3. Amidon TM, Chou TM, Rankin JS, Ports TA. Mitral and aortic paravalvular leaks with hemolytic anemia. Am Heart J 1993; 125:266–8.
4. Brown MR, Hasaniya NW, Dang CR. Hemolytic anemia secondary to a porcine mitral prosthetic valve leaflet dissection. Ann Thorac Surg 1995; 59:1573–4.
5. Mecozzi G, Milano D, De Carlo M, et al. Intravascular hemolysis in patients with new-generation prosthetic heart valves: a prospective study. J Thorac Cardiovasc Surg 2002; 123:550–6.
6. Cerfolio R, Orszulak T, Daly R, Schaff H. Reoperation for hemolytic anaemia complicating mitral valve repair. Eur J Cardiothorac Surg 1997; 11:479–84.
7. De Cesare W, Rath C, Hufnagel C. Hemolytic anemia of mechanical origin with aortic-valve prostheses. N Engl J Med 1965; 272:1045–50.
8. Lillehei C. Hemolysis and the St Jude medical valve. Eur J Cardiothorac Surg 1989; 3:90–1.
9. Birnbaum D, Laczkovics A, Heidt M, et al. Examination of hemolytic potential with the On-X(R) prosthetic heart valve. J Heart Valve Dis 2000; 9:142–5.
10. Rao K, Learoyd P, Rao R, Rajah S, Watson D. Chronic haemolysis after Lillehei–Kaster valve replacement. Comparison with the findings after Björk–Shiley and Starr–Edwards mitral valve replacement. Thorax 1980; 35:290–3.
11. Vongpatanasin W, Hillis L, Lange R. Prosthetic heart valves. N Engl J Med 1996; 335:407–16.
12. Ismeno G, Renzulli A, Carozza A, et al. Intravascular hemolysis after mitral and aortic valve replacement with different types of mechanical prostheses. Int J Cardiol 1999; 69:179–83.
13. Grigioni M, Daniele C, D'Avenio G, Barbaro V. The influence of the leaflets' curvature on the flow field in two bileaflet prosthetic heart valves. J Biomech 2001; 34:613–21.
14. Yacoub MH, Keeling DH. Chronic hemolysis following insertion of ball valve prostheses. Br Heart J 1968; 30:676–8.
15. Falk RH, Mackinnon J, Wainscoat J, Mellkin V, Bignell AHC. Intravascular hemolysis after valve replacement: comparative study between Starr–Edwards (ball valve) and Björk–Shiley (disk valve) prosthesis. Thorax 1979; 34:746–8.
16. Febres-Roman PR, Bourg WC, Crone RA, Davis RC, Williams TH. Chronic intravascular hemolysis after aortic valve replacement with Ionescu–Shiley Xenograft: comparative study with Björk–Shiley prosthesis. Am J Cardiol 1980; 46:735–8.
17. Kloster F. Diagnosis and management of complications of prosthetic heart valves. Am J Cardiol 1975; 35:872–85.
18. Jindani A, Neville E, Venn G, William B. Paraprosthetic leak: a complication of cardiac valve replacement. J Cardiovasc Surg 1991; 32:503–8.
19. Pyeritz R. Genetics and cardiovascular disease. In: Company WS, ed. Heart disease: a textbook of cardiovascular medicine, 5th edn. Philadelphia: WB Saunders, 1992: 1643.
20. Kastor JA, Buckley MJ, Sanders CA, Austen WG. Paravalvular leaks and hemolytic anemia following insertion of Starr–Edwards aortic and mitral valves. J Thorac Cardiovasc Surg 1968; 56:279–88.
21. Dhasmana J, Blackstone E, Kirklin J, Kouchoukos N. Factors associated with periprosthetic leakage following primary mitral valve replacement: with special consideration of the suture technique. Ann Thorac Surg 1983; 35:170–8.

22. Dameshek W, Roth S. Case records of the Massachusetts General Hospital – weekly clinicopathological exercises. Case 52. N Engl J Med 1964; 271:898.

23. Shulman L, Braunwald E, Rosenthal D. Affezioni ematologiche ed oncologiche e malattie cardiache. In: Braunwald E, ed. Malattie del cuore. Philadelphia: Piccin, 1998: 2505.

24. Ellis J, Wick T, Yoganathan A. Prosthesis-induced hemolysis: mechanisms and quantification of shear stress. J Heart Valve Dis 1998; 7:376–86.

25. Bettadapur MS, Griffin BP, Asher CR. Caring for patients with prosthetic heart valves. Cleve Clin J Med 2002; 69(1):75–87.

26. Kuypers FA. Red cell membrane damage. J Heart Valve Dis 1998; 7:387–95.

27. Mohandas N, Chasis J, Shohet S. The influence of membrane skeleton on red cell deformability, membrane material proprieties, and shape. Semin Hematol 1983; 20:225–42.

28. Yoganathan A, Wick T, Reul H. Influence of flow characteristics of prosthetic valves on thrombus formation. In: Butchart EG, Bodnar E, eds. Current issues in heart valve disease; thrombosis, embolism and bleeding. London: ICR Publishers; 1992: 123–47.

29. Sutera S, Joist J. Hematologic effects of turbulent blood flow. In: Butchart EG, Bodnar E, eds. Current issues in heart valve disease; thrombosis, embolism and bleeding. London: ICR Publishers; 1992: 149–59.

30. Sung H, Cape E, Yoganathan A. In vitro fluid dynamic evaluation of the CarboMedics bileaflet valve prosthesis in the aortic and mitral positions. J Heart Valve Dis 1994; 3:673–83.

31. Tanaka Y, Schroit A. Insertion of fluorescent phosphatidylserine into the plasma membrane of red blood cells: recognition by autologous macrophages. J Biol Chem 1983; 258:11335–43.

32. Schroit A, Madsen J, Tanaka Y. In vivo recognition and clearance of red blood cells containing phosphatidylserine in their plasma membranes. J Biol Chem 1985; 260:5131–8.

33. Connor J, Pak C, Schroit A. Exposure of phosphatidylserine in the outer leaflet of human red blood cells. Relationship to cell density, cell age, and clearance by mononuclear cells. J Biol Chem 1994; 269:2399–404.

34. Sgambati MT, Kon ND, Cruz JM. Mitral valve replacement in sickle cell disease. Clin Cardiol 1998; 21:602–3.

35. Sutton SW, Hunley EK, Duncan MA, Rodriguez R, Meyers TP. Sickle cell disease and aortic valve replacement: use of cardiopulmonary bypass, partial exchange transfusion, platelet sequestration, and continuous hemofiltration. Tex Heart Inst J 1999; 26:283–8.

36. Hirawat S, Lichtman S, Allen S. Recombinant human erythropoietin use in hemolytic anemia due to prosthetic heart valves: a promising treatment. Am J Hematol 2001; 66:224–6.

37. Krantz S, Jacobson L. Erythropoietin and the regulation of erythropoiesis. Chicago: University of Chicago Press, 1970.

38. Dessypris E, Graber S, Krantz S, Stone W. Effects of recombinant erythropoietin on the concentration and cycling status of human marrow hematopoietic progenitor cells in vivo. Blood 1988; 72:2060–2.

39. Shapira Y, Bairey O, Vatury M, et al. Erythropoietin can obviate the need for repeated heart valve replacement in high-risk patients with severe mechanical hemolytic anemia: case reports and literature review. J Heart Valve Dis 2001; 10:431–5.

40. Carabello B, De Leon A, Edmunds L, et al. ACC/AHA guidelines for the management of patients with valvular heart disease. J Am Coll Cardiol 1998; 32:1486–588.

41. Tyers GF, Jamieson WR, Munro AA, et al. Reoperation in biological and mechanical valve populations: fate of the reoperative patient. Ann Thorac Surg 1995; 60(2 Suppl):S464–8.

12

Prevention of prosthetic valve endocarditis

Pilar Tornos, Benito Almirante and Manuel J Antunes

Introduction

Prosthetic valve endocarditis (PVE) is a serious, often fatal complication, even when adequate medical and/or surgical treatments are instituted. The disease is caused by an infection of the prosthesis and surrounding tissues that can generate vegetations, periannular abscesses, pseudoaneurysms and fistulae. As a consequence, patients can experience embolism, prosthetic dysfunction leading to heart failure, and all the clinical manifestations and complications of the septic process,[1,2] as described in Chapter 13.

Prevention of this complication includes both hygienic care and antibiotic prophylaxis during the valve surgery and, thereafter, before any medical and/or surgical instrumentation. Patients and health professionals must be aware that any potential cause of bacteraemia should be avoided, especially when this is caused by microorganisms that are usually involved in prosthetic endocarditis. Therefore, every effort is required to maintain good oral and cutaneous hygiene in patients with prosthetic valves, as well as to avoid unnecessary cutaneous punctures or intravenous lines. The importance of these measures is being increasingly recognised.[3]

The real efficacy of routine antibiotic prophylaxis to prevent prosthetic valve endocarditis is a matter of continuous debate and this is, in fact, an empirical practice characterised by uncertainty.[4,5] Case–control studies suggest that the efficacy of antibiotic prophylaxis is far from being clinically proven.[6–8] However, recommendations for the routine use of prophylactic antibiotics have been proposed worldwide since 1954 and regularly updated.[3,9–14] The initial differences between national and international recommendations have been attenuated over time and most authorities agree that the principle and modalities of antibiotic prophylaxis should remain, but its indications should be limited to high-risk patients and high-risk procedures. Individuals who have prosthetic cardiac valves, including bioprostheses and homograft valves, are considered high-risk individuals in most guidelines on prophylaxis of endocarditis.[3,9–14]

Prosthetic valve endocarditis has been classified into two types, early and late, which are defined in Chapter 13. Each has specificities which require specific measures that are the subject of this chapter.

Prevention of early prosthetic valve endocarditis

General measures

The dental health of the patient must be evaluated before elective valve replacement, and any necessary dental work completed with appropriate antibiotic coverage.[15] Any other focus of infection should be looked for and eradicated, if possible.

Patients who are nasal carriers of *Staphylococcus aureus* have an increased risk of surgical wound infections caused by that organism. It has recently been shown that intranasal treatment with mupirocin decreases the rate of nosocomial infections among patients who were *S. aureus* carriers, including wound infection in those submitted to cardiothoracic surgery.[16–19] Although these data seem encouraging, the impact of this treatment in the prevention of early PVE needs further evaluation.[20,21]

Utmost care must be exercised in the preparation of the skin and in the operating room, the use of meticulous surgical technique, as well as attention to haemostasis on closure to avoid the formation of haematomas. The role of pretreatment of the prosthetic sewing ring with antibiotics was studied experimentally,[22] but was never proven effective in clinical practice. The same recommendations apply to any subsequent cardiac and non-cardiac operations, however minor they may appear to be. If the wound becomes infected, the risk of PVE increases enormously.

Antibiotic prophylaxis

Back in 1963, Geraci et al[23] demonstrated that the incidence of early prosthetic valve endocarditis diminished if

Table 12.1 Micro-organisms causing early and late prosthetic valve endocarditis (PVE)

Microorganism	Early PVE (<12 months) n = 149	Late PVE (>12 months) n =102	p-value
Coagulase-negative staphylococci	83 (56%)	14 (14%)	<0.05
Staphylococcus aureus	14 (10%)	17 (16%)	ns
Streptococci and enterococci	13 (9%)	47 (46%)	<0.05
Gram-negative bacilli	8 (5%)	12 (12%)	<0.05
Diphtheroid	5 (3%)	1 (1%)	ns
Fungi	15 (10%)	2 (2%)	<0.05
Other	3 (2%)	3 (3%)	ns
Culture negative	8 (5%)	6 (6%)	ns

perioperative antibiotics were used. Most surgeons believe that the use of antibiotics has contributed to reduce the incidence of early PVE; hence, the use of antibiotics during open heart surgery has become standard practice.[24] But because early PVE can be caused by a variety of micro-organisms (Table 12.1), there is not a single antibiotic that could be efficacious against all and the use of more than one broad-spectrum antibiotic would not only fail to increase the efficacy of prevention but also could favour the appearance of multiresistant bacteria.

Therefore, there is a consensus that prophylaxis during surgery should be directed against staphylococci, which are the most common pathogens, and should be of short duration.[9,25,26] The most widely used antibiotics are first- or second-generation cephalosporins. Vancomycin or teicoplanin should be used in cases of allergy to beta-lactams or

in hospitals with a high prevalence of methicillin-resistant *S. aureus* (MRSA) infections. Patients who have been in hospital for a prolonged period of time prior to surgery are at higher risk of MRSA infections. Antibiotics should be started 30–60 minutes prior to skin incision, repeated to maintain intraoperative levels and continued for no more than 24 hours postoperatively (Table 12.2).

During the early postoperative period, scrupulous care must be taken in the handling of intravenous lines, drains and urethral catheters, and in care of the surgical wound, to avoid potential portals of entry for infection.

Prevention of late prosthetic valve endocarditis

General measures and education

Prosthetic valve patients should be taught about the importance of prevention of endocarditis. They should be instructed regarding oral hygiene and the need for regular dental care, twice a year, and receive information regarding antibiotic prophylaxis.

Considering that early diagnosis is of utmost importance to improve prognosis, patients should also be educated about the early manifestations of endocarditis. In particular, they should know that any fever that lasts for more than 2 or 3 days should be a matter for medical consultation and they must be instructed to avoid self-administration of antibiotics before blood cultures have been drawn.

Patients with prosthetic valves subjected to any medical instrumentation, such as placement of intravenous lines or urethral catheterisation, should be considered at risk. All indications for instrumentation should be seriously questioned and these procedures should be performed only when absolutely essential and carried out with extreme caution, especially in diabetic or renal patients.

Table 12.2 Prophylactic regimen before open heart surgery

Situation	Agent	Regimen
Standard	Cefazolin	1 g iv 30–60 minutes prior to skin incision, followed by 1 g 8-hourly during the first 24 hours (overall 3 doses)
Hospitals with high prevalence of *S. aureus* with beta-lactamase hyperproduction	Cefuroxime	1.5 g iv at the beginning of the intervention followed by 0.75 g 8-hourly during the first 24 hours (overall 3 doses)
MRSA and hypersensitivity to beta-lactams	Vancomycin	1 g iv (1 hour infusion) at the beginning of the intervention, followed by 1 g iv 12-hourly (overall 3 doses)

Antibiotic prophylaxis

Procedures that require antibiotic prophylaxis

Antibiotic prophylaxis is recommended in prosthetic valve patients when submitted to medical and/or surgical procedures or instrumentations that carry a substantial risk of bacteraemia. These procedures include dental work and some instrumentations or surgeries of the ear, nose and throat, upper respiratory tract, gastrointestinal tract, genitourinary tract and procedures involving infected tissues. A list of procedures that require antibiotic prophylaxis is given in Table 12.3.

Prophylaxis is recommended before dental, oral procedures, tonsillectomy, adenoidectomy, surgical operations that involve the respiratory mucosa, bronchoscopy with a rigid bronchoscope, sclerotherapy for oesophageal varices and dilatation of oesophageal strictures. Other procedures involving the upper respiratory tract, such as intubation or nasotracheal suction, or percutaneous dilatation of tracheostomy, as well as transoesophageal echocardiography, do not need antibiotic prophylaxis because the risk of bacteraemia is extremely low.

In dental procedures, prophylaxis is recommended when the procedure is associated with significant bleeding, such as dental extractions and periodontal procedures. Recommendations from the American Heart Association and the French recommendations list a number of dental procedures in which prophylaxis is recommended.[3,12,27]

Antibiotic prophylaxis is recommended before endoscopic retrograde cholangiography with biliary obstruction, biliary tract surgery and surgical operations that involve intestinal mucosa. It is also recommended before prostatic surgery, cystoscopy and urethral dilatation. The risk of endocarditis after gastrointestinal endoscopy, including mucosal biopsy or polypectomy, is very small, as is the risk after transoesophageal echocardiography. The American Heart Association recommendations and the new French recommendations consider that in these cases the use of prophylaxis is optional, even in patients with prosthetic valves.[12,27] However, it seems wise that high-risk prosthetic valve patients (diabetic patients, patients in renal failure or heart failure and patients with a previous episode of endocarditis) receive prophylaxis in some situations, especially in cases of colonoscopy when removal of polyps or biopsies are likely to be undertaken.

Antibiotic prophylaxis is considered unnecessary in uninfected cases before urethral catheterisation, hysterectomy or vaginal delivery, sterilisation procedures, caesarean section, therapeutic abortion, insertion of intrauterine devices and circumcision.

Table 12.3 Procedures for which endocarditis prophylaxis is recommended in patients with mechanical valves, bioprostheses and homografts

Oral and dental procedures
Tooth extraction
Dental work associated with gingival bleeding

Respiratory tract
Tonsillectomy
Adenoidectomy
Surgical operations that involve the respiratory mucosa
Bronchoscopy with a rigid bronchoscope
Bronchoscopy with a flexible bronchoscope[a]

Gastrointestinal tract
Sclerotherapy for oesophageal varices
Oesophageal stricture dilatation
Endoscopic retrograde cholangiopancreatography with biliary tract obstruction
Biliary tract surgery
Surgical operations that involve the intestinal mucosa
Endoscopy with or without biopsy[a]

Genitourinary tract
Prostatic surgery
Cystoscopy
Urethral dilatation
Vaginal hysterectomy[a]
Vaginal delivery[a]

Procedures involving infected tissues
Urethral catheterisation
Uterine dilatation and curettage
Therapeutic abortion
Insertion or removal of intrauterine devices
Incision or drainage of infected tissue

---

[a]Prophylaxis in these cases is considered optional in the French guidelines.[3] It probably should be given in high-risk prosthetic valve patients (diabetes, renal or heart failure and patients with a previous episode of endocarditis). In cases of colonoscopy, prophylaxis is recommended for polypectomy or difficult examinations.

Antibiotic regimens

Streptococci of the viridans group are the most common cause of endocarditis following dental, oral, upper respiratory tract and oesophageal procedures and prophylaxis should be directed against these organisms. Antibiotics should be given as a single dose before the procedure. To prolong antibiotic treatment does not add efficacy to the prophylaxis, may lead to the emergence of resistant organisms and places the patient at an additional risk of adverse reactions.

Amoxicillin is the preferred antibiotic and the recommended dose varies between 2 and 3 g, taking into account

Table 12.4 Prophylactic regimens for dental, oral, respiratory tract or oesophageal procedures

Situation	Agent	Regimen
Standard	Amoxicillin	2 or 3 g orally 1 hour before procedure
Hypersensitivity to penicillin	Clindamycin	600 mg 1 hour before procedure
	or	
	Azithromycin[a]	500 mg 1 hour before procedure
Unable to take oral medications	Ampicillin	2 g iv or im (30 min before procedure)
Hypersensitivity to penicillin and unable to take oral medications	Clindamycin	600 mg iv (30 min before procedure)
	or	
	Cefazolin[b]	1 g iv (30 min before procedure)
	or	
	Vancomycin[c]	1 g iv (1 hour infusion)

[a]See text for this recommendation.
[b]Not to be used in individuals with immediate-type hypersensitivity reactions to penicillin.
[c]In cases of severe hypersensitivity to beta-lactams.

the weight of the patient and a previous intolerance to the highest dose[12] (Table 12.4). Individuals who are allergic to penicillins should be treated with clindamycin.[28] Azithromycin or clarithromycin may also be used, but the high cost and the fact that some failures have been reported make them the worse alternative.[29,30] In patients who are unable to take oral medications, intravenous amoxicillin or ampicillin can be used. Intravenous clindamycin, vancomycin or cefazolin may be utilised in patients who are allergic to penicillin. In patients who are taking antibiotics before the visit to the dentist, it is wise to select a different drug rather than increase the dose of the current antibiotic. This is the case for patients who receive antibiotics to prevent acute rheumatic fever in whom clindamycin, azithromycin or clarithromycin should be chosen.

Bacterial endocarditis that follows genitourinary or gastrointestinal instrumentation is most often caused by *Enterococcus faecalis*. In these cases, parenteral administration of antibiotics is recommended and includes ampicillin, 2 g, plus gentamicin (1.5 mg/kg), intravenously 30 minutes before starting the procedure, and a second dose of ampicillin or amoxicillin, either parenterally or orally, must be given 6 hours after the procedure. In patients allergic to penicillin, vancomycin plus gentamicin should be used (Table 12.5).

In patients with abscesses and in procedures involving infected tissues, prophylaxis should be carried out if the patient is not already on antibiotics and should be directed to the most likely pathogen causing the infection. In cellulitis and bone or joint infections, an antistaphylococcal penicillin, or clindamycin in allergic patients, should be used. In urinary tract infections, when urethral catheterisation is needed, agents which are active against enteric bacilli, such as ampicillin and gentamicin, are recommended.

Table 12.5 Prophylactic regimens for gastrointestinal (non-oesophageal) and genitourinary procedures

Situation	Agents	Regimen
Standard	Ampicillin or amoxicillin	2 g iv 30 minutes before procedure and amoxicillin 1 g orally 6 hours later
	+	
	Gentamicin	1.5 mg/kg iv 30 minutes before procedure (maximum 120 mg)
Allergic to penicillin	Vancomycin	1 g iv (1 hour perfusion)
	+	
	Gentamicin	1.5 mg/kg iv 30 minutes before procedure (maximum 120 mg)

References

1. Wilson WR, Jaumin TM, Danielson GK, et al. Prosthetic valve endocarditis. Ann Intern Med 1975; 82:751–6.
2. Rutledge R, Kim J, Applebaum RE. Actuarial analysis of the risk of prosthetic valve endocarditis in 1598 patients with mechanical and bioprosthetic valves. Arch Surg 1995; 120:469–72.
3. Selton-Suty C, Duval X, Brochet E, et al. [New French recommendations for the prophylaxis of infectious endocarditis]. Arch Mal Coeur Vaiss 2004; 97:626–31 [in French].
4. Durack DT. Prevention of infective endocarditis. N Engl J Med 1995; 332:38–44.
5. Chemoprophylaxis for infective endocarditis: faith, hope and charity challenged. Editorial. Lancet 1992; 339:525–6.
6. Lacassin F, Hoen B, Leport C, et al. Procedures associated with

infective endocarditis in adults. A case control study. Eur Heart J 1995; 16:1968–74.

7. van der Meer JTM, van Wijk W, Thompson J, et al. Efficacy of antibiotic prophylaxis for prevention of native valve endocarditis. Lancet 1992; 339:135–9.

8. Oliver R, Roberts GJ, Hooper L. Penicillins for the prophylaxis of bacterial endocarditis in chemistry. Cochrane Database Syst Rev 2004; 2:CD003813.

9. Durack DT. Prophylaxis of infective endocarditis. In: Mandell GL, Douglas RG, Dolin R, eds. Principles and practice of infectious diseases. New York: Churchill Livingstone, 2005: 1004–52.

10. Antibiotic prophylaxis of infective endocarditis. Recommendations from the endocarditis working party of the British Society for Antimicrobial Chemotherapy. Lancet 1990; 335:88–9.

11. Leport C, Hortskotte D, Burckhardt D, et al. Antibiotic prophylaxis from an international group of experts towards a European Consensus. Eur Heart J 1995; 16(Suppl B):126–31.

12. Dajani AS, Taubert KA, Wilson W, et al. Prevention of bacterial endocarditis. Recommendations by the American Heart Association. JAMA 1997; 277:1794–801.

13. Leport C and the Group of Experts of the International Society for Chemotherapy. Antibiotic prophylaxis for infective endocarditis. Clin Microb Infect 1998; 4:S56–61.

14. Horstkotte D, Follath F, Gutschik E, et al. Guidelines on prevention, diagnosis and treatment of infective endocarditis executive summary; the task force on infective endocarditis of the European Society of Cardiology. Eur Heart J 2004; 25:267–76.

15. Terezhalmy GT, Safadi TJ, Longworth DL, et al. Oral disease burden in patients undergoing prosthetic heart valve implantation. Ann Thorac Surg 1997; 63:402–4.

16. Perl TM, Cullen JJ, Wenzel RP, et al. Intranasal mupirocin to prevent postoperative Staphylococcus aureus infections. N Engl J Med 2002; 346:1871–7.

17. Kluytmans JA, Mouton JW, Vanderberg MFQ, et al. Reduction of surgical-site infections in cardiothoracic surgery by elimination of nasal carriage of Staphylococcus aureus. Infect Control Hosp Epidemiol 1996; 17:780–5.

18. Cimochowski GE, Harostock MD, Brown R, et al. Intranasal mupirocin reduces sternal wound infection after open heart surgery in diabetics and non-diabetics. Ann Thorac Surg 2001; 71:1572–9.

19. Haas JP, Evans AM, Preston KE, Larson EL. Risk factors for surgical site infection after cardiac surgery: the role of endogenous flora. Heart Lung 2005; 32:108–14.

20. Banbury MK. Experience in prevention of sternal wound infections in nasal carriers of Staphylococcus aureus. Surgery 2003; 134 (Suppl 5):18–22.

21. Kluytmans JA, Werheim HF. Nasal carriage of Staphylococcus aureus and prevention of nosocomial infections. Infection 2005; 33:3–8.

22. Karck M, Siclari F, Wahlig H, et al. Pretreatment of prosthetic valve sewing-ring with the antibiotic/fibrin sealant compound as a prophylactic tool against prosthetic valve endocarditis. Eur J Cardiovasc Surg 1990; 4:142–6.

23. Geraci JE, Dale ADJ, McGoon DC. Bacterial endocarditis and endarteritis following cardiac operations. Wis Med J 1963; 62:302–15.

24. Hyde JAJ, Darouiche RO, Costerton JW. Strategies for prophylaxis against prosthetic valve endocarditis: a review article. J Heart Valve Dis 1998; 7:316–26.

25. Conte JE, Cohen SN, Roe BD, Elashoff RM. Antibiotic prophylaxis in cardiac surgery. A prospective double-blind comparison of single-dose versus multiple-dose regimens. Ann Intern Med 1972; 76:943–9.

26. Goldmann DA, Hopkins CC, Karchmer AW, et al. Cephalotin prophylaxis in cardiac valve surgery. A prospective double blind comparison of two-day and six-day regimens. J Thorac Cardiovasc Surg 1977; 73:470–9.

27. Prophylaxie de l'endocardite infectieuse. Revision de la conference de consensus de Mars 1992. Recomandations 2002. Med Mal Inf 2002; 22:533–644.

28. Hall G, Nord CE, Heimdahl A. Elimination of bacteraemia after dental extraction: comparison of erythromycin and clindamycin for prophylaxis of infective endocarditis. J Antimicrob Chemother 1996; 37:83–95.

29. Rouse MS, Steckelberg JM, Brandt CM, et al. Efficacy of azithromycin or clarithromycin for prophylaxis of viridans group streptococcus experimental endocarditis. Antimicrob Agents Chemother 1997; 41:1673–6.

30. Durack DT, Kaplan EL, Bisno AL. Apparent failures of endocarditis prophylaxis: analysis of 52 cases submitted to a national registry. JAMA 1983; 250:2318–22.

13

Management of prosthetic valve endocarditis

Manuel J Antunes and Pilar Tornos

Patients with prosthetic heart valves are permanently at risk of developing infection of the prosthesis. The risk of infection is higher in the first 3–6 months, but remains relatively constant thereafter. Hence, antibiotic prophylaxis is mandatory after cardiac valve replacement. But because of better antibiotic prophylaxis at the time of the initial surgery and improved prophylaxis during dental, endoscopic or other surgical procedures, the incidence of prosthetic valve endocarditis (PVE) has been decreasing. The guidelines for antibiotic prophylaxis in patients with prosthetic heart valves are discussed in Chapter 12.

PVE is a serious and often fatal condition, with a reported mortality in the range of 10–30%.[1] The in-hospital mortality of reoperations for PVE has declined in recent years. With the use of extensive debridement of infected tissue and postoperative antibiotic therapy, the extent and activity of the infection does not appear to have a major impact on late outcome, and the majority of patients with this complication survive for 10 years after the operation.[2,3]

Incidence

Prosthetic valve endocarditis occurs at a rate ranging from 0.2% to 1.4% per patient-year.[4–29] Rutledge and colleagues[8] found that the overall incidence was 3.2% at 5 years and 5% at 10 years. It is considerably more common in the aortic than in the mitral valve.[9,10] In their more recent series, Gordon et al,[11] from the Cleveland Clinic, found that the incidence of early-onset PVE (EO-PVE; see definition below) was 1% and that the incidence decreased during the study period from 1.5% (1992–94) to 0.7% (1995–97). The incidence for annuloplasty rings (0.2%) was significantly lower than for mechanical (1.6%) and bioprosthetic valves (1.1%). Finally, the incidence of EO-PVE was also significantly lower for the mitral valve than for the aortic valve (0.6% vs 1.4%). Published linearised rates of late PVE for both mechanical and bioprosthetic valves are shown in Figure 13.1.

Renzulli et al[30] found that recurrent endocarditis developed in 22.5% of patients operated on for native valve endocarditis (NVE). Variables predicting recurrence were positive valve culture and persistence of fever by the seventh postoperative day. They concluded that correct protocols of guided antibiotic therapy may cure the infection or reduce its virulence to allow for surgery on sterile tissues and thus prevent prosthetic infection. A similar approach may be justified in some cases of PVE.

Definition and classification

Classically, prosthetic valve endocarditis has been divided into two categories:

- early-onset, occurring less than 60 days after valve replacement
- late-onset, occurring after 60 days.

This classification is justified because the mode of infection and the infecting agents are different. However, it is possible that infection in many cases of 'late-onset' PVE that occur up to the first year after surgery is acquired at the time of implantation of the artificial heart valve. This may be particularly true when the infection is caused by bacteria of the HACEK group. Hence, some authors have called for the early period to be extended to 6 months and even to 1 year. The Centers for Disease Control and Prevention (CDC) consider that an infection involving an implanted prosthetic device within the first 12 months of an operative procedure is considered to be a nosocomial infection and is more likely to have been acquired at the time of operation. However, the infectious disease groups at the Massachusetts General Hospital and the Mayo Clinic, as well as the Alabama and Stanford cardiovascular surgeons, have all come up with a now fairly generally accepted definition of 3 months after

PVE rates for AVR

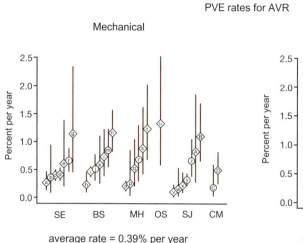

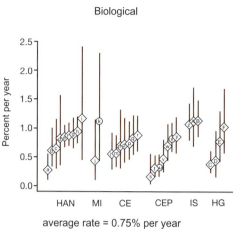

Figure 13.1
Incidence of PVE for both aortic and mitral prostheses (mechanical and biological). Modified from Vlessis et al, J Heart Valve Dis 1997; 6:443–65.

PVE rates for MVR

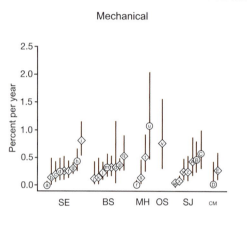

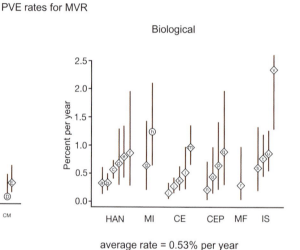

implantation of the prosthesis (Miller DC in discussion of Lytle et al[2]).

The microbiology of prosthetic aortic valve endocarditis is different from that of the native valve.[31–35] Early prosthetic endocarditis is caused by contamination at the time of implantation or by perioperative bacteraemia. *Staphylococcus aureus*, *S. epidermidis* and *Enterococcus faecalis* are the causative microorganisms in more than two-thirds of the patients,[31,33–37] and are usually associated with extensive tissue destruction. Coagulase-negative staphylococci are able to adhere to the surfaces of the prostheses and produce an antibiotic-resistant biofilm.[38,39] Fungi are the second most prevalent pathogen associated with EO-PVE, accounting for up to 13% of the cases and may be especially associated with a contaminated aortic valve homograft.[40]

Bacteraemia is the principal cause of late endocarditis but the port of entry is often difficult to determine. Streptococci and staphylococci are the most commonly cultured agents but a very large number of different microorganisms may cause late PVE.[17,20,21]

Pathology

Infection usually begins in the sewing ring of the prosthesis.[16,21,26] In a bioprosthesis, it may also involve the leaflets.[17,18,22] Depending on the virulence of the microorganism and the resistance of the host, the infection may spread into the annulus and surrounding structures, with abscess formation (Figure 13.2). Extension of the infection to and beyond the valve annulus occurs in 56–100% of patients,[27] probably because the sewing ring is the most common primary site of the infection.[22] Progression of periannular infection with formation of abscesses can create fistulae, which may rupture into the pericardial cavity, or result in intracardiac shunts or in ventriculo-aortic dehiscence.

Infection in aortic valve homografts and pulmonary autografts, now sometimes used in primary aortic valve replacement, resembles that of the native aortic valve, destroying the leaflets to produce aortic insufficiency, but may also extend into the annulus and the surrounding structures.

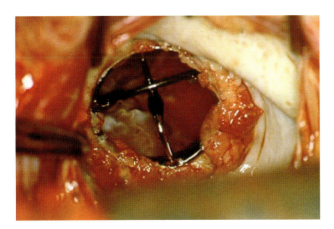

Figure 13.2
Intraoperative photograph in a patient with fungal mitral PVE, occurring only 3 weeks after valve replacement. Fungal agents are very virulent and rapidly lead to destruction of the periannular tissues.

Diagnosis

The diagnosis of prosthetic endocarditis is based on the clinical picture, the microbiological findings and the echocardiographic findings. The clinical picture is similar to that of native endocarditis and consists of fever, vascular phenomena including arterial embolism, mycotic aneurysms, central nervous system haemorrhages, Osler's nodes or Roth's spots and immunological phenomena such as immune complex glomerulonephritis. There are no clear differences in the clinical presentation between early and late endocarditis. In early cases, the diagnosis can be difficult because fever may be attributed to other infections that are common in the immediate postoperative period, such as wound and urinary infections or catheter sepsis. In late cases, the severity of the clinical picture relates to the infecting agent: in infections due to *S. aureus*, the clinical presentation is usually acute, with hectic fever, prostration and early complications such as embolism or heart failure, whereas in cases due to streptococci the disease is usually subacute, presenting with low-grade and well-tolerated fever. Sometimes, prosthetic endocarditis can occur without fever, and the diagnosis is suspected after discovering new prosthetic valve dysfunction on the echocardiogram. Some cases of PVE proven intraoperatively by the macroscopic signs of infection, especially tissue destruction and abscess formation, may have had a completely silent course, without fever or any other signs of infection, including negative blood cultures. When a periprosthetic leak occurs late in a patient with a previously normal-functioning prosthesis, PVE must be considered as a possible diagnosis and appropriately treated.

Blood cultures are an essential part of the diagnosis. In order to be considered as a major criterion for the diagno-sis, bacteraemia has to be continuous and blood cultures have to be positive for microorganisms that normally cause endocarditis, mainly streptococci and staphylococci. In the early postoperative period, patients can have positive cultures to other organisms, such as Gram-negative bacilli: in most cases, this bacteraemia does not cause endocarditis and can be cured by catheter removal and antibiotics for 2 weeks. However, if fever reappears and blood cultures become positive again, the diagnosis of endocarditis should be considered and appropriate treatment instituted. In patients with a clinical suspicion of endocarditis and negative blood cultures, serology for the more unusual microorganisms that can cause endocarditis needs to be performed. These include *Coxiella burnetii*, and *Legionella*, *Chlamydia*, *Bartonella*, *Brucella* and *Mycoplasma* species.

Echocardiographic findings include vegetations, paraprosthetic abscesses or pseudoaneurysm, a new periprosthetic leak or an intracardiac fistula. In the investigation of prosthetic valve endocarditis, the use of transoesophageal echocardiography is recommended because of its greater sensitivity and better definition of paraprosthetic anatomy.[28,29] Echocardiography is extremely sensitive for detecting paravalvular abscesses and cardiac fistulae. Abnormal (rocking) motion of the prosthesis is commonly seen on the echocardiogram (see also Chapter 4).

Because heart catheterisation with coronary angiography increases the risk of embolisation in patients with vegetations, it should be avoided, unless there is a strong suggestion of coronary artery disease, in which case it is strongly advised.

Medical treatment

An appropriate antibiotic regimen is the most important therapy in the management of patients with infective endocarditis, in PVE as in NVE.[30,31] Generally, antibiotic treatment of PVE follows the lines of treatment of NVE and depends on the infecting agent. The initial choice of antibiotics is based on the clinical circumstances, the suspected source of infection and the sensitivity of the organisms, and therapy should be started soon after obtaining several blood cultures (Table 13.1). Once the agent is identified and its sensitivity is known, antibiotic therapy is adjusted accordingly, if necessary. The antibiotic regimens recommended for the most common types of infection are shown in Tables 13.2 and 13.3. Intravenous antibiotic therapy is continued for 4–6 weeks. If the patient needs surgery during the active phase of the disease, the length of antibiotic therapy after surgery depends on the culture of the surgical specimen. If the culture is negative, it is enough to finish the previous antibiotic regimen. If the culture is positive, a full antibiotic regimen should be continued for a further 6 weeks.

Table 13.1 Empirical antibiotic treatment (before results of the blood cultures)

Type of PVE	Standard regimen	Alternative regimen
Early PVE	Vancomycin 1 g per 12 h iv + Gentamicin 1 mg/kg per 8 h iv + Rifampicin 300 mg per 8 h po	Teicoplanin 12 mg per 12 h (3 doses) and then 24 h iv + Gentamicin 1 mg/kg per 8 h iv + Rifampicin 300 mg per 8 h po
Late PVE	Vancomycin 1 g per 12 h iv + Gentamicin 1 mg/kg per 8 h iv + Rifampicin 300 mg per 8 h po	Cloxacillin 2 g per 4 h iv + Ampicillin 2 g per 4 h iv + Gentamicin 1 mg/kg per 8 h iv

Table 13.2 Antibiotic regime for streptococcal and enterococcal PVE

Microorganism	Standard regimen[a]
S. viridans sensitive to penicillin, S. bovis, other streptococci with penicillin CMI <0.1 mg/L	Penicillin G 2 million units iv per 4 h × 6 weeks + Gentamicin 1 mg/kg per 8 h iv × 2 weeks
Streptococci with intermediate sensitivity to penicillin (CMI between 0.1 and 0.5 mg/L)	Penicillin G 3 million units iv per 4 h × 6 weeks + Gentamicin 1 g/kg per 8 h iv × 4 weeks
Streptococcus spp. with CMI >0.5 mg/L, Enterococcus spp., Abiotrophia spp.	Penicillin 4 million units per 4 h iv × 6 weeks or ampicillin 2 g per 4 h iv × 6 weeks + Gentamicin 1 mg/kg per 8 h iv × 6 weeks

[a]In penicillin allergy, vancomycin 15 mg/kg per 12 h iv (total dose ≤2 g).

Some patients with bioprosthetic valvular endocarditis may be 'cured' of low-potency organisms such as streptococcus.[15,32] This is especially the case when there is no evidence of prosthetic dysfunction or periprosthetic leakage.

However, it is unlikely that antibiotics alone can sterilise more virulent infections, particularly those caused by staphylococcus. For these reasons and because of the possibility of invasion of the cardiac skeleton, which may cause ventriculo-aortic or atrioventricular disruption, and the involvement of the conduction system, these infections usually require urgent, and sometimes emergency, surgery in up to 70% of the patients.[16,21,30]

There is no evidence that anticoagulation has any useful therapeutic effect on the course of endocarditis. However, oral anticoagulation should be maintained in patients with mechanical valves. Some groups have recommended the use of heparin in the first 2 weeks of treatment because embolic episodes or the necessity for surgery are likely to

Table 13.3 Antibiotic regime for staphylococcal prosthetic valve endocarditis

Microorganism	Standard regimen
Methicillin sensitive	Cloxacillin 2 g per 4 h iv × 6 weeks + Rifampicin 300 mg per 8 h iv × 6 weeks + Gentamicin 1 mg/kg per 8 h iv × 2 weeks
Methicillin resistant (MRSA)	Vancomycin 15 mg/kg per 12 h iv × 6 weeks + Rifampicin 300 mg per 8 h po × 6 weeks + Gentamicin 1 mg/kg per 8 h iv × 2 weeks

occur in this time period. In endocarditis caused by *S. aureus*, in which cerebral complications are common, it has been suggested to avoid any anticoagulation in the very early septic phase of the disease in order to avoid early cerebral haemorrhage that would preclude surgery, which is needed by most patients. However, this is likely to increase the risk of valve thrombosis, particularly as patients with endocarditis who have evidence of increased coagulation activation are at a greater risk of thromboembolism.

Surgery
Indications

The surgical indications for prosthetic valve endocarditis are persistent sepsis, congestive failure, significant perivalvular leak, large vegetations, intracardiac fistulae or systemic infected emboli.[33–35] Once these complications appear, medical therapy alone is usually insufficient to cure the disease. However, in some situations, under stable clinical and haemodynamic conditions, there may be some advantages in attempting to control the infection before surgery is undertaken. In the case of endocarditis of the mitral valve which accompanies aortic PVE, conservative surgery may be possible if the infection is controlled. However, there are conflicting data as to the advantage or otherwise of such a policy.

Technique

During reoperation, the sternotomy can be complicated by right ventricular injury, but femoral artery and vein cannulation are usually unnecessary. Sternotomy performed with a vibrating saw is usually uneventful. Although some surgeons fully mobilise the heart, limited dissection of adhesions to expose only the ascending aorta, a portion of the right atrium and the right superior pulmonary vein are sufficient for aortic valve reoperations. Complete dissection of the external walls of the right and left atria, down to the interatrial groove and right pulmonary veins, are essential for mitral valve reoperations. Cardiopulmonary bypass is conducted with an ascending aorta and a single or two-stage venous cannulae, and, in aortic surgery, a left-sided vent placed via the right superior pulmonary vein. After cardiopulmonary bypass is started, the remainder of the operation is conducted as for routine cardiac operations,[36] but myocardial protection is of utmost importance because the reoperations are often complex and require long aortic cross-clamp times.

Coronary ostial antegrade and/or continuous or intermittent retrograde cardioplegia is used for aortic valve

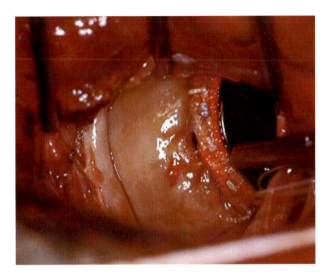

Figure 13.3
Periprosthetic leak in a patient reoperated 3 months after initial valve replacement. PVE was suspected pre-operatively and the patient treated with antibiotics. The infection was considered cured and the leak closed by a direct suture.

surgery.[36,37] Particular care is exerted to ensure right ventricular protection. For the mitral valve,[36] intermittent cold cardioplegia is recommended to avoid compromising visualisation. Myocardial temperature is maintained between 10 and 15°C and systemic temperature between 28 and 32°C.

The general principles of operation for PVE are identical for the mitral and the aortic positions and consist of removing the prosthesis from the infected site and meticulous and extensive debridement of the annulus and abscesses to remove all infected and non-viable tissue.[16,21,27,36,38–40] Samples of the infected tissues removed must be sent for microbiological and histological diagnosis, the latter also with a request for identification of the infective agent. Local application of an antiseptic (povidone-iodine) or antibiotic solution is recommended.

Occasionally, cured infections may be treated by direct closure of periprosthetic leaks (Figure 13.3). In cases of extensive destruction, especially in the mitral valve, with atrioventricular disruption, the annulus should be reconstructed using autologous or heterologous pericardium, because they are more resistant to colonisation by the offending microorganism.[16,21,38,40] Artificial materials such as Dacron or Teflon should be avoided. To obtain secure anchorage of the new prosthesis, the sutures must be placed through healthy tissue or pericardial patches. Several operative techniques for closure and repair of local abscesses and infectious destruction of the mitral valve annulus have been proposed.[41]

Anatomy and pathology determine the type of prosthesis to be used. Mechanical valves are preferred for younger patients (<65–70 years), but porcine bioprostheses are

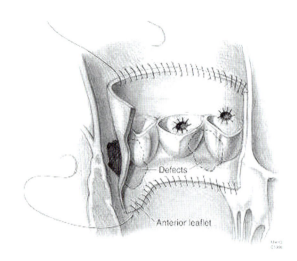

Figure 13.4
Use of an aortic homograft for aortic valve replacement in a patient with root abscesses. The homograft is sutured proximally to the upper rim of the ventricular endocardium; thus, the abscesses, potentially still infected, are excluded from the circulation.

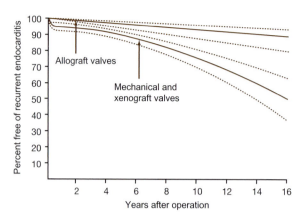

Figure 13.5
Homograft aortic valve replacement has consistently shown better freedom from recurrent endocarditis when compared with either mechanical valves or bioprostheses. Reproduced with permission from McGiffin et al. J Thorac Cardiovasc Surg 1992; 104:511–12.

more suitable for the elderly, because durability is better in these cases.[42–47] Mitral bioprostheses have a lower durability than aortic bioprostheses, but, as observed by Grunkemeier et al,[48] some patients may not outlive their prosthetic valves because of co-morbid disease. Stentless porcine bioprostheses are currently implanted in elderly patients because they have reduced fatigue-related stress and potentially extended durability.

Severe disruption of the aortic annulus with ventriculoaortic discontinuity may be repaired with pericardium, as indicated for the mitral annulus, but when there is extensive destruction of the aortic root it may be necessary to use a valved conduit of Dacron, using the Bentall technique or one of its modifications. However, in recent years, 'fresh' antibiotic-sterilised or cryopreserved homografts have been preferentially used for aortic valve replacement, mostly as aortic root or mini-root, because of their greater resistance to infection (Figure 13.4).[49–51]

Homograft root replacement is indicated for any abnormality of the aortic valve or aortic wall that distorts the aortic sinuses. The technique is facilitated by implanting the graft in a subannular position, in the upper rim of the ventricular endocardium. If necessary, the retained anterior leaflet of the mitral valve may be used to repair periannular defects. A pulmonary autograft may be used in children or adolescents to facilitate growth and in young adults for extended durability.[52] All aortic root reconstructions require coronary arterial anastomoses. In less-extensive lesions, subcoronary (free-hand) implantation of the homograft valve alone may be used.[53,54] In these cases, sizing is particularly important for an allograft to fit a dilated,

pressurised aortic root without incompetence (see also Chapter 6). Nonetheless, O'Brien and colleagues[51,54] provided evidence that cryopreserved allograft root replacements are preferable, because immediate and late results are the same as for non-root procedures. Besides, root procedures are technically easier.

One of the most important advantages of a homograft is the ease of use because of its compliance and adaptability to the host annulus. The use of homografts has been associated with a lower incidence of recurrence of infection (Figure 13.5). In special circumstances, heterografts (stentless porcine valves) may be similarly used, but there is, as yet, insufficient information about their advantage with regard to the incidence of recurrence of infection.[55] Recently, unstented homograft[56] and heterograft[57,58] mitral valve replacements have been done, but medium-term results have fallen short of expectations.[59,60]

However, the use of homografts, and probably of heterografts, has some potential drawbacks. Homografts deteriorate progressively once implanted, and reoperation, technically challenging, will eventually be required. Moreover, an irregular base for the proximal suture line can distort and render the homograft insufficient (see also Chapter 6).

Finally, for patients with destruction of the curtain between the mitral and aortic valves, with endocarditis involving both valves, extensive reconstruction is required, which may include excision of part of the anterior mitral valve leaflet and of the roof of the left atrium. Pericardial reconstruction of the mitro-aortic curtain, extending to and including the base of the anterior leaflet, may be possible. The retained anterior mitral valve leaflet in aortic homografts may be used in this reconstruction. Otherwise, replacement of the mitral valve may be necessary.

De-airing of the heart is especially critical in the presence of adhesions between the heart and the pericardium. The left ventricular and aortic root vents must remain under strong suction until normal ejection occurs. Intermittent inflation of the lungs and vigorous agitation of the chest helps to displace the air entrapped in the left-side cavities.

Secondary mitral valve involvement

Secondary mitral valve endocarditis may occur in parallel with aortic PVE. This may be the result of direct extension or be caused by jet lesions from the aortic valve. Often, the damage to the valve is limited and involves mainly the

anterior leaflet and chordae tendinae. The most frequent pathology includes chordal rupture, leaflet perforation and vegetations. Valvuloplasty techniques have been used recently in cases of mitral valve endocarditis that cause limited damage to the valve. Its advantages are well known, especially the avoidance of new prosthetic material. This is another good reason for attempting control of the infection preoperatively. Short-term results are excellent.[61,62] Dreyfus et al[61] reported repair in 80% of all patients. Autologous pericardium, preferably glutaraldehyde-treated, is used to repair perforations or to extend leaflets (Figure 13.6). Ruptured chordae may be replaced with artificial chordae made of PTFE (polytetrafluoroethylene).[63] In the vast majority of cases the annulus is normal, thus making the use of an annuloplasty ring unnecessary but if annuloplasty is required, autologous pericardium can be used.

Results

Results of surgery for PVE are shown in Table 13.4.

Mortality

Hospital mortality depends on the preoperative clinical condition of the patients and on the degree of destruction of cardiac structures, especially in the presence of aortic root abscesses.[16,38,64,65] In recent series of surgically treated patients, operative mortality for the prosthetic valve was still 20–30%,[16,21,30,38,65] but there are many reports of much lower mortalities.[1,66,67] Mortality rates in the order of 10% are more acceptable today and some teams have reported even lower rates.

Failure to eradicate the local infection and subsequent recurrent perivalvular leak, ongoing sepsis and multi-organ failure are the most common causes of death.[34] In the experience of Alexiou et al,[1] coagulase-negative staphylococcus and annular or myocardial infectious invasion were the critical determinants of adverse late outcome. With the possible exception of homografts, there is no evidence of superiority with regards to recurrence of infection of either mechanical or biological prostheses.

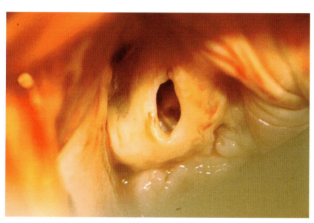

A

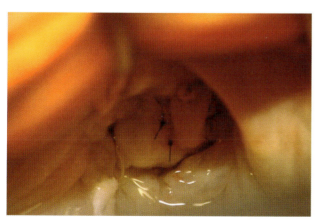

B

Figure 13.6
Intraoperative photographs of the mitral valve in a patient treated for aortic PVE. Perforation of the anterior leaflet (A) was treated by an autologous pericardial patch (B).

Other complications

After surgery for active infective endocarditis, complications are common and may include haemorrhage, because of severe coagulopathy, which may require treatment with antifibrinolytic drugs and clotting factors. Atrioventricular block may result from radical resection of an aortic root

Table 13.4 Results of surgery for prosthetic valve endocarditis

Author	Year	No. of cases	Early mortality (%)	Late survival (%) 5Y	10Y	15Y	Recurrence (%)	Survival free from reoperation for recurrence at 10 years (%)
Lyttle	1996	146	13	82	60			50
Edwards	1998	322	19.9	55	38			87
Delay	2000	27	0		55(7A)		18.5	
Alexiou	2000	35	16.6		61		17.1	
Moon	2001	97	29	41			2.5 ± 0.7% per patient-year	
Romano	2004	95	24.2	64	34	34		59

abscess and requires implantation of a permanent pacemaker. In some patients, prophylactic implantation of a pacemaker must be considered because of the possibility of progression of left bundle branch block to complete heart block.

Patients with prosthetic endocarditis who need surgery are often very sick and may develop multi-organ failure. Ischaemic and haemorrhagic neurological infarcts are common postoperative complications. Preoperative cerebral, pulmonary, splenic, hepatic and other organ abscesses may require surgical intervention. Appropriate intravenous antibiotic therapy should be continued for at least 6 weeks postoperatively, but in some cases this may be reduced, taking into account the duration of preoperative antibiotic treatment, especially if intraoperative observation suggests control of the infection.

Dossche et al[68] found that the 5-year actuarial survival was 87.3% and the 5-year freedom from recurrent endocarditis was 96.5% for allograft aortic root replacement in the complex setting of PVE with involvement of the periannular tissues. However, Hagl et al,[69] from Mount Sinai, New York, report that prosthetic root replacement may be superior to the use of a homograft for acute aortic PVE, with only a 4% incidence of recurrent endocarditis and reoperations.

PVE of fungal aetiology carries a poorer prognosis, but Muehrcke et al[25] found that preoperative treatment with amphotericin B, radical resection of all infected tissue, cardiac reconstruction using biological tissue when possible and lifelong oral antifungal therapy are effective for fungal prosthetic valve endocarditis.

Late results

In one series, Delay et al reported that 5-year survival following surgery for PVE was lower than for NVE, averaging 66% ± 12% following aortic valve replacement and 43% ± 19% following mitral valve replacement, vs 75% ± 9% and 79% ± 9%, respectively, for NVE.[67]

Lytle et al[2,3] observed a late survival of 82% at 5 years and 60% at 10 years. Older age was the only factor associated with late death. Reoperation-free survival was 75% at 5 years and 50% at 10 years postoperation, respectively. In another two reports from the same institution, these authors found that aortic valve and root replacement had better late results, especially freedom from recurrent infection (95% freedom from recurrent PVE at ≥2 years).[2,68]

References

1. Alexiou C, Langley SM, Stafford H, et al. Surgery for active culture-positive endocarditis: determinants of early and late outcome. Ann Thorac Surg 2000; 69:1448–54.
2. Lytle BW, Priest BP, Taylor PC, et al. Surgical treatment of prosthetic valve endocarditis. Thorac Cardiovasc Surg 1996; 111:198–210.
3. Lytle BD, Sabik JF, Blackstone EH, et al. Reoperative cryopreserved root and ascending aorta replacement for acute aortic prosthetic valve endocarditis. Ann Thorac Surg 2002; 74:S1754–7.
4. David TE, Armstrong S, Sun Z. The Hancock II bioprosthesis at 10 years. Ann Thorac Surg 1995; 60(Suppl):S229.
5. Khan S, Chaux A, Matloff J, et al. The St. Jude Medical valve experience with 1,000 cases. J Thorac Cardiovasc Surg 1994; 108:1010–19.
6. O'Brien MF, Stafford EG, Gardner MAH, et al. A comparison of aortic valve replacement with viable cryopreserved and fresh allograft valves, with a note on chromosomal studies. J Thorac Cardiovasc Surg 1987; 94:812–23.

7. Kratz JM, Crawford FA Jr, Sade RM, Crumbley AJ, Stroud MR. St. Jude prosthesis for aortic and mitral valve replacement: a ten-year experience. Ann Thorac Surg 1993; 56:462–8.

8. Rutledge R, Kim BJ, Applebaum RE. Actuarial analysis of the risks of prosthetic valve endocarditis in 1,598 patients with mechanical and bioprosthetic valves. Arch Surg 1985; 120:469–72.

9. Edwards MJ, Richardson JD, Klamer TW. Management of aortic prosthetic infections. Am J Surg 1988; 155:327–30.

10. de Luca L, Vitale N, Giannolo B, et al. Mid-term follow-up after heart valve replacement with CarboMedics bileaflet prostheses. J Thorac Cardiovasc Surg 1993; 106:1158–65.

11. Gordon SM, Serkey JM, Longworth DL, Lytle BW, Cosgrove DM. Early onset prosthetic valve endocarditis: the Cleveland Clinic Experience 1992–1997. Ann Thorac Surg 2000; 69:1388–92.

12. Sarris GE, Robbins RC, Miller DC, et al. Randomized, prospective assessment of bioprosthetic valve durability: Hancock versus Carpentier–Edwards valves. Circulation 1993; 88(5 pt 2):II-55.

13. Louagie Y, Noirhomme P, Aranguis E, et al. Use of the Carpentier–Edwards porcine bioprosthesis: assessment of a patient selection policy. J Thorac Cardiovasc Surg 1992; 104:1013–24.

14. Bortolotti U, Milano A, Mossuto E, et al. Porcine valve durability: a comparison between Hancock standard and Hancock II bioprostheses. Ann Thorac Surg 1995; 60:S216–20.

15. Antunes MJ, Wessels A, Sadowski RG, Schultz JG. Medtronic Hall valve replacement in a third-world population group. A review of the performance of 1000 prostheses. J Thorac Surg 1988; 95:980–93.

16. David TE. The surgical treatment of patients with prosthetic valve endocarditis. Semin Thorac Cardiovasc Surg 1995; 7:47–53.

17. Sett SS, Hudon MPJ, Jamieson WRE, Chow AW. Prosthetic valve endocarditis. Experience with porcine bioprostheses. J Thorac Cardiovasc Surg 1993; 105:428–34.

18. Nunez L, de la Llana R, Aguado MG, et al. Bioprosthetic valve endocarditis: indicators for surgical intervention. Ann Thorac Surg 1983; 35:262–70.

19. Watanakunakorn C, Burkert T. Infective endocarditis at a large community teaching hospital, 1980–1990: a review of 210 episodes. Medicine (Baltimore) 1993; 72:90–102.

20. Fang G, Keys TF, Gentry LO, et al. Prosthetic valve endocarditis resulting from nosocomial bacteremia. A prospective, multicenter study. Ann Intern Med 1993; 119:560–7.

21. David TE, Bos J, Christakis GT, et al. Heart valve operations in patients with active infective endocarditis. Ann Thorac Surg 1990; 49:701–5.

22. Fernicola DJ, Roberts WC. Frequency of ring abscess and cuspal infection in active infective endocarditis involving bioprosthetic valves. Am J Cardiol 1993; 72:314–23.

23. Zimmerli W. Experimental models in the investigation of device-related infections. J Antimicrob Chemother 1993; 31:97–102.

24. Horstkotte D, Weist K, Rueden H. Better understanding of the pathogenesis of prosthetic valve endocarditis: recent perspectives for prevention strategies. J Heart Valve Dis 1998; 7:313–15.

25. Muehrcke DD, Lytle BW, Cosgrove DM 3rd. Surgical and long-term antifungal therapy for fungal prosthetic valve endocarditis. Ann Thorac Surg 1995; 60:538–43.

26. Blumberg EA, Karalis DA, Chandrasekaran K, et al. Endocarditis-associated paravalvular abscesses: do clinical parameters predict the presence of abscess? Chest 1995; 107:898–903.

27. Buda AJ, Zotz RJ, LeMire MS, Bach DS. Prognostic significance of vegetations detected by two-dimensional echocardiography in infective endocarditis. Am Heart J 1986; 112:1291–6.

28. Lowry RW, Zoghbi WA, Baker WB, Wray RA, Quinones MA. Clinical impact of transesophageal echocardiography in the diagnosis and management of infective endocarditis. Am J Cardiol 1994; 73:1089–91.

29. Larbalestier RJ, Kinchla NM, Aranki SF, et al. Acute bacterial endo-carditis. Optimizing surgical results. Circulation 1992; 86(Suppl): II68–74.

30. Renzulli A, Carozza A, Romano GP, et al. Recurrent infective endocarditis: a multivariate analysis of 21 years of experience. Ann Thorac Surg 2001; 72:39–43.

31. Romano G, Carozza A, Della Corte A, et al. Native versus primary prosthetic valve endocarditis: comparison of clinical features and long-term outcome in 353 patients. J Heart Valve Dis 2004; 13:200–8.

32. Bayliss R, Clarke C, Oakley CM, et al. The microbiology and pathogenesis of infective encocarditis. Br Heart J 1983; 50:513–19.

33. Aranki SF, Adams DH, Rizzo RJ, et al. Determinants of early mortality and late survival in mitral valve endocarditis. Circulation 1995; 92(Suppl):II43–9.

34. Miller DC. Determinants of outcome in surgically treated patients with native valve infective endocarditis (NVE). J Card Surg 1989; 4:331–9.

35. Verheul HA, Van den Brink RBA, van Vreeland T, et al. Effects of changes in management of active infective endocarditis on outcome in a 25-year period. Am J Cardiol 1993; 72:682–7.

36. Buckberg GD, Beyersdorf F, Allen BS. Integrated myocardial management in valvular heart disease. J Heart Valve Dis 1995; 4(Suppl 2):S198–212.

37. Menasché P, Tronc F, Nguyen A, et al. Retrograde warm blood cardioplegia preserves hypertrophied myocardium: a clinical study. Ann Thorac Surg 1994; 57:1429–34.

38. Ralph-Edwards A, David TE, Bos J. Infective endocarditis in patients who had replacement of the aortic root. Ann Thorac Surg 1994; 58:429–32.

39. Fiore AC, Ivey TD, McKeown PP, et al. Patch closure of aortic annulus mycotic aneurysms. Ann Thorac Surg 1986; 42:372–9.

40. David TE, Komeda M, Brofman PR. Surgical treatment of aortic root abscess. Circulation 1989; 80(3 Pt 1):I269–74.

41. Cachera JP, Loisance D, Mourtada A, Castanie JB, Heurtemette Y. Surgical techniques for treatment of bacterial endocarditis of the mitral valve. J Card Surg 1987; 2:265–74.

42. Burr LH, Jamieson WRE, Munro AI, Miyagishima RT, Germann E. Porcine bioprostheses in the elderly: clinical performance by age groups and valve positions. Ann Thorac Surg 1995; 60:S264–9.

43. Culliford AT, Galloway AC, Colvin SB, et al. Aortic valve replacement for aortic stenosis in persons aged 80 years and over. J Am Coll Cardiol 1991; 67:1256–60.

44. Gehlot A, Mullany CJ, Ilstrup D, et al. Aortic valve replacement in patients aged eighty years and older: early and long-term results. J Thorac Cardiovasc Surg 1996; 111:1026–36.

45. Holper K, Wottke M, Lewe T, et al. Bioprosthetic and mechanical valves in the elderly: benefits and risks. Ann Thorac Surg 1995; 60:S443–6.

46. Pupello DF, Bessone LN, Hiro SP, et al. Bioprosthetic valve longevity in the elderly: an 18-year longitudinal study. Ann Thorac Surg 1995; 60:S270–4.

47. Sintek CF, Fletcher AD, Khonsari S. Stentless porcine aortic root: valve of choice for the elderly patient with small aortic root? J Thorac Cardiovasc Surg 1995; 109:871–6.

48. Grunkemeier GL, Jamieson WR, Miller DC, Starr A. Actuarial versus actual risk of porcine structural valve deterioration. J Thorac Cardiovasc Surg 1994; 108:709–18.

49. O'Brien MF, Stafford EG, Gardner MAH, et al. Allograft aortic valve replacement: long-term follow-up. Ann Thorac Surg 1995; 60:S65–70.

50. Rubay JE, Raphael D, Sluysmans T, et al. Aortic valve replacement with allograft/autograft subcoronary versus intraluminal cylinder or root. Ann Thorac Surg 1995; 60:S78–82.

51. O'Brien MF. Allograft aortic root replacement: standardization and simplification of technique. Ann Thorac Surg 1995; 60:S92–4.

52. Elkins RC, Knott-Craig CJ, Ward KE, McCue C, Lane MM. Pulmonary autograft in children: realized growth potential. Ann Thorac Surg 1994; 57:1387–93.

53. Jones EL, Shah VB, Shanewise JS, et al. Should the freehand allograft be abandoned as a reliable alternative for aortic valve replacement? Ann Thorac Surg 1995; 59:1397–403.

54. O'Brien MF, Finney RS, Stafford EG, et al. Root replacement for all allograft aortic valves: preferred technique or too radical? Ann Thorac Surg 1995; 60:S87–91.

55. Sakaguchi T, Sawa W, Ohtake S, Hirata N, Matsuda H. The freestyle stentless bioprosthesis for prosthetic valve endocarditis. Ann Thorac Surg 1999; 67:533–5.

56. Acar C, Iung B, Cormier B, et al. Double mitral homograft for recurrent bacterial endocarditis of the mitral and tricuspid valves. J Heart Valve Dis 1994; 3:470–2.

57. Deac RFP, Simionescu D, Deac D. New evolution in mitral physiology and surgery: mitral stentless pericardial valve. Ann Thorac Surg 1995; 60:S433–8.

58. Vrandecic MDP, Fantini FA, Gontijo BF, et al. Surgical technique of implanting the stentless porcine mitral valve. Ann Thorac Surg 1995; 60:S439–42.

59. Chauvaud SM, Waldmann T, d'Attellis N, et al. Homograft replacement of the mitral valve in young recipients: mid-term results. Eur J Cardiothorac Surg 2003; 23:560–6.

60. McGiffin DC, O'Brien MF, Galbraith AJ, et al. An analysis of risk factors for death and mode-specific death after aortic valve replacement with allograft, xenograft, and mechanical valves. J Thorac Cardiovasc Surg 1993; 106:895–911.

61. Dreyfus G, Serraf A, Jebara VA, et al. Valve repair in acute endocarditis. Ann Thorac Surg 1990; 49:706–11.

62. Hendren WG, Morris AS, Rosenkranz ER, et al. Mitral valve repair for bacterial endocarditis. J Thorac Cardiovasc Surg 1992; 103:124–8.

63. David TE, Bos J, Rabowski H. Mitral valve repair by replacement of chordae tendineae with polytetrafluoroethylene sutures. J Thorac Cardiovasc Surg 1991; 101:495–501.

64. Davenport J, Hart RG. Prosthetic valve endocarditis, 1976–1987. Antibiotics, anticoagulation, and stroke. Stroke 1990; 21:993–9.

65. Jault F, Gandjbakhch I, Chastre JC, et al. Prosthetic valve endocarditis with ring abscesses. Surgical management and long-term results. J Thorac Cardiovasc Surg 1993; 105:1106–13.

66. Delay D, Pellerin M, Carrier M, et al. Immediate and long-term results of valve replacement for native and prosthetic valve endocarditis. Ann Thorac Surg 2000; 70:1219–23.

67. Sabik J, Lytle BW, Blackstone EH, et al. Aortic root replacement with cryopreserved allograft for prosthetic valve endocarditis. Ann Thorac Surg 2002; 74:650–9.

68. Dossche KM, Defauw JJ, Ernst SM, et al. Allograft aortic root replacement in prosthetic aortic valve endocarditis: a review of 32 patients. Ann Thorac Surg 1997; 63:1644–9.

69. Hagl C, Galla JD, Lansman SL, et al. Replacing the ascending aorta and aortic valve for acute prosthetic valve endocarditis: is using prosthetic material contraindicated? Ann Thorac Surg 2002; 74:S1781–5.

14

Management of pregnant women who have had previous heart valve surgery

Dawn L Adamson and Roger JC Hall

Introduction

Managing the pregnant woman who has undergone previous cardiac surgery requires a multidisciplinary approach and close cooperation between cardiologists, obstetricians, obstetric physicians and obstetric anaesthetists. It is important that this joint antenatal care is carried out in collaboration with a high-risk pregnancy obstetric team. Women should be managed throughout their pregnancy so that all necessary areas of expertise are covered. This may require referral to a more specialised unit, which may be at a distance, but the inconvenience of this is outweighed by the advantages for the mother and baby. Pregnancy presents a specific set of problems when considering the management of an individual patient. Broadly these are:

- the effect of pregnancy on the maternal condition
- the effect of the maternal condition on the pregnancy
- what effects, if any, concurrent drug use may have on the fetus
- what effects the condition has on the timing and mode of delivery.

There is often a conflict between the interests of the mother and that of the fetus and, consequently, management decisions may be difficult.

The commonest problem in the developed world is managing a pregnancy in a woman who has a prosthetic valve. The outcome is usually satisfactory for the mother, although problems may develop, and most but not all babies do well. However, there is a small but significant incidence of severe maternal complication and death, and pregnancy is more risky than normal for the baby. The main aim of management is to minimise the occurrence of these problems, and treat them promptly if they occur (see Box 14.1).

> **Box 14.1** General considerations
>
> There are two patients, the mother and child, who may have competing medical interests
>
> These patients have complex problems
>
> About 80% of pregnancies will have a satisfactory outcome
>
> Anticoagulation remains the largest source of problems

Before pregnancy
Counselling

Many women of childbearing age have undergone previous valvular surgical intervention. It is imperative that these women are counselled prior to conception if at all possible so that they understand the risks both to themselves and the fetus of undergoing a pregnancy. This allows an informed decision as to whether they want to proceed with a pregnancy. Most women with prosthetic valves have more than adequate cardiovascular reserve to undergo pregnancy; however, if there is doubt, investigation with exercise testing and echocardiography are recommended prior to conception.

Areas of particular concern are women taking potentially teratogenic drugs, e.g. warfarin and ACE (angiotensin-converting enzyme) inhibitors, which are required for the ongoing well-being of the mother. Since there are no clinical trials and what data are available are often from animal studies, it is impossible to define the individual risk precisely.

However it is often possible to stop potentially harmful drugs that are not essential before conception (e.g. statins) or convert the woman to a safer alternative, e.g. changing an ACE inhibitor given for hypertension to a more acceptable alternative.

Although many women contemplating pregnancy who have had previous cardiac surgery for valve disease have adequate exercise tolerance to look after a child, and a life expectancy that is sufficiently long for them to expect to see the child grow up, there are a few who do not. This is an extremely delicate area to tackle in pre-pregnancy counselling, since the woman may not be completely aware of her true prognosis or prefer not to confront it.

Other difficult ethical problems arise which often do not have a 'correct' answer and these are outside the remit of this chapter. Just one example is the advisability of surrogacy when the mother may not be able to adequately look after a child and is unlikely to survive long enough to see the child grow up.

Choice of valve

There are no clear-cut answers as to the best valve for a woman of childbearing age. Many women choose tissue valves in the hope that they can avoid the potential complications of anticoagulation in pregnancy. This may be confounded particularly in patients with mitral prostheses, since they may still need anticoagulation because of atrial fibrillation and left atrial enlargement. The situation may change somewhat if the recent trend for surgical procedures to maintain sinus rhythm after valve surgery prove to be successful. If this is the case, then tissue valves will have an attraction since maintenance of sinus rhythm will reduce the need for anticoagulants. The other downside of tissue valves is their limited durability, with a second valve operation often being needed within a few years. Figures of 80% re-replacement have been suggested.[1,2] This risk may be worthwhile if pregnancy is likely within a short term, but may be questionable if the patient is known to have fertility problems already. This is increasingly an issue with older primagravidae. Although it was thought that pregnancy itself brings forward tissue valve failure,[2–4] more recent studies[1,5] have found no evidence of accelerated valve failure as a result of pregnancy. Thus, the high failure rate of tissue valves in this group of patients is likely to be mainly a function of their young age.

Over the last few decades, the Ross procedure (the patient's own pulmonary valve moved to the aortic position – i.e. a pulmonary autograft, and a tissue valve implanted in the pulmonary position) has been increasingly popular in some cardiac surgical centres for young patients requiring aortic valve replacement.[6] A recent prospective evaluation of pulmonary autografts in middle-aged patients (mean 37 years old) confirmed a significant reduction in 5-year major complications in patients having a pulmonary autograft compared with those who had a bioprosthetic valve.[7] To date, only limited data are available on the durability of pulmonary autografts in pregnant women. Two studies in a total of 55 pregnancies have found no evidence of pregnancy-related structural deterioration,[8,9] while a third found that pregnancy did not influence loss in aortic homografts.[1] At present, there are limited long-term data on the Ross procedure; however, if ongoing experience reflects early success, the Ross procedure may become the preferred valve operation of choice in young women requiring aortic valve surgery, particularly if they are contemplating pregnancy.

Contraception

It is important to discuss contraception with women following valve surgery so that, hopefully, subsequent pregnancy will be planned and thus will have less risk. Intrauterine contraceptive devices (IUCDs) are associated with a significant bleeding frequency (35%) in patients having undergone cardiac surgery, predominantly as a result of concomitant anticoagulant therapy.[10] There is also the concern that IUCDs may pose a risk for endocarditis and are therefore often avoided, although there is little or no evidence to support this view. Barrier methods are unreliable and the oral contraceptive pill is associated with the side-effects of fluid retention and hyperlipidaemia, contraindicating their use in women with pre-existing hypertension, thromboembolic disorders, cerebrovascular disease and coronary artery disease. A further contraindication to the oral contraceptive pill is the presence of more than one cardiac risk factor (smoking, diabetes, hypertension, hyperlipidaemia and obesity). More recently, the single-rod intrauterine contraception implant (Implanon) containing etonogestrel (i.e. progesterone-only) has gained favour, particularly for cardiac patients, as it is highly effective (some quote a greater efficacy than sterilisation). As yet, there have been no systematic studies of this method in patients who have had previous valve surgery but since it has none of the oestrogen side-effects and does not promote coagulation[11] in seems very suitable for this group of patients. Furthermore, as a subcutaneous implant, it avoids the possibility of vagal stimulation or possible bacteraemia that may occur when inserting a progesterone-only IUCD through the cervix and into the uterus.

Valve assessment before pregnancy (see Box 14.2)

If possible, valve function should be assessed clinically and by echocardiography before pregnancy or as early as possible in pregnancy. Often the cardiologist is presented with a *fait accompli*: the woman is already pregnant and her problems must be dealt with as they occur. If, however, a woman with deteriorating valve function or a developing new lesion presents before pregnancy, then it is sensible to consider correcting the valve situation before embarking on pregnancy. An elective valve operation in an otherwise-fit young woman usually has a very low risk. An emergency in an unwell woman with an advanced pregnancy has a high mortality for both mother and fetus. Recently, a group from Toronto, looking at nearly 600 pregnancies in women with many different cardiac conditions, found that primary cardiac events could be predicted by the presence of one or more of the following four risk factors: prior cardiac event or arrhythmia, baseline NYHA (New York Health Association) functional class II or below or the presence of cyanosis, left heart obstruction (mitral valve area <2 cm², aortic valve area <1.5 cm²) or peak outflow gradient >30 mmHg on echo and reduced left ventricular function (ejection fraction <40%).[12]

Outcome of pregnancy

The limited retrospective studies available show that women with a prosthetic heart valve have a higher rate of fetal morbidity and mortality than normal pregnancies. Some groups report an up to 23% miscarriage rate and the majority of these occurred in women on anticoagulant therapy.[13,14] Between 70 and 85% of pregnancies resulted in a baby who did well and there was no difference between those babies born to mothers with bioprosthetic valves compared with mechanical valves. The incidence of still-births ranged between 2 and 8%.[2,3,15]

Box 14.2 Before pregnancy

Pre-pregnancy counselling is important but often not possible

Ensure early discussions with the pregnant woman to plan management

Manage the patient with an experienced multidisciplinary team

Assess the patient as early as possible to establish baseline cardiovascular status

Identify risk factors for poor outcome for either mother or fetus

The possibility of pregnancy must be considered when deciding on the timing and type of valve surgery in young women

---

During pregnancy

Complications of previous valve surgery

The majority of women who have had previous valve surgery and become pregnant have had prior valve replacement. In worldwide terms, the majority of these patients originally had rheumatic fever and rheumatic valve lesions. Consequently, because rheumatic fever often involves multiple valves and in particular the mitral initially, followed by the aortic valve, such patients may have had previous mitral valve surgery and be developing an aortic lesion when they become pregnant. Patients who have prosthetic valves may have normal prosthetic function or have prosthetic valve dysfunction. Patients may also have impaired left ventricular function. Finally, those who have had a previous mitral valvotomy (operative or balloon) may have restenosis.

By far the most common and often extremely difficult problem is the question of how to manage anticoagulants during pregnancy.[16] This is discussed separately elsewhere (Chapter 15). Published data show that maternal thromboembolic events (TE) are worryingly common in pregnant women with prosthetic valves,[3,13] and these may be fatal. They tend to be associated with alteration of the anticoagulant regimen and tend to occur when heparin is used rather than when the patient is on oral anticoagulants. Serious bleeding may also be a problem, particularly while the mother is on heparin.

Prosthetic valve thrombosis

Mechanical valves are far more likely than tissue valves to thrombose in women of childbearing age,[1] and this complication is particularly likely when the prosthetic valve is in the mitral position. The St Jude Medical mechanical prosthesis, one of a new generation of bileaflet prosthetic valves, has a relatively low thrombogenicity compared with earlier monoleaflet disc valves, e.g. the Björk–Shiley valve. A group in Turkey reviewed 46 pregnancies in 32 women who had received such a valve.[14] A wide variety of anticoagulant regimens were employed, including uninterrupted warfarin, low molecular weight heparin, unfractionated heparin at the beginning and end of pregnancy, with warfarin the rest of the time. A small group (8 patients) stopped anticoagulation against medical advice. There were no maternal deaths. There was a high incidence of abortion (18 therapeutic and 8 spontaneous) and there were 20 live births. Eight patients stopped anticoagulation against medical advice and, although 7 had normal term deliveries, four (50%) developed prosthetic valve thrombosis in the postpartum period. This timing is not unexpected, as thromboembolism is highest in the puerperium and greatest in women who have undergone Caesarean section. One patient who was on heparin in the third trimester developed left atrial thrombus that resolved when warfarin was reintroduced. Overall, this modern type of valve showed a low level of thrombo-embolism events despite a wide range of different anticoagulation regimens; however, complete cessation of anticoagulants still carries a high risk of valve thrombosis.

Prosthetic valve thrombosis should be considered in patients with unexpected dyspnoea. Clinically, the normal metallic valve clicks are muffled or lost, reflecting a lack of normal closure of the valve, and there is often but not always a regurgitant murmur. Valves usually stick in a half-open (or half-closed) position, which is why they are not usually associated with sudden death. The patient may also develop new physical signs of a stenotic lesion. It is therefore important when booking such women for their antenatal care that they have a thorough clinical and echocardiographic cardiovascular examination in order both to identify problems early and to provide a baseline against which any changes can be assessed. This can be difficult, as the changes in the cardiovascular system in pregnancy mean new flow murmurs are heard and pre-existing murmurs are often more intense. Patients with valve thrombosis usually develop pulmonary oedema, and may be hypotensive and extremely unwell. Confirmation of valve thrombosis is obtained with both echo and colour flow Doppler and screening of valve motion with X-ray.

Treatment of valve thrombosis provides a management dilemma at the best of times and its occurrence in pregnancy is complicated by the potential for harming the baby while treating the mother. Thrombolysis is accepted as the treatment of choice for tricuspid valve thrombosis,[17] and there is increasing experience of successful outcomes when used to treat left-sided prosthetic valve thrombosis.[18] However, thrombolysis poses a high risk of retroplacental haemorrhage and may result in fetal loss. Emergency cardiac surgery is at least as risky for the baby and may also carry a substantial risk to the mother. Consequently, it is difficult to decide the right course of action. Every case is different, but in reality the risk for the fetus is much the same whether treatment is by thrombolysis or surgery, but in the opinion of the authors the risk to the mother is less with thrombolysis. However, there are no scientific data to favour one approach over another and the decision has to come down to individual clinical judgement and patient preference in the individual case.

Development of a new valve lesion in pregnancy

Most commonly, a patient with a previous mitral valve operation develops a new aortic lesion (usually stenosis). Many of these patients have moderate lesions and, with careful conservative management and with a well-managed labour involving minimal stress to the mother, the pregnancy will proceed normally and a vaginal delivery will be possible. In a few patients it may be decided that Caesarean section may be a better option.

If intervention on the valve is required before the baby can be delivered safely, then (if possible) a technique not involving cardiopulmonary bypass surgery should be employed. In addition, the simple measure of beta-blocking the patient with recurrent mitral stenosis will often be sufficient to get the patient through pregnancy. There is a theoretical risk of fetal growth retardation, but in the context of the higher risks of intervention, particularly if the valve does not look suitable for balloon valvuloplasty, these risks become insignificant. Mitral balloon valvuloplasty often produces good results,[19] and in some cases of aortic stenosis, if the valve is not severely calcified, balloon valvuloplasty is also feasible and may give enough relief to tide the patient through the pregnancy. It is possible to shield the baby effectively from any radiation involved by using lead aprons over the abdomen, and in some centres mitral balloon valvuloplasty has been performed under ultrasound guidance alone. If cardiopulmonary bypass is required, it may lead to fetal loss (see section Timing of Delivery).

Patients with regurgitant lesions generally have less problems than those with stenotic lesions during pregnancy, particularly since pregnant women are naturally vasodilated. They can frequently be managed conservatively. The value of bedrest should not be forgotten and vasodilators will improve the situation. In pregnancy, the vasodilator should if possible be with a drug other than an ACE inhibitor because of the potentially harmful effect of these agents on the fetus, and hydralazine is probably the best choice in most cases. Very occasionally, women require surgical correction of regurgitant lesions in pregnancy and this procedure will carry the usual risk for the fetus of cardiopulmonary bypass.

Prosthetic valve dysfunction

The commonest form of valve dysfunction is thrombosis, and this has been discussed above. A few patients develop increasing regurgitation during pregnancy. Infective endocarditis should be excluded; in its absence the situation is dealt with in exactly the same way as a leaking native valve. If endocarditis occurs, this is a very serious situation. If the infected valve is prosthetic, it is almost certain surgery will be required. Unless it is sufficiently late in pregnancy for the baby to be delivered either vaginally or by Caesarean section at the same time as dealing with the infected valve, the outlook for the fetus is poor, even with the best management.

Impaired left ventricular function

Some patients who have undergone previous valve surgery have impaired left ventricular (LV) function. This is one of the indicators that a pregnancy will be high risk; a large study of pregnancy in heart disease (not specifically post valve surgery) showed that an LV ejection of less than 40% carried a significantly increased chance of a complication during pregnancy although maternal mortality was very low.[12] However, many patients with LV function at this level will get through pregnancy safely. It is extremely difficult to set limits at which LV function is too poor for pregnancy to be safe. In reality, the functional status of the mother is far more important than the measured LV function. If a patient is limited significantly by cardiac symptoms before pregnancy, then the wisdom of proceeding with pregnancy has to be considered very carefully and the option of termination discussed. As usual, every case is different.

The mainstay of treatment is medical and, again, the benefits of resting the patient should not be underestimated. ACE inhibitors should be replaced by hydralazine and nitrates if at all possible. If the patient has a broad QRS or other evidence of dyssynchrony, then biventricular pacing to resynchronise the ventricles should be considered. There are no data on this approach as yet, but theoretically it has no major disadvantages and potentially has significant advantages for the patient.

In some patients with very poor ventricular function and intractable heart failure, termination of pregnancy may have to be considered (see Box 14.3).

> **Box 14.3** During pregnancy
>
> Despite earlier beliefs, pregnancy is probably not associated with increased deterioration in prosthetic tissue valves – accelerated degeneration is simply a function of the young age of this group
>
> Cardiopulmonary bypass is bad for the fetus (20%+ mortality)
>
> If possible, use approaches that avoid cardiopulmonary bypass
>
> Stenotic lesions are generally more of a problem than regurgitant lesions
>
> Valve thrombosis is the commonest major complication. It may occur after delivery and can often be treated successfully with thrombolysis
>
> Don't forget:
> - beta-blockers in recurrent MS, since slowing the rate can produce major benefits
> - the value of bedrest

Delivery

Timing of delivery

When complications occur during pregnancy, a common dilemma is when to deliver the baby. Furthermore, there is concern about the effect on the fetus of a valve procedure carried out on the mother. In general, with modern neonatal care, there is little advantage in allowing pregnancy to go beyond 32 weeks if the mother requires urgent surgery to deal with her cardiac problem. If a surgical approach involving cardiopulmonary bypass is needed to treat the mother, this leads to death of the fetus in about 20% of cases.[20] Therefore, it is preferable to either use a procedure not involving bypass, e.g. balloon valvuloplasty for recurrent mitral stenosis (MS), even if the conditions for the procedure are not perfect. Another strategy that may be very useful in extreme situations is to deliver the baby by Caesarean section and replace or repair the offending valve (natural or prosthetic) under the same anaesthetic once the baby is delivered.

Mode of delivery

For most cardiac conditions a normal vaginal delivery with good analgesia and a low threshold for forceps or vacuum assistance is the safest mode of delivery for the mother; it is associated with less blood loss, lower risk of venous thromboembolism and less rapid haemodynamic changes than occur with Caesarean section.[21] Patients with Marfan's syndrome, dilated aortic root or aortic aneurysm of any cause should be delivered electively by Caesarean section with cardiothoracic surgical cover in order to reduce the risk of aortic dissection as a result of blood pressure surges during the physical efforts of normal labour in case of acute aortic dissection. Women with a mechanical Björk–Shiley mitral valve prosthesis may be considered for elective Caesarean section to reduce the time off warfarin, since valve thrombosis is probably more likely with this type of valve than with more modern bileaflet valves. However, this indication is still debatable among cardiologists. Clearly, in patients where there is concern that delivery may be associated with deterioration in the maternal condition, the availability and coordination of experienced specialists to cover all aspects of care for both mother and baby is paramount. It must also be remembered that unwell mothers are often delivered prior to term, and therefore provision needs to be made for the availability of a neonatal cot. Furthermore, it is important to take into account the size of family a mother wants, as repeated Caesarean sections are associated with increased operative risks, particularly haemorrhage.[22] Whereas physicians often favour the Caesarean section because they assume there is more control of the situation, this often means all future pregnancies may require the same mode of delivery since vaginal birth after Caesarean (VBAC) is only successful in 75–85% of pregnancies and is associated with an increased risk of major complications.[23,24]

Endocarditis

Premature ruptures of membranes prior to the onset of labour, perineal laceration during vaginal delivery and bladder catheterisation for Caesarean section are all potential causes of bacteraemia, but despite this the incidence of endocarditis is very low and recommendations are made in the hope rather than the knowledge that they will benefit the mother and baby. The ESC guidelines state that prosthetic heart valves are an indication for antibiotic prophylaxis to cover delivery.[25] Obstetric textbooks[26] now go as far as to say that antibiotic prophylaxis at the time of delivery in patients with prosthetic valves is 'mandatory'. The current recommendations[25] are 2 g iv amoxicillin or ampicillin and 2.5 mg/kg iv gentamicin at the onset of labour or rupture of membranes with a further 1 g oral amoxicillin/ampicillin 6 hours later. For women who are allergic to penicillin, 1 g iv vancomycin plus 1.5 mg/Kg gentamicin can be substituted. Despite the lack of evidence, the catastrophic consequence of prosthetic valve endocarditis makes this the most reasonable approach in the presence of a prosthetic valve.

Box 14.4 Delivery

There is little to gain in maintaining the pregnancy beyond 32 weeks if the mother is becoming increasingly compromised

Under most circumstances, a normal vaginal delivery is the safest mode of delivery for the mother

Although evidence is lacking, antibiotic prophylaxis against endocarditis is recommended when the patient has a prosthetic valve

Remember that high-level input is needed at delivery and that an intensive care cot may be needed for the baby

---

Conclusion

An understanding of the effects of the haemodynamic changes of pregnancy on the valve lesion, and good communication and planning involving all team members and the mother, should lead to a successful pregnancy in most circumstances. This is an area of medicine that needs high-level input and must not be left to junior doctors.

References

1. North RA, Sadler L, Stewart AW, et al. Long-term survival and valve-related complications in young women with cardiac valve replacements. Circulation 1999; 99:2669–76.
2. Badduke BR, Jamieson WR, Miyagishima RT, et al. Pregnancy and childbearing in a population with biologic valvular prostheses. J Thorac Cardiovasc Surg 1991; 102(2):179–86.
3. Sbarouni E, Oakley CM. Outcome of pregnancy in women with valve prostheses. Br Heart J 1994; 71:196–201.
4. Vongpatanasin W, Hillis LD, Lange RA. Prosthetic heart valves. N Engl J Med 1996; 335(6):407–16.
5. Emir M, Uzunonat G, Yamak B, et al. Effects of pregnancy on long-term follow-up of mitral valve bioprostheses. Asian Cardiovasc Thorac Ann 1998; 6:174–8.
6. Ross D, Yacoub MH. Homograft replacement of the aortic valve, a critical review. Prog Cardiovasc Dis 1969; 11(4):275–93.
7. Concha M, Aranda PJ, Casares J, et al. Prospective evaluation of aortic valve replacement in young adults and middle-aged patients: mechanical prosthesis versus pulmonary autograft. J Heart Valve Dis 2005; 14(1):40–6.
8. Dore A, Sommerville J. Pregnancy in patients with pulmonary autograft valve replacement. Eur Heart J 1997; 18:1659–62.
9. Sadler L, McCowan L, White H, et al. Pregnancy outcomes and cardiac complications in women with mechanical, bioprosthetic and homografts valves. BJOG 2000; 107:245–53.
10. Abdalla MY, el Din Mostafa E. Contraception after heart surgery. Contraception 1992; 45(1):73–80.
11. Lindqvist PG, Rosing J, Malmquist A, Hillarp A. Etonogesterel implant use is not related to hypercoagulable changes in anticoagulant system. J Thromb Haemost 2003; 1(3):601–2.
12. Siu SC, Sermer M, Colman JM, et al; Cardiac Disease in Pregnancy (CARPREG) Investigators. Prospective multicenter study of pregnancy outcomes in women with heart disease. Circulation 2001; 104:515–21.
13. Hanania G, Thomas D, Michel PL, et al. Pregnancy and prosthetic heart valves: a French cooperative retrospective study of 155 cases. Eur Heart J 1994; 15(12):1651–8.
14. Vural KM, Ozatik MA, Uncu H, et al. Pregnancy after mechanical mitral valve replacement. J Heart Valve Dis 2003; 12(3):370–6.
15. Bhutta SZ, Aziz S, Korejo R. Pregnancy following cardiac surgery. J Pak Med Assoc 2003; 53(9):407–13.
16. Hanania G. Management of anticoagulants during pregnancy. Heart 2001; 86:125–6.
17. Shapira Y, Sagie A, Jortner R, Adler Y, Hirsch R. Thrombosis of bileaflet tricuspid valve prosthesis: clinical spectrum and the role of nonsurgical treatment. Am Heart J 1999; 137(4 Pt 1):721–5.
18. Birdi I, Angelini GD, Bryan AJ. Thrombolytic therapy for left sided prosthetic heart valve thrombosis. J Heart Valve Dis 1995; 4:154–9.
19. Fawzy ME, Kinsara AJ, Stefadorous M, et al. Long-term outcome of mitral balloon valvotomy in pregnant women. J Heart Valve Dis 2001; 10:153–7.
20. Pomini F, Mercogliani D, Calvetti C, et al. Cardiopulmonary bypass in pregnancy. Ann Thorac Surgery 2000; 61:259–68.
21. Thorne SA. Pregnancy in heart disease. Heart 2004; 90(4):450–6.
22. Makoha FW, Felimban HM, Fathuddien MA, Roomi F, Ghabra T. Multiple cesarean section morbidity. Int J Gynaecol Obstet 2004; 87(3):227–32.
23. Macones GA, Cahill A, Pare E, et al. Obstetric outcomes in women with two prior cesarean deliveries: is vaginal birth after cesarean delivery a viable option ? Am J Obstet Gynecol 2005; 192(4):1223–8.
24. Lieberman E, Ernst EK, Rooks JP, Stapleton S, Flamm B. Results of the national study of vaginal birth after cesarean in birth centres. Obstet Gynecol 2004; 104:933–42.
25. Horstkotte D, Follath F, Gutschik E, et al; Task Force Members on Infective Endocarditis of the European Society of Cardiology; ESC Committee for Practice Guidelines (CPG); Document Reviewers. Guidelines on prevention, diagnosis and treatment of infective endocarditis executive summary; the Task Force on Infective Endocarditis of the European Society of Cardiology. Eur Heart J 2004; 25(3):267–76.
26. Nelson-Piercy C. Handbook of obstetric medicine, 2nd edn. London: Martin Dunitz, 2002.

15

Anticoagulation during pregnancy

Christa Gohlke-Bärwolf and Roger JC Hall

The optimal management of anticoagulation during pregnancy has been and remains controversial. During pregnancy, vitamin K antagonists have been considered contraindicated by the manufacturers as well as by the majority of expert groups. The rationale for this contraindication is the fact that vitamin K antagonists cross the placenta and can lead to embryopathy and an increased risk of fetal haemorrhage.

Heparin has been proposed as an alternative anticoagulant. It has been assumed that it offers the same protection for the mother as oral anticoagulants during pregnancy. This assumption has not been evaluated in any randomised controlled study, but observational studies suggest that this is not the case.[1–4]

Because pregnancy induces a series of haemostatic changes, with an increased concentration of coagulation factors, fibrinogen and platelet adhesiveness as well as diminished fibrinolysis, hypercoagulability and an increased risk of thromboembolic events are associated with it.[5] In addition, obstruction to venous return by the enlarging uterus leads to stasis and further increases the risk for venous thrombosis and pulmonary emboli. This relative prothrombotic state represents a higher risk for women with pre-existing thrombophilia and for women who already have an indication for anticoagulation in the non-pregnant state, such as women with prosthetic heart valves.

In addition to the medical problems associated with anticoagulation during pregnancy, this therapy raises psychological, emotional and forensic issues. The mother's safety must be weighed against that of the fetus. Pregnant patients with prosthetic heart valves have a much higher risk of valve thrombosis, arterial embolism and mortality during their pregnancy if the anticoagulation regimen employed is less effective than their usual anticoagulation.

Because there are no randomised controlled studies available, there are no universally accepted guidelines on the management of anticoagulation during pregnancy; in fact, the presently available guidelines differ in their recommendations.[6–8] The information available comes from retrospective analyses of treatment series and case reports. The statements by the manufacturers and the majority of expert groups that oral anticoagulants are contraindicated during pregnancy due to possible embryopathy considers the child's safety more important than the safety of the mother. Four different anticoagulation therapy regimens have been recommended in the literature:.[3,9,10]

1. Heparin during the whole pregnancy.
2. Heparin during the first trimester, followed by oral anticoagulation up to the 36th week of pregnancy, with subsequent replacement by heparin. The dose of heparin is controlled by the activated partial thromboplastin time (aPTT), with the target of >1.5 times the control valve.
3. Oral anticoagulants throughout pregnancy up to the 36th week, followed by heparin until birth or delivery by programmed Caesarean section at the 38th week, controlled by aPTT.
4. Low molecular weight heparin (LMWH) throughout pregnancy.

Heparin therapy

Heparin has the advantage of not crossing the placenta and therefore does not cause teratogenicity or embryopathy. However, it can lead to retroplacental bleeding and thereby to abortions, premature birth and stillbirth. Furthermore, it causes an increased risk of maternal bleeding. A further problem is that of laboratory control, together with uncertainty about optimal dose. Heparin is relatively less effective during pregnancy as a result of increased protein binding and increased neutralisation by platelet factor 4, levels of which are elevated during pregnancy. Inadequate heparin therapy thus leads to a higher rate of thromboembolic complications in comparison to warfarin.

There are also uncertainties concerning the aPTT itself as a measure of heparin activity during pregnancy. The aPTT reagents commercially available vary in their sensitivity towards heparin and the concentration of the clotting factors increases during pregnancy. During the 3rd trimester there is a discrepancy between heparin concentration and the aPTT, as shown by simultaneous measurement of the aPTT and anti-factor Xa activity.[11] Consequently, an aPTT ratio of >2 times the control valve is necessary in order to achieve a sufficiently high heparin concentration of >0.55 Xa units in 90% of patients.[12] Hence, a ratio of >2 as a target aPTT has been recommended during pregnancy,[13] but not prospectively evaluated. A safer approach would be to assess the anti-factor Xa activity to guide heparin therapy during pregnancy.[14]

Because of the short half-life of unfractionated heparins and the variable bioavailability, subcutaneous injections three times a day and laboratory controls are necessary. Close control of the aPTT or anti-factor Xa activity and an augmentation of the dose in the second half of pregnancy is required, because of the increasing concentration of the clotting factors and platelet activity in the uteroplacental circulation.[5]

Long-term therapy with heparin is associated with a 2–3% risk of osteoporosis with spontaneous fractures[15] as well as the risk of thrombocytopenia in about 3% of patients.[16] Thrombocytopenia with paradoxical thrombosis is an uncommon but potentially dangerous complication of heparin therapy.[17]

Low molecular weight heparin

As a result of problems associated with oral anticoagulants and unfractionated heparins, LMWH was initially considered as an alternative anticoagulant.[18] LMWH does not cross the placenta and therefore does not directly affect the fetal clotting system.[19] However, in animal experiments a prolongation of the fetal aPTT was found, even though the LMWH did not cross the placenta. It was assumed that endogenous substances similar to dermatan were induced. The longer half-life allows a reduction in subcutaneous injections, and the greater bioavailability allows a more stable form of anticoagulation. Furthermore, thrombocytopenia and osteoporosis occur rarely. A disadvantage is that LMWH is less sensitive to reversal with protamine. Because of the longer half-life, this may be a problem prior to delivery, if labour starts while the patient is still under therapeutic heparinisation. LMWH has not been approved in any country for anticoagulation during pregnancy.

No large experience in patients with mechanical heart valve prostheses is available yet. There are single favourable case reports,[20,21] but several reports of valve thromboses in patients treated with LMWH.[22–27] In a recent review of 81 pregnancies in 75 patients with mechanical valves prostheses treated with LMWH a total maternal thromboembolic rate of 12.3% was found (valve thrombosis 8.61%, stroke 2.5%, peripheral emboli 1.2%). The fetal complications rate was 8.6%.[27a]

During pregnancy there is an increase in dose requirement.[27b] The therapeutic dose required during pregnancy is still unclear and safe anti-Xa activity levels have not been determined yet. The therapeutic dose required during pregnancy is still unclear. Controlled studies, randomised against oral anticoagulants, are necessary, with accurate monitoring of the intensity of anticoagulation, measured with the anti-factor Xa activity.

Because of concern about cases of valve thrombosis, the US Food and Drug Administration (FDA) Safety Information and Adverse Event Reporting Program issued a warning not to use LMWH in patients with prosthetic heart valves.

Oral anticoagulant therapy

The main risk of all oral anticoagulants is the development of an embryopathy that was described in detail in 1975.[28,29] The critical time of exposure for the fetus is in the 6th–9th week of pregnancy.[30,31] Oral anticoagulants cross the placenta and exert a profound effect on the relatively immature liver. The embryopathy is caused by bleeding into the developing cartilage and by an interference with calcium metabolism, leading to retarded growth of long bones and nasal hypoplasia.

The reported incidence of embryopathy ranges from 0%[4,32–35] through 4–6%[36,37] to 30%,[20,30] and is associated with high intensities of anticoagulation and warfarin doses over 5 mg/day.[35,38] There is also a 3% risk of fetal central nervous system abnormalities, including intracerebral haemorrhage and microcephaly.[30] At the time of delivery, the international normalised ratio (INR) of the umbilical cord blood is higher than the mother's INR when warfarin is discontinued 2 days before.[38] The fetus or neonate may remain anticoagulated 8–10 days after discontinuation of the oral anticoagulant.

Comparison of different anticoagulation regimens

Fetal and maternal risks associated with the different anticoagulation regimens are shown in Boxes 15.1 and 15.2.[1,4,36,37]

Valve thrombosis during pregnancy is associated with a mortality of 40%.[4] Patients with mechanical valve prostheses in the mitral position have a particularly high risk of valve thrombosis and thromboembolism with heparin therapy.

Box 15.1 Fetal complications in % (*n*) with different anticoagulation regimens

Regimen	Spontaneous abortions	Embryopathy	Fetal death or spontaneous abortion
1. UF heparin total	23.8 (5/21)	0.0 (0/17)	42.9 (9/21)
2. UF heparin 1st trimester	24.8 (57/230)	3.4 (6/174)	26.5 (61/230)
3. OAC total	24.7 (196/792)	6.4 (35/549)	33.6 (266/792)

UF = unfractionated, total = during whole pregnancy, OAC = oral anticoagulation.

Box 15.2 Maternal complications in % (*n*), with different anticoagulation regimens

Regimen	Thromboembolic complications	Death
1. UF heparin total	33.3 (7/21)	15.0 (3/20)
2. UF heparin 1st trimester	9.2 (57/230)	4.2 (7/167)
3. OAC total	3.9 (31/788)	1.8 (10/561)

UF = unfractionated, total = during whole pregnancy, OAC = oral anticoagulation.

Anticoagulation recommendations

Oral anticoagulants applied throughout pregnancy provide the greatest protection against valve thromboses and thromboembolism, which are the most frequent causes of maternal mortality. Therefore, this regimen is recommended. If the daily dose of warfarin required to achieve a therapeutic INR of 2.5–3.0 is not more than 5 mg, this regimen should be used up to the 36th week of pregnancy. If the patient who needs higher doses of warfarin opts for heparin to avoid embryopathy after having been informed in detail about her own increased risk, heparin should be given only for the first 12 weeks under strict aPTT control, prolonged to twice normal. Thereafter, oral anticoagulants should be resumed. From the 36th week of pregnancy, treatment should be changed to heparin under hospital conditions, because premature birth often occurs among these patients. Heparin should be discontinued at the onset of labour. Four to six hours after delivery, heparin therapy can be restarted. After 24 hours, oral anticoagulation may be resumed.[39,40]

If labour occurs preterm while the patient is still on oral anticoagulants, a Caesarean section should be performed after reducing the INR to 2.0 or less. A vaginal delivery should be avoided under oral anticoagulation because of the danger of fetal intracranial bleeding.

Mode of delivery

Other than issues relating to anticoagulation management, discussed above, choice of the mode of delivery is an area in which close collaboration is required between the cardiologist, obstetrician and obstetric anaesthetist. In the past many cardiologists recommended Caesarean section under general anaesthesia for patients with any significant haemodynamic compromise. This was on the basis that most patients with cardiac problems can usually withstand general anaesthesia without difficulty. Although this approach may sometimes be taken nowadays, advances in anaesthetic techniques mean that a specialist obstetric anaesthetist can produce extremely stable circulatory conditions using modern techniques of epidural and spinal anaesthesia to assist vaginal delivery. In a recent survey from South Africa of 59 pregnancies in 38 women with prosthetic valves, all but 6 deliveries were vaginal.[41]

Breast-feeding and anticoagulation

Unfractionated and low molecular weight heparins are not excreted in the breast milk and thus present no problem for breast-feeding.[42] Oral anticoagulants are excreted in the milk but in clinically non-significant amounts and as inactive metabolites. They can therefore also be taken during breast-feeding.[43]

References

1. Hanania G, Thomas D, Michel PL, et al. Pregnancy and prosthetic heart valves: a French cooperative retrospective study of 155 cases. Eur Heart J 1994; 15:1651–8.

2. Hanania G. Management of anticoagulants during pregnancy. Heart 2001; 86:125–6.

3. Salazar E, Izaguirre R, Verdejo J, Mutchinick O. Failure of adjusted doses of subcutaneous heparin to prevent thromboembolic phenomena in pregnant patients with mechanical cardiac valve prostheses. J Am Coll Cardiol 1996; 27:1698–703.

4. Sbarouni E, Oakley CM. Outcome of pregnancy in women with valve prostheses. Br Heart J 1994; 71:196–201.

5. Bonnar J. Haemostasis and coagulation disorders in pregnancy. In: Bloom AL, Thomas DP, eds. Haemostasis and thrombosis. London: Churchill Livingstone, 1994: 570–83.

6. Gohlke-Bärwolf C, Acar J, Oakley CM, et al. Guidelines for prevention of thromboembolic events in valvular heart disease. Eur Heart J 1995; 16:1320–30.

7. Bonow RO, Carabello B, De Leon AC, et al. ACC/AHA guidelines for the management of patients with valvular heart disease. J Am Coll Cardiol 1998; 32:1486–588.

8. Bates S, Greer I, Hirsh J, Ginsberg J. Use of antithrombotic agents during pregnancy; The Seventh ACCP Conference on Antithrombotic and Thrombolytic Therapy. Chest 2004; 126:627–44S.

9. Iturbe-Alessio I, Fonseca MC, Mutchinik O, et al. Pregnant women with artificial heart valves. N Engl J Med 1986; 315:1390–3.

10. Oakley CM. Anticoagulants in pregnancy. Br Heart J 1995; 74:107–11.

11. Brancazio LR, Roperti KA, Stierer R, et al. Pharmacokinetics and pharmacodynamics of subcutaneous heparin during the early third trimester of pregnancy. Am J Obstet Gynecol 1995; 173:1240–5.

12. McGehee W. Anticoagulation in pregnancy. In: Elkayam U, Gleicher N, eds. Cardiac problems in pregnancy, 3rd edn. New York: Wiley-Liss, 1998: 407–17.

13. Ginsberg JS, Greer I, Hirsh J. Use of antithrombotic agents during pregnancy. Chest 1998; 114(Suppl):S524–30.

14. Elkayam U. Pregnancy through a prosthetic heart valve. J Am Coll Cardiol 1999; 33:1642–5.

15. Barbour LA, Kick SD, Steiner JF, et al. A prospective study of heparin-induced osteoporosis in pregnancy using bone densitometry. Am J Obstet Gynecol 1994; 170:862–9.

16. Warkentin TE, Levine MN, Hirsh J, et al. Heparin-induced thrombocytopenia in patients treated with low-molecular weight heparin or unfractionated heparin. N Engl J Med 1995; 332:1330–5.

17. Cimo PL, Moake JL, Weinger RS, et al. Heparin-induced thrombocytopenia associated with platelet aggregating antibodies and arterial thrombosis. Am J Hematol 1979; 6:125–33.

18. Messmore H, Kundur R, Wehrmacher W, et al. Anticoagulant therapy of pregnant patients with prosthetic heart valves: rationale for a clinical trial of low molecular weight heparin. Clin Appl Thromb Hemost 1999; 5:73–7.

19. Omri A, Delaloye JF, Anderson H, Bachmann F. Low molecular weight heparin Novo (LHN-1) does not cross the placenta during the second trimester of pregnancy. Thromb Haemost 1989; 61:55–6.

20. Lee LH, Liauw PCY, Ng AS. Low molecular weight heparin for thromboprophylaxis during pregnancy in 2 patients with mechanical mitral heart valve replacement. Thromb Haemost 1996; 76:628–30.

21. Lindhoff-Last E, Schinzel H, Erbe M, et al. Antikoagulation in der Schwangerschaft bei mechanischem Herzklappenersatz. Z Kardiol 2001; 90(Suppl 6):125–30.

22. Idir M, Madonna F, Roudaut R. Collapse and massive pulmonary edema secondary to thrombosis of a mitral mechanical heart valve prosthesis during low molecular weight heparin therapy. J Heart Valve Dis 1999; 8:303–4.

23. Lev-Ran O, Kramer A, Gurevitch J, et al. Low-molecular-weight heparin for prosthetic heart valves: treatment failure. Ann Thorac Surg 2000; 69:264–6.

24. Anbarasan C, Kumar VS, Latchumanadhas K, et al. Successful thrombolysis of prosthetic mitral valve thrombosis in early pregnancy. J Heart Valve Dis 2001; 10:393–5.

25. Leyh RG, Fischer S, Ruhparwar A, et al. Antikoagulation bei schwangeren Frauen nach künstlichem Herzklappenersatz: Ist niedermolelulares Heparin eine alternative? Z Kardiol 2002; 91:297–303.

26. Behrendt P, Schwartzkopff B, Perings S, et al. Successful thrombolysis of St. Jude medical aortic prosthesis with tissue-type plasminogen activator in a pregnant woman: a case report. Cardiol Rev 2002; 10:349–53.

27. Mahesh B, Evans S, Bryan AJ. Failure of low-molecular-weight heparin in the prevention of prosthetic mitral valve thrombosis during pregnancy: case report and a review of options for anticoagulation. J Heart Valve Dis 2002; 11:745–50.

27a. Oran B, Lee-Parritz A, Ansell J. Low molecular weight heparin for the prophylaxis of thromboembolism in women with prosthetic mechanical heart valves during pregnancy. Thromb Haemost 2004; 92(4):747–51.

27b. Barbour LA, Oja JL, Schultz LK. A prospective trial that demonstrates that dalteparin requirements increase in pregnancy to maintain therapeutic levels of anticoagulation. Am J Obstet Gynecol 2004; 191(3):1024–9.

28. Pettifor JM, Benson R. Congenital malformations associated with administration of oral anticoagulants during pregnancy. J Pediatr 1975; 86:459–62.

29. Shaul WL, Emery H, Hall JG. Chondrodysplasia punctata and maternal warfarin use during pregnancy. Am J Dis Child 1975; 129:360–2.

30. Hall JG, Pauli RM, Wilson KM. Maternal and fetal sequelae of anticoagulation during pregnancy. Am J Med 1980; 68:122–40.

31. Pauli RM. Mechanism of bone and cartilage maldevelopment in the warfarin embryopathy. Pathol Immunopathol Res 1988; 7:107–12.

32. Ben Ismail M, Abid F, Trabeisi S, et al. Cardiac valve prostheses, anticoagulation and pregnancy. Br Heart J 1986; 55:101–5.

33. Chen WWC, Chan CS, Lee PK, et al. Pregnancy in patients with prosthetic heart valves: an experience with 45 pregnancies. Q J Med 1982; 51:358–65.

34. Pavankumar P, Venugopal P, Kaul U, et al. Pregnancy in patients with prosthetic cardiac valves. A 10-year experience. Scand J Thorac Cardiovasc Surg 1988; 22:19–22.

35. Vitale N, De Feo M, De Sant LS, et al. Dose-dependent fetal complications of warfarin in pregnant women with mechanical heart valves. J Am Coll Cardiol 1999; 33:1637–41.

36. Chan WS, Anand S, Ginsberg JS. Anticoagulation of pregnant women with mechanical heart valves. A systematic review of the literature. Arch Intern Med 2000; 160:191–6.

37. Meschengiesser SS, Fondevila CG, Santarelli MT, et al. Anticoagulation in pregnant women with mechanical heart valve prostheses. Heart 1999; 82:23–6.

38. Cotrufo M, de Luca TSL, Calabro R, et al. Coumarin anticoagulation during pregnancy in patients with mechanical valve prostheses. Eur J Cardiothorac Surg 1991; 3:300–5.

39. Gohlke-Bärwolf C. Aktuelle Empfehlungen zur thromboembolieprophylaxe bei Herzklappenprothesen. Z Kardiol 2001; 90(Suppl 6)112–17.

40. Butchart EG, Gohlke-Barwolf C, Antunes MJ, et al. Recommendations for the management of patients after heart valve surgery. Eur Heart J 2005; 26:2463–71.

41. Hall FDR, Oliver J, Rossouw GJ, et al. Pregnancy outcome in women with prosthetic valves. J Obst Gynaecol 2001; 21:149–53.

42. Greer IA. Thrombosis in pregnancy: maternal and fetal issues. Lancet 1999; 353:1258–65.

43. McKenna R, Cale ER, Vasan U. Is warfarin sodium contraindicated in the lactating mother? J Pediatr 1983; 103:325–7.

16

Management during non-cardiac surgery

Bernard D Prendergast and Pilar Tornos

Introduction

Patients with prosthetic heart valves undergoing non-cardiac surgery share the risks of all patients with cardiac disease and are also threatened by the hazards of infective endocarditis, increased bleeding risk and the possibility of acute/subacute valve thrombosis or systemic thromboembolism associated with any interruption in anticoagulation. This chapter addresses these general issues briefly but focuses specifically on anticoagulant treatment in this difficult area.

General measures

The general principles of management broadly follow those of all patients with cardiovascular disease undergoing noncardiac surgery (Table 16.1). Preprocedural cardiac assessment should be undertaken in a centre with appropriate facilities and expertise. Operative risks are principally governed by underlying left ventricular function and the presence or absence of coronary artery disease. This

---

Table 16.1 Preprocedural checklist for patients with prosthetic valves undergoing non-cardiac surgery

Recent cardiological and/or echocardiographic assessment:
  Prosthetic valve function?
  Left ventricular function?
  Coronary artery disease?
  Rhythm management?
Preprocedural transthoracic echocardiography if high thromboembolic risk
Infective endocarditis prophylaxis
Withdrawal of antiplatelet therapy
Perioperative anticoagulant regimen

---

information is usually readily available from previous documentation and update echocardiography or coronary angiography are not routinely required. However, preprocedural echocardiography is strongly recommended to guide management in those patients at high thromboembolic risk (see below) in whom special measures may be necessary and transoesophageal imaging may be required in patients with an abnormal transthoracic study. Patients taking aspirin, or alternative antiplatelet agents, should discontinue this treatment 1 week before the procedure and restart it when bleeding risk ceases. An exception applies in patients with a recently implanted coronary stent in whom withdrawal of antiplatelet therapy may result in stent thrombosis. Management is difficult in this situation and should be determined after multidisciplinary discussion. Patients with prosthetic valves are at high risk of infective endocarditis and require appropriate pre- and perioperative prophylactic antibiotic regimens (see Chapters 11 and 12). Instrumentation should be reduced to the minimum necessary in order to reduce systemic bacteraemia. Similarly, intramuscular injections and unnecessary traumatic medical procedures, e.g. urethral catheterisation and central line insertion, should be avoided in anticoagulated patients.

A detailed discussion of general perioperative haemodynamic management is beyond the scope of this chapter. Perioperative risk of ischaemic events in patients with coronary artery disease is reduced by beta-blockade[1,2] and best assessed using dobutamine stress echocardiography.[3] Special attention should be paid to fluid balance, particularly in those with left ventricular impairment.

Patients with prosthetic valves who require major surgical treatment or surgery for major trauma (e.g. fracture of the femoral neck) should ideally be managed in a major centre equipped for cardiology and cardiac surgery, which not only permits experienced anticoagulation management, cardiological advice and echocardiographic surveillance but also provides the necessary facilities if there are postoperative cardiac complications. In patients with impaired cardiac function who are on multiple medications, the involvement of an anaesthetist skilled in cardiac anaesthesia should be sought, together with the availability

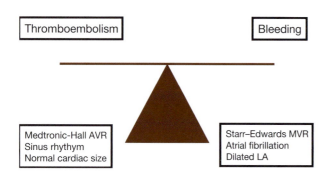

Figure 16.1
The balance of risk and benefit requires careful clinical evaluation in all patients for whom anticoagulation is considered. Patients with mechanical prosthetic valves require oral anticoagulation, although thromboembolic risks vary according to the type of prosthesis, its position and other clinical variables (see text for details). AVR = aortic valve replacement, MVR = mitral valve replacement, LA = left atrium.

of postoperative ITU (intensive therapy unit) care if required.

Patients with bioprosthetic valves require no special precautions other than those described above. In the small minority of patients who require anticoagulation for other reasons, e.g. coexistent atrial fibrillation or left ventricular impairment, management should adhere to the recommendations below.

Perioperative anticoagulation

International guidelines[4,5] and a series of scientific statements[6–10] provide a basis for anticoagulant management in patients with prosthetic valves undergoing non-cardiac surgery but are centred on clinical judgement and common sense rather than robust clinical evidence.[11] In any patient requiring anticoagulant treatment, the risk of increased bleeding during a procedure has to be weighed against the increased risk of thromboembolism caused by stopping the therapy (Figure 16.1). Thromboembolic risk for patients with prosthetic valves without anticoagulation has been estimated at 8–22% per annum (equivalent to 0.02–0.06% per day).[12] Theoretically, therefore, withdrawal of anticoagulation to allow a surgical procedure with a subtherapeutic international normalised ratio (INR) for 4–6 days exposes the patient to a thromboembolic risk of approximately 0.08–0.36%.

Current perioperative anticoagulation regimens for patients with prosthetic heart valves undergoing non-cardiac surgery are effective, but in practice there is little consensus as to their application. Consequently, perioperative

anticoagulation is often haphazard and retrospective reviews have demonstrated that mortality and morbidity remain high.[13] In the limited clinical studies on non-cardiac surgery in patients with mechanical valves, the incidence of thromboembolic events (manifesting as valve thrombosis and failure, cerebral ischaemia or infarction, or more peripheral embolism) varied between 0–2% in patients with aortic valve replacements and 11–20% in those with mitral valve replacements.[5,12,13] In one institutional review of 235 consecutive patients with mechanical prosthetic valves undergoing non-cardiac surgery using a variety of anticoagulant regimens,[13] in-hospital mortality was 2.9%. Thromboembolism occurred up to 1 month following surgery, affecting 7% and was more frequent in patients in atrial fibrillation with a mitral prosthesis. The rate of significant haemorrhage was 8%. Approximately 20% of major thromboembolic episodes are fatal and 40% result in major disability. A small proportion (3%) of episodes of major postoperative bleeding are fatal, but most patients make a full recovery, despite the need for

Table 16.2 Thromboembolic risk assessment for non-cardiac surgical procedures

Procedure	Low risk	High risk
Clinical factors		
Atrial fibrillation		+
Previous thromboembolism		+
Hypercoagulable condition		+
Left ventricular dysfunction		+
>3 thromboembolic risk factors[a]		+
Prosthesis design		
Ball valve		+
Tilting disc	+	
Bileaflet	+	
Prosthesis position		
Mitral		+
Aortic	+	
Procedure		
Dental, ophthalmic	+	
Skin	+	
Gastrointestinal		+
Pathology		
Malignancy		+
Infection		+

[a]Risk factors for thromboembolism: hypertension, atrial fibrillation, diabetes mellitus, previous thromboembolism, hypercoagulable condition, left ventricular impairment, left atrial enlargement, mitral stenosis and documented left atrial/left ventricular thrombus.

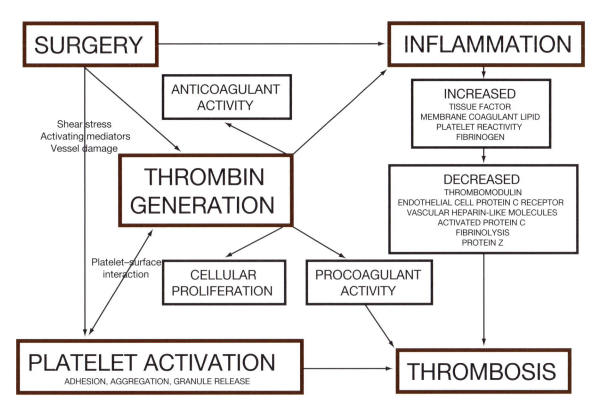

Figure 16.2
Mechanisms underlying the prothrombotic effects of surgery.

reoperation in as many as 50%. Rarely (about 1.5%), episodes of major postoperative bleeding result in permanent disability.[14]

Risk assessment

Overall, thromboembolic risk is governed by a number of clinical characteristics (Table 16.2) including not only the type and position of the prosthesis but also the presence of left ventricular impairment and atrial fibrillation, the procedure undertaken and the underlying pathology, and the innate susceptibility to thrombosis.[15–17] The chosen perioperative anticoagulant regimen should be tailored to the individual patient, this assessment being based on thromboembolic risk, the duration of lowered anticoagulant levels and the risk of haemorrhage conferred by the procedure. Haemostatic mechanisms are disrupted during and after surgery, with increased platelet aggregation and activation, conversion of fibrinogen to fibrin and depressed fibrinolysis, thereby increasing thromboembolic risk (Figure 16.2). Prothrombotic tendency correlates with the magnitude and duration of surgery, the presence of complications (e.g. infection) and underlying pathology (e.g. malignancy).[18] Interruption of anticoagulation is

Table 16.3 Surgical procedures which may be undertaken with relative safety under continued oral anticoagulation (selected procedures only)

Dental surgery
Minor dermatological procedures
Ophthalmic surgery
   Trabeculectomy
   Vitreoretinal surgery
   Cataract extraction
Cardiac catheterisation
Balloon mitral valvuloplasty
Upper and lower gastrointestinal endoscopy
Transurethral resection of the prostate
Abdominal surgery (unless exposed raw surfaces)

clearly an important additional factor in the genesis of thromboembolism, particularly since a period of rebound hypercoagulability occurs after withdrawal of oral anticoagulation; this may be compounded by substitution with heparin, which has platelet proaggregatory effects.[19,20] In many cases, subsequent valve thrombosis may develop slowly and insidiously and may not become clinically

Table 16.4 Anticoagulation recommendations before diagnostic and surgical procedures (see text for details)

Procedure	INR
Dental surgery	<4.5
Left heart catheterisation	
Percutaneous femoral/brachial approach	<2.0
Percutaneous radial approach	<4.0
Brachial arteriotomy	<2.5
Trans-septal puncture/pericardiocentesis	<1.2
Replace with heparin when INR:	<2.5 (high risk)
	<2.0 (low risk)
Percutaneous balloon mitral valvuloplasty	<2.0
Minor surgical procedure	<2.0
Major surgical procedure	<1.5
Replace with heparin when INR:	<2.5 (high risk)
	<2.0 (low risk)

INR = international normalised ratio.

apparent for several months, especially in patients with tilting-disc prostheses.[15] Careful follow-up with a high index of clinical suspicion for symptoms suggestive of valve thrombosis is therefore necessary in this setting and seamless anticoagulation using continued oral anticoagulation is preferred whenever possible.

The risks and consequences of significant haemorrhagic complications related to non-cardiac surgery vary, but are more severe in the presence of large raw surfaces and when the procedure is a major one. Older small studies have demonstrated that minor surgery, including some abdominal procedures,[21] dental[22] and ophthalmic surgery,[23] and even transurethral resection of the prostate,[24] may be performed under continued anticoagulation (Table 16.3), but similar data in patients undergoing more major surgery are unavailable. The following guidelines are therefore applicable (Table 16.4).

Dental surgery

Dental surgery has a low risk of thromboembolic complications and in a recent review of 2014 procedures, thromboembolism occurred in 5 (0.9%) of 493 patients in whom

Perclose

Duett

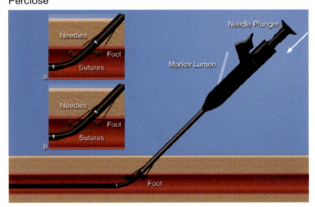

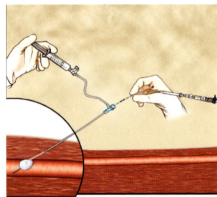

Angioseal

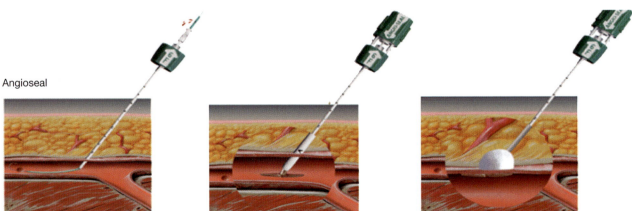

Figure 16.3
Percutaneous closure devices employed following cardiac catheterisation via femoral arterial puncture.

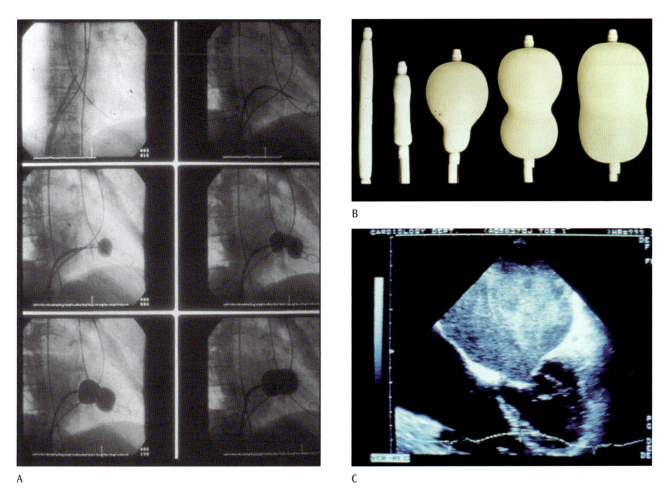

A   C

Figure 16.4
Percutaneous balloon mitral valvuloplasty performed via an antegrade approach using the femoral vein and interatrial septal puncture (A) with the Inoue balloon (B). Left atrial dilatation and haemostasis in mitral stenosis (C) increase the risk of thromboembolism during the procedure and many experienced operators recommend continued oral periprocedural anticoagulation despite the risks of trans-septal puncture.

anticoagulation was discontinued at the time of surgery and proved fatal in 4. In contrast, continued anticoagulation proved safe in 774 patients, with a 1.6% incidence of bleeding complications (all of which occurred with an INR >4.5).[25]

Dental surgery therefore does not require major alteration in the intensity of anticoagulation. Even complete dental extractions have a low risk of bleeding, which can be easily treated using local measures supplemented by tranexamic acid mouthwash if necessary.[26] Continued oral anticoagulation with an INR <4.5 on the day of the procedure is recommended as the safest approach, and heparin is not required.

Cardiac catheterisation

Oral anticoagulation can be continued at modified doses in the majority of patients. Percutaneous puncture of the femoral or brachial arteries to allow left heart catheterisation is safe with an INR <2.0. Experienced investigators may proceed with catheterisation via the femoral approach if the INR exceeds this threshold and employ a percutaneous closure device at the end of the procedure (Figure 16.3). Alternatively, recent experience suggests that percutaneous access via the radial artery is safe in the fully anticoagulated patient (INR <4.0),[27] and this approach may be adopted if appropriate expertise is available. Catheterisation via the brachial approach using surgical cutdown and arteriotomy under direct vision is safe with an INR <2.5.

In the rare patient who requires trans-septal catheterisation, direct left ventricular puncture or pericardiocentesis, the INR should be less than 1.2. Patients at high risk of thromboembolism should receive intravenous heparin when the INR is <2.5 in high-risk patients and <2.0 in those at lower risk (Table 16.2). Heparin may then be discontinued 6 hours before the procedure and recommenced 6 hours after its completion (see section on Major Surgical Procedures). An exception is the patient with mitral stenosis requiring trans-septal catheterisation to allow percutaneous balloon mitral valvuloplasty when left atrial stasis increases thromboembolic risk (Figure 16.4). Many investigators with considerable experience of the procedure recommend continued oral anticoagulation with a threshold INR <2.0, supplemented by a bolus of 5000 IU heparin immediately after trans-septal puncture.

Minor surgical procedures

Anticoagulation should not be stopped for procedures in which bleeding is unlikely or inconsequential (Table 16.3), e.g. minor dermatological procedures or selected eye surgery, including trabeculectomy, vitreoretinal surgery and cataract extraction (bleeding risk is higher following complex lid, lacrimal and orbital surgery).[28] Other minor surgical procedures, including upper and lower gastrointestinal endoscopy, can be performed while the INR is around 2.0, and oral anticoagulation can be resumed on the day of surgery.

Major surgical procedures

With careful technique and modern surgical management, many major surgical procedures can be performed safely while oral anticoagulation is continued. When this approach is deemed inappropriate, current guidelines[4,5,18,29] recommend that major surgical procedures require withdrawal of oral anticoagulation 72 hours (or more for agents with long half-lives) before surgery to lower the INR to <1.5 and maintain anticoagulation with unfractionated heparin (Figure 16.4). Heparin should be started when the INR is <2.5 in high-risk patients and <2.0 in those at lower risk (Table 16.2). The activated partial thromboplastin time (aPPT) should be maintained at 1.5–2.0 times the control value. Falls in platelet count associated with unfractionated heparin are usually transient and occur within the first few days of treatment. Life-threatening thrombocytopenia is rare. Heparin should be discontinued 6 hours before surgery and resumed 6 hours after, when surgically feasible, until the INR is >2.5 in high-risk patients and >2.0 in those at lower risk. Oral anticoagulation should be resumed as soon as possible and, if feasible, on the day of the procedure, although this may be delayed in exceptional circumstances when bleeding carries excess risk, e.g. following neurosurgery. Intravenous warfarin is available in some nations (e.g. the UK), and its use may be considered in patients unable to take oral medication.

Rapid decreases in INR are undesirable and may create a hypercoagulable condition. In elective situations, therefore, oral anticoagulation should be withdrawn to allow the INR to fall spontaneously. Alternative measures may be considered in emergency situations or following trauma (see below). Hospital admission or delay in discharge to give heparin may be considered unnecessary in low-risk patients,[5] and home administration and management of heparin and oral anticoagulation can be arranged to minimise time in hospital and provide cost-effective management.[30] The determination of which patients require prolonged regimens of overlapping heparin and oral anticoagulants may be difficult. Clinical judgement is required but these regimens are strongly recommended for those at highest risk of thromboembolism. With strict adherence to these guidelines, the incidence of thromboembolic and haemorrhagic complications is low.[4,14,31,32]

Trauma, bleeding and emergency surgery

Patients with prosthetic valves may present with bleeding problems following trauma or as a late sequel to previous non-cardiac surgery. Bleeding may also complicate coexistent medical conditions, e.g. peptic ulcer disease, and in some situations may be life-threatening, e.g. intracerebral haemorrhage. Indeed, in some instances the hazards of anticoagulation may exceed those of potential valve thrombosis, and in these situations an INR of 1.5 may be accepted. In most cases, however, the broad principles of anticoagulant management described above remain applicable, although the rapid achievement of a 'safe' INR is clearly desirable. High-dose parenteral vitamin K_1, e.g. 10 mg, should be avoided, since overcorrection increases the risk of a hypercoagulable state and prolongs resistance to oral anticoagulants, which is difficult to manage over the ensuing days. Lower doses of intravenous[33] or oral[34] vitamin K_1, e.g. 0.5–2 mg, have been recommended, but may be potentially dangerous for patients with prosthetic valves (see Chapter 8).

Follow-up

Patients with prosthetic valves who have had a period of anticoagulation interruption for another surgical procedure or following trauma require particularly close follow-up for the next few months. Ideally, they should undergo echocardiography prior to leaving hospital and again at 3 months to ensure that there is no thrombus on the prosthesis. In the case of high-risk patients with mitral prostheses, transoesophageal echocardiography is advisable (see also Chapters 4 and 10).

Future alternatives

The low molecular weight heparins (LMWH) offer several advantages over conventional unfractionated heparin (Table 16.5). Outpatient administration without labora-

Table 16.5 Advantages of low molecular weight heparins over unfractionated heparin

Easy to use
Effective anticoagulation
High bioavailability
Long half-life
Predictable dose response
Lower incidence of complications:
   Thrombocytopenia
   Haemorrhage
   Osteoporosis
Outpatient use feasible

tory monitoring is safe and feasible, with obvious implications for bed occupancy and overall cost.[30] These advantages have been confirmed in recent studies of patients in atrial fibrillation undergoing cardioversion[35] and in large trials of patients with unstable manifestations of ischaemic heart disease[36–38] in which LMWH was at least as effective as unfractionated heparin in preventing death, myocardial infarction and recurrent angina, and have now become the standard of care.

In contrast, the use of LMWH in patients with prosthetic heart valves is a relatively unexplored and unlicensed indication. In one study, Montalescot et al[39] reported 2 major episodes of bleeding and no thromboembolic events in 102 patients receiving the LMWH, enoxaparin, immediately after valve surgery. Anticoagulation was more predictable and rapidly and easily achieved with the LMWH, and there was no statistical difference in outcome in comparison with historical controls receiving unfractionated heparin. However, the study was non-randomised and terminated at 14 days with no long-term follow-up or echocardiographic surveillance. In the only published observational prospective study,[40] enoxaparin was used as a replacement for oral anticoagulation in 82 consecutive patients with mechanical heart valves, either to allow a variety of scheduled surgical procedures or because of bleeding complications. Anticoagulation was managed according to a strict protocol supervised by a local haematologist. There were 8 minor and 1 major bleeding events during treatment with enoxaparin and no clinical thromboembolic complications were noted during hospitalisation or at mean 3-month follow-up. Similar data are available for the alternative LMWH, dalteparin, although such information is currently available in abstract form only;[41,42] otherwise, experience has been limited to institutional audit[13,43] or isolated case reports.[44–46]

Randomised clinical trials examining the role of LMWH in the management of patients with prosthetic heart valves are long overdue, but for the time being their routine use cannot be recommended until further data are available.

Indeed, a recent statement from the US Food and Drug Administration (FDA) discouraged this management strategy in the light of adverse events in pregnant patients with prosthetic valves, although this has generated considerable controversy.[47] Similarly, ximelagatran, a recently developed oral thrombin inhibitor, has shown promise in the management of patients with venous thromboembolic disease and 'lone' atrial fibrillation.[48] However, concerns have been expressed regarding abnormalities of liver function associated with this drug and there are no data in patients with prosthetic valves or native valve disease.

Conclusions

Non-cardiac surgery poses major hazards to patients with prosthetic heart valves. Seamless oral anticoagulation is preferred whenever possible and aggressive overlapping regimens of unfractionated heparin and oral anticoagulation are recommended for major surgery, especially in those at the highest risk of thromboembolism. In view of the lack of available evidence, LMWH is not yet routinely recommended in this situation. Ultimately, the chosen management should be tailored and based upon thromboembolic risk, the duration of lowered anticoagulation and the risk of haemorrhage.

Summary

- Overall, thromboembolic risk is governed by a number of clinical characteristics
- The chosen perioperative anticoagulant regimen should be tailored and based on thromboembolic risk, the duration of lowered anticoagulation and the risk of haemorrhage
- Dental and most minor surgical procedures (including cardiac catheterisation) can be performed safely with continued oral anticoagulation
- Most major surgical procedures require withdrawal of oral anticoagulation for 72 hours and maintenance with unfractionated heparin
- Low molecular weight heparins and new direct thrombin inhibitors offer potential advantages, although their role is experimental and uncertain

References

1. Poldermans D, Boersma E, Bax JJ, et al. The effect of bisoprolol on perioperative mortality and myocardial infarction in high-risk patients undergoing vascular surgery. N Engl J Med 1999; 341:1789–94.

2. Mangano DT, Layug EL, Wallace A, et al. Effect of atenolol on mortality and cardiovascular morbidity after noncardiac surgery. N Engl J Med 1996; 335:1713–20.

3. Kertai MD, Boersma E, Bax JJ, et al. A meta-analysis comparing the prognostic accuracy of six diagnostic tests for predicting perioperative cardiac risk in patients undergoing major vascular surgery. Heart 2003; 89:1327–34.

4. Gohlke-Barwolf C, Acar J, Oakley C, et al. Guidelines for prevention of thromboembolic events in valvular heart disease. Study Group of the Working Group on Valvular Heart Disease of the European Society of Cardiology. Eur Heart J 1995; 16:1320–30.

5. Bonow RO, Carabello B, de Leon AC, et al. ACC/AHA guidelines for the management of patients with valvular heart disease. J Am Coll Cardiol 1998; 32:1486–582.

6. Hirsh J, Fuster V. Guide to anticoagulant therapy. Part 2: oral anticoagulants. American Heart Association. Circulation 1994; 89:1469–80.

7. Cannegieter SC, Rosendaal FR, Wintzen AR, et al. Optimal oral anticoagulant therapy in patients with mechanical heart valves. N Engl J Med 1995; 333:11–17.

8. Stein PD, Grandison D, Hua TA. Therapeutic levels of oral anticoagulation with warfarin in patients with mechanical prosthetic heart valves: review of the literature and recommendations based on international normalised ratio. Postgrad Med J 1994; 70:S72–83.

9. Stein PD, Alpert JS, Copeland J, et al. Antithrombotic therapy in patients with mechanical and biological prosthetic heart valves. Chest 1995; 108:371–9S.

10. Tiede DJ, Nishimura RA, Gastineau DA, et al. Modern management of prosthetic valve anticoagulation. Mayo Clin Proc 1998; 73:665–80.

11. Bryan AJ, Butchart EG. Prosthetic heart valves and anticoagulant management during non-cardiac surgery. Br J Surg 1995; 82:577–8.

12. Cannegieter SC, Rosendaal FR, Briet E. Thromboembolic and bleeding complications in patients with mechanical heart valve prostheses. Circulation 1994; 89:635–41.

13. Carrel TP, Klingenmann W, Mohacsi PJ, Berdat P, Althaus U. Perioperative bleeding and thromboembolic risk during non-cardiac surgery in patients with mechanical prosthetic heart valves: an institutional review. J Heart Valve Dis 1999; 8:392–8.

14. Kearon C, Hirsh J. Management of anticoagulation before and after elective surgery. N Engl J Med 1997; 336:1505–11.

15. Butchart EG. Thrombogenesis and its management. In: Acar J, Bodnar E, eds. Textbook of acquired heart valve disease. London: ICR Publishers, 1996.

16. Butchart EG. Anticoagulation management during non-cardiac surgery – time for common sense. J Heart Valve Dis 1994; 3:313–14.

17. Butchart EG, Ionescu A, Payne N, et al. A new scoring system to determine thromboembolic risk after heart valve replacement. Circulation 2003; 108 (Suppl II):II68–74.

18. Gohlke-Barwolf C. Anticoagulation in valvar heart disease: new aspects and management during non-cardiac surgery. Heart 2000; 84:567–72.

19. Grip L, Blomback MS, Schulman S. Hypercoagulable state and thromboembolism following warfarin withdrawal in post-myocardial infarction patients. Eur Heart J 1991; 12:1225–33.

20. Genewein U, Haeberli A, Straub PW, et al. Rebound after cessation of oral anticoagulant therapy: the biochemical evidence. Br J Haematol 1996; 92:479–85.

21. Rustad H, Myrhe E. Surgery during anticoagulant treatment. The risk of increased bleeding in patients on oral anticoagulant treatment. Acta Med Scand 1963; 173:115–19.

22. McIntyre H. Management during dental surgery of patients on anticoagulants. Lancet 1966; ii:99–100.

23. Robinson GA, Nylander A. Warfarin and cataract extraction. Br J Ophthalmol 1989; 73:702–3.

24. Parr NJ, Loh CS, Desmond AD. Transurethral resection of the prostate and bladder tumour without withdrawal of warfarin therapy. Br J Urol 1989; 64:623–5.

25. Wahl MJ. Dental surgery in anticoagulated patients. Arch Intern Med 1998; 158:1610–16.

26. Sindet-Pedersen S, Ramstrom G, Bernvil S, et al. Hemostatic effect of tranexamic acid mouthwash in anticoagulated patients undergoing oral surgery. N Engl J Med 1989; 320:840–3.

27. Hildick-Smith DJR, Walsh JT, Lowe MD, et al. Coronary angiography in the fully anticoagulated patient: the transradial route is successful and safe. Cathet Cardiovasc Intervent 2003; 58:8–10.

28. McCormack P, Simcock PR, Tullo AB. Management of the anticoagulated patient for ophthalmic surgery. Eye 1993; 7:749–50.

29. British Society of Haematology. British Committee for Standards in Haematology. Guidelines on oral anticoagulation. Br J Haematol 1998; 101:374–87.

30. Eckman MH, Beshansky JR, Durand-Zaleski I, et al. Anticoagulation for non-cardiac procedures in patients with prosthetic heart valves: does low risk mean high cost? JAMA 1990; 263:1513–21.

31. Darmon D, Enriquez-Sarano M, Acar J. Cardiac complications after subsequent non-cardiac operations in patients with non-biological prosthetic heart valves. Eur Heart J 1983; 4 (Suppl I):30.

32. Katholi RE, Nolan SP, McGuire LB. The management of anticoagulation during noncardiac operations in patients with prosthetic heart valves: a prospective study. Am Heart J 1978; 96:163–5.

33. Shetty HG, Backhouse G, Bentley DB, Routledge PA. Effective reversal of warfarin-induced excessive anticoagulation with low dose vitamin K_1. Thromb Haemost 1992; 67:13–15.

34. Weibert RT, Le DT, Kayser SR, et al. Correction of excessive anticoagulation with low-dose oral vitamin K_1. Ann Intern Med 1997; 126:959–62.

35. Stellbrink C, Nixdorff U, Hofmann T, et al. Safety and efficacy of enoxaparin compared with unfractionated heparin and oral anticoagulants for prevention of thromboembolic complications in cardioversion of nonvalvular atrial fibrillation. The Anticoagulation in Cardioversion using Enoxaparin (ACE) trial. Circulation 2004; 109:997–1003.

36. Klein W, Buchwald A, Hillis WS, et al. Fragmin in unstable angina pectoris or in non-Q wave acute myocardial infarction (the FRIC study). Am J Cardiol 1997; 80:30–4E.

37. Cohen M, Demers C, Gurfinkel E, et al. A comparison of low molecular weight heparin with unfractionated heparin for unstable coronary artery disease. N Engl J Med 1997; 337:447–52.

38. The ASSENT-3 investigators. Efficacy and safety of tenecteplase in combination with enoxaparin, abciximab, or unfractionated heparin: the ASSENT-3 randomised trial in acute myocardial infarction. Lancet 2001; 358:605–13.

39. Montalescot G, Polle V, Collet JP, et al. Low molecular weight heparin after mechanical heart valve replacement. Circulation 2000; 101:1083–6.

40. Ferreira I, Dos L, Tornos P, et al. Experience with enoxaparin in patients with mechanical heart valves who must withhold acenocumarol. Heart 2003; 89:527–30.

41. Kovacs M, Kahn S, Solymoss S, et al. Prospective multicentre trial of bridging therapy with dalteparin for patients who require temporary discontinuation of OAC for prosthetic heart valves or high risk atrial fibrillation. Blood 2002; 100(11):149a.

42. Douketis JD, Johnson JA, Turpie AG. Low-molecular-weight heparin as bridging anticoagulation during interruption of warfarin: assessment of a standardized periprocedural anticoagulation regimen. Arch Intern Med 2004; 164:1319–26.

43. Harenberg J, Huhle G, Piazolo L, et al. Long term anticoagulation of outpatients with adverse events to oral anticoagulants using low molecular weight heparin. Semin Thromb Hemost 1997; 23:167–72.

44. Lee LH, Liauw PC, Ng AS. Low molecular weight heparin for thromboprophylaxis during pregnancy in 2 patients with mechanical mitral valve replacement. Thromb Haemost 1996; 76:628–30.

45. De Paulis R, Fleury JP, Veyssie L, et al. Acute massive postoperative atrial thrombosis in a patient undergoing low molecular weight heparin anticoagulation. J Cardiovasc Vasc Anesth 1993; 7:332–4.

46. Manley HJ, Smith JA, Garris RE. Subcutaneous enoxaparin for outpatient anticoagulation therapy in a patient with an aortic valve replacement. Pharmacotherapy 1998; 18: 408–12.

47. Ginsberg JS, Chan WS, Bates SM, et al. Anticoagulation of pregnant women with mechanical heart valves. Arch Intern Med 2003; 163:694–8.

48. Olsson SB; Executive Steering Committee on behalf of the SPORTIF III Investigators. Stroke prevention with the oral direct thrombin inhibitor ximelagatran compared with warfarin in patients with non-valvular atrial fibrillation (SPORTIF III): randomised controlled trial. Lancet 2003; 362:1691–8.

17

Prevention of rheumatic fever: primary and secondary prophylaxis

Edward L Kaplan

Introduction

Despite the fact that it has been acknowledged for more than half a century that infection with group A beta-haemolytic streptococci (*Streptococcus pyogenes*) is responsible for the development of acute rheumatic fever and rheumatic heart disease, the pathogenetic mechanism(s) remain incompletely defined. Stollerman proposed the term 'rheumatogenic streptococci,' implying that there are specific strains of group A streptococci that have an increased propensity for causing this non-suppurative sequel of group A streptococcal infection, rheumatic fever and rheumatic heart disease.[1] At the time a relatively limited number of serotypes (M-types 1, 3, 5, 6, 18 and 24) was incriminated, almost solely on the basis of epidemiologically associated data. However, a 'rheumatogenic' factor was not identified.

Despite many subsequent hypotheses that attempted to explain the roles of the organism and the human host in the pathogenesis, the precise mechanism remains unknown at the beginning of the 21st century, even though it is generally accepted that it is an immunologically mediated entity. With the advent of molecular technologies, allowing more sophisticated approaches to the pathogenesis of disease, important increases in knowledge about the anatomy and physiology of the group A streptococcus and the relationship to non-suppurative sequelae have resulted. Detailed reviews have summarised currently available data.[2] As it pertains to the prevention of rheumatic fever and rheumatic heart disease, the objective of this quest for understanding is to gain necessary knowledge that can assist in developing a cost-efficient group A streptococcal vaccine, which would not only theoretically prevent infection but, by doing so, virtually eliminate the risk of development of rheumatic fever and rheumatic heart disease. However, to date, important perplexing riddles remain. It is likely that several years will pass before the efficacy of a vaccine is confirmed and a group A streptococcal vaccine approved by regulatory agencies.

With that being the case, the only current way for preventing rheumatic fever after streptococcal infection is by prompt recognition and appropriate medical management of the preceding infection. There are two current methodologies for attempting to prevent attacks of rheumatic fever. The first, known as *primary prophylaxis*, involves recognition and appropriate antibiotic treatment of the group A streptococcal upper respiratory tract infection to prevent an initial attack of rheumatic fever. The other technique, known as *secondary prophylaxis*, involves continuous administration of an antibiotic (most often penicillin) to prevent streptococcal colonisation/infection of those human hosts who have previously experienced an initial attack of rheumatic fever.

Data supporting the efficacy of these two methods of prevention have been available for more than 50 years. The sentinel studies were carried out in the late 1940s and early 1950s and, in fact, are the only controlled studies confirming the efficacy of primary prophylaxis.[3] In those studies in military recruits with streptococcal pharyngitis, the attack rate of acute rheumatic fever in untreated controls was many times larger than the attack rate in those subjects promptly treated with penicillin. It should be recognised that those studies involved the use of a parenteral penicillin; a proper controlled study has not been successfully carried out using oral penicillin. In fact, since those initial studies there have been no confirmative studies carried out, in large part due to ethical reasons. Those initial studies also showed clearly that treatment could be postponed for as long as 9 days after onset of the group A upper respiratory tract infection and development of rheumatic fever could still be prevented.[4] Furthermore, those important studies demonstrated that eradication of the group A streptococcus from the upper respiratory tract was essential to the success of primary prophylaxis.[5] (Available evidence suggests that while acute post-streptococcal glomerulonephritis may follow either group A streptococcal infection of the throat or of the skin (pyoderma/impetigo), acute rheumatic fever follows only infection of the throat.)

Guidelines for the diagnosis and management of patients with acute group A streptococcal pharyngitis have changed little in the half century since recommendations were initially described. Several authoritative scientific bodies have issued guidelines recently for primary rheumatic fever prophylaxis.[6–8]

The principles involved include timely diagnosis utilising the clinical microbiology laboratory whenever possible to confirm the presence of group A streptococci. Clinical diagnosis is often difficult. Whereas the throat culture remains the 'gold standard' for determining the presence of group A streptococci in the upper respiratory tract, new rapid antigen detection techniques that require only 10–20 minutes are commercially available. Their specificity exceeds the sensitivity of these rapid tests, and many experts agree that the presence of a negative rapid test is cause for a back-up throat culture.

Since there has never been a clinical isolate of group A streptococcus that is resistant to penicillin,[9] the drug has remained the antibiotic of choice for primary prophylaxis. Penicillin (or one of its analogues such as amoxicillin) may be given orally for treatment of the acute streptococcal pharyngitis; this has been proven to be effective. However, the intramuscular injection of repository benzathine penicillin G significantly reduces the problem of patient compliance and continues to be preferred by many medical and public health authorities.

In recent years numerous other antibiotics have been shown to be equivalent to penicillin in their ability to eradicate group A streptococci from the upper respiratory tract. Most current guidelines indicate that first-generation cephalosporins are acceptable substitutes.[6,7] For those patients allergic to penicillin, the classical alternative therapy has been erythromycin. However, because of the threat of erythromycin resistance which has been demonstrated to be as high as 40% in some countries around the world at the present time, care must be taken when selecting either erythromycin or one of the other macrolides (or the close relative, the azalides) for treatment of group A streptococcal pharyngitis or tonsillitis.[10]

Supporting studies suggested that either a single intramuscular injection of repository benzathine penicillin G or 10 full days of oral therapy are more likely to result in eradication of the organism from the throat. Oftentimes, clinicians may be misled by the fact that patients tend to improve clinically after only 2 or 3 days of antibiotics, and this has led to the error of insufficiently long oral treatment courses. However, carefully done studies indicate that patients improve clinically even without antibiotics. Thus, uniform recommendations by national societies, as well as by the World Health Organisation, recommend 10 full days of oral therapy if this route of administration for primary prophylaxis is selected by the physician.[6–8]

Concern about the duration of antibiotic therapy in primary prophylaxis has been re-emphasised by the recent introduction of several 'new' antibiotics that have been recommended and, in some cases, approved for shorter courses (less than 10 days) of therapy. However, some authoritative groups recommending antibiotics for primary prevention of rheumatic fever have urged caution in selecting short-course therapy for eradication of group A streptococci.[7] Indeed, there are data in the literature suggesting that short-course therapy may not be as effective as a full 10-day course of primary prophylaxis.[11] Shorter courses of penicillin have also been shown not to be as effective as the full 10-day course.

Most authorities do not believe that it is necessary to reculture individuals after completing appropriate antibiotic therapy for streptococcal pharyngitis, particularly in view of the fact that there has never been a group A streptococcus resistant to penicillin.[9] On the other hand, under special epidemiological circumstances such as there being a known rheumatic fever patient in the household or in close contact or in the situation of an epidemic, many feel more comfortable performing post-therapy cultures.

Table 17.1 contains a summary of current recommendations and doses for treatment of streptococcal upper respiratory tract infection (primary prophylaxis). This table represents a compilation/modification of several available guidelines.

Secondary prophylaxis of rheumatic fever

Secondary prophylaxis of rheumatic fever refers to the *continuous* administration of specific antibiotics to prevent colonisation and/or infection with group A streptococci. This form of prevention is reserved for those patients who have had a previous attack of rheumatic fever; it is different from treatment of individuals who have acute streptococcal infection and have no history of a previous attack of rheumatic fever. One of the most important advances in secondary prophylaxis was the formulation of long-acting repository benzathine penicillin G approximately 50 years ago. Intramuscular administration of benzathine penicillin G virtually eliminates the issue of compliance in taking oral penicillin. In fact, studies have shown that even in those patients for whom oral penicillin compliance has been documented, there is a statistical advantage in using intramuscular benzathine penicillin G.[12]

The original studies suggested that adequate levels of penicillin necessary to kill streptococci remained in the serum of patients for approximately 4 weeks after an injection of benzathine penicillin G, and thus the original recommendations for secondary prophylaxis were that the appropriate dose be given every 4 weeks.[13] This was clinically translated into once a month administration. More

Table 17.1 Suggestions for primary prophylaxis for prevention of rheumatic fever

Antibiotic	Administration	Dose	Comments
Penicillins			
Penicillin V	Oral	For children: 250 mg tid–qid for 10 days. For adolescents/adults: 250 mg to 500 mg bid to tid for 10 days	Twice-daily doses have been shown to be efficacious in some studies, but many prefer three times daily doses
Benzathine (penicillin G)	Intramuscular	Single dose 600 000 units for children weighing less than 27 kg. 1 200 000 units for larger children and for adults	Preparations which contain mixtures of benzathine penicillin G and other formulations of penicillin should not be used unless the total dose is based only upon the amount of benzathine penicillin G present
Amoxicillin	Oral	For children: 25–50 mg/kg/day in two or three doses for 10 days. Total adult dose is 750–1500 mg/day	This has been effective for children and is used because of its less-offensive taste
Erythromycin	Oral	Orally 3 to 4 times/day for 10 days. Dosage varies with formulation	Several preparations are available. Other macrolides and azalides are available. The physician should be aware of local macrolide resistance rates of group A streptococci
First-generation cephalosporins	Oral	2–3 times/day for 10 days. Dose varies with preparation	The use of sulfa drugs or tetracyclines is not recommended for treatment of acute streptococcal infections because of the high incidence of resistance

Modified from References 6, 7 and 8.

recently, carefully performed studies have shown that giving this antibiotic every 3 weeks has a distinct advantage in preventing recurrences of attacks of rheumatic fever because serum levels remain higher for longer periods of time.[14] Thus, most recommendations now indicate that for high-risk patients (e.g. multiple previous attacks of rheumatic fever) in high-risk situations (e.g. disadvantaged socioeconomic living conditions), intramuscular benzathine penicillin G should be given every 3 weeks.[6]

Studies have suggested that some manufactured formulations of benzathine penicillin G result in lower serum levels.[15] Studies have shown that these preparations of benzathine penicillin G have lower serum levels for shorter periods of time. This is an important consideration for the clinician and public health physician when purchasing benzathine penicillin G for use in public health secondary prophylaxis programmes. Use of such substandard preparations could result in inadequate protection for patients.

Some physicians and public health authorities have been reluctant to recommend intramuscular benzathine penicillin G secondary prophylaxis for two reasons. The first reason is that it is painful; this pain may last 24 hours or longer. Some children are reluctant to accept repeated painful injections, especially teenagers. This can be a major hurdle for patients and their parents, even though there is

evidence that the injections are more protective. The second reason, and one of more concern among some physicians, is the perceived threat of anaphylaxis associated with injectable penicillin. It has been shown that anaphylaxis is more common in the adult age group than in the paediatric age group, but the risk of anaphylaxis, be it very small, remains finite. However, a multi-country study carried out in the early 1990s reported the risk of anaphylaxis is extremely rare, being in the neighbourhood of approximately 1 per 30 000 injections.[16] Furthermore, in individuals reported to have had severe anaphylaxis or in those rare instances where death occurred, it almost exclusively has occurred in individuals with severe decompensated rheumatic valvular heart disease. This raises the question as to whether the incidents actually represented bona fide anaphylaxis or perhaps could be the result of an exaggerated vagal response in decompensated patients with unstable cardiovascular status. Nevertheless, it is important to recognise the possibility of anaphylactic reactions. Consequently, it is recommended that appropriate resuscitative equipment be available in clinics where injections are given.

A practical clinical question about secondary prophylaxis relates to the recommended duration of prophylaxis. There are few firm data to support clinical recommendations. Since group A streptococcal infections are more

Table 17.2 Suggestions for secondary prophylaxis for prevention of rheumatic fever

Antibiotic	Administration	Dose	Comments
Penicillin V	Oral	250 mg orally twice a day	Compliance is a potentially significant problem
Benzathine penicillin G	Intramuscular	1 200 000 units every 3 or 4 weeks (see text)	For patients who are receiving warfarin, care must be taken with any intramuscular injection
Erythromycin	Oral	250 mg twice daily	Several preparations available. If local resistance rates are significant, this must be taken into consideration
Sulfonamides (e.g. sulfadiazine, sulfisoxazole)	Oral	For patients weighing more than 30 kg, 1 g daily. For children weighing less than 30 kg, 500 mg daily	

Modified from References 6 and 8.

common in children, some believe that those over the age of 18 or 21 do not require long-term secondary prophylaxis. However, although the risk of developing recurrences decreases remarkably after 5 years since the most recent attack, the risk of recurrence is still greater than in individuals who have not had a previous bout of rheumatic fever. Similarly, in certain populations, the risk is higher because the incidence of streptococcal infection is higher. Such information must be taken into consideration when making a decision. Finally, in those individuals who have documented rheumatic heart disease, the risk of recurrence cannot be overlooked and many of these patients are given prophylaxis well into adulthood, some even for life. Thus, most experienced clinicians are reluctant to adopt rigid rules about the duration of secondary prophylaxis, but they prefer to tailor the individual prophylaxis to the patient's cardiac/valvular status, the number of previous rheumatic fever recurrences and the risk of the individual to have recurrent streptococcal infections (e.g. patients who are schoolteachers or work in hospitals or other medical care facilities). Many believe that the risk of not receiving long-term secondary prophylaxis is greater than the risk of side-effects and adverse reactions.[16] It also must be recalled that, even after replacement of a valve damaged by rheumatic fever, these patients remain at risk for rheumatic fever recurrences and require continuing secondary prophylaxis.

It must also be remembered that neither primary nor secondary prophylaxis for prevention of rheumatic fever is a substitute for antibiotic prophylaxis for prevention of infective endocarditis.

Table 17.2 reflects a compilation/modification of current recommendations for secondary rheumatic fever prophylaxis. These are adapted from guidelines of representative professional societies and are those in general use in countries around the world.

Summary

In the absence of an approved effective vaccine for prevention of group A streptococcal infections, prevention of rheumatic fever and rheumatic heart disease is dependent upon prompt recognition and therapy of the group A streptococcal infection (*primary prophylaxis*). For those individuals who have experienced a previous rheumatic fever attack, continuous compliance with antibiotic administration (*secondary prophylaxis*) is the optimal way for prevention of recurrent attacks resulting in further valvular damage. Hopefully, if and when a cost-effective group A streptococcal vaccine becomes available and effective distribution can be implemented, more effective prevention of rheumatic fever will result.

References

1. Stollerman GH. Rheumatogenic streptococci and autoimmunity. Clin Immunol Immunopathol 1991; 61:131–42.
2. Ayoub EM, Kotb M, Cunningham MW. Rheumatic fever pathogenesis. In: Stevens DL, Kaplan EL, eds. Streptococcal infections. Clinical aspects, microbiology, and molecular pathogenesis. New York: Oxford University Press, 2000: 102–33.
3. Wannamaker LW, Rammelkamp CH Jr, Denny FW, et al. Prophylaxis of acute rheumatic fever by treatment of the preceding streptococcal infection with various amounts of depot penicillin. Am J Med 1951; 10:673–95.
4. Chamovitz R, Catanzaro FJ, Stetson CA, Rammelkamp CH Jr. Prevention of rheumatic fever by treatment of previous streptococcal infections. N Engl J Med 1954; 251:466–70.
5. Catanzaro FJ, Rammelkamp CH Jr, Chamovitz R. Prevention of rheumatic fever by treatment of streptococcal infections. II. Factors responsible for failures. N Engl J Med 1958; 259:51–7.
6. Report of a WHO Expert Consultation. WHO Technical Report Series 923. Rheumatic fever and rheumatic heart disease. Geneva: World Health Organization, 2004.

7. Bisno AL, Gerber MA, Gwaltney JM Jr, Kaplan EL, Schwartz RH; Infectious Diseases Society of America. Practice guidelines for the diagnosis and management of group A streptococcal pharyngitis. Infectious Diseases Society of America. Clin Infect Dis 2002; 35:113–25.

8. Dajani A, Aubert K, Ferrieri P, Peter G, Shulman ST. Treatment of acute streptococcal pharyngitis and prevention of rheumatic fever: a statement for health professionals. Pediatrics 1995; 96:758–64.

9. Macris MH, Hartman N, Murray B, et al. Studies of the continuing susceptibility of group A streptococcal strains to penicillin during eight decades. Pediatr Infect Dis J 1998; 17:377–81.

10. Kaplan EL, Cornaglia G. Persistent macrolide resistance among group A streptococci: the lack of accomplishment after 4 decades. Clinic Infect Dis 2005; 41:609–11.

11. Kaplan EL, Gooch III WM, Notario GF, Craft JC. Macrolide therapy of group A streptococcal pharyngitis: 10 days of macrolide therapy (clarithromycin) is more effective in streptococcal eradication than 5 days (azithromycin). Clin Infect Dis 2001; 32:1798–802.

12. Wood HF, Feinstein AR, Taranta A, et al. Rheumatic fever in children and adolescents. A long-term epidemiologic study of subsequent prophylaxis, streptococcal infections, and clinical sequelae. III. Comparative effectiveness of three prophylaxis regimens in preventing streptococcal infections and rheumatic recurrences. Ann Intern Med 1964; 60(Suppl 5):31–46.

13. Stollerman GH, Rusoff H. Prophylaxis against group A streptococcal infections in rheumatic fever patients: use of a new repository penicillin preparation. JAMA 1952; 150:1571–5.

14. Lue HC, Wu MH, Hsieh KH, et al. Rheumatic fever recurrences: controlled study of 3-week versus 4-week benzathine penicillin prevention programs. J Pediatr 1986; 108:299–304.

15. Zaher SR, Kassem AS, Abou-Shleib H, et al. Differences in serum penicillin concentrations following intramuscular injection of benzathine penicillin G (BPG) from different manufacturers. J Pharmacol Med 1992; 2:17–23.

16. Markowitz M, Kaplan EL, Cuttica R, et al. Allergic reactions to long-term benzathine penicillin prophylaxis for rheumatic fever. Lancet 1991; 337:1308–10.

18

Follow-up and management in children

Peter Pastuszko and Thomas L Spray

Infants and children who require valve surgery represent a patient population with a unique set of challenges. Although some of these mirror the difficulties facing clinicians treating adult patients having valve surgery, many are distinctly different. Unlike developing countries where rheumatic valve disease is prevalent, in developed countries valve disease leading to surgery in an infant or a small child is often a result of a congenital defect and is associated with a number of other anatomical abnormalities. Frequently, this results in cardiopulmonary physiology that is different from that observed in adult patients, requiring different early as well as late postoperative management. Finally, the valve surgery, in particular valve replacement surgery, is often the last of many interventions a particular patient may undergo.

Valve replacement surgery in a young patient faces several distinct limitations, including size restrictions, with fewer options for the smallest patients, as well as the issue of somatic growth, with the same individuals frequently requiring multiple operations over the course of a lifetime. In addition, there is the risk associated with a lifetime of anticoagulation in a young patient after a mechanical valve replacement versus the problem of early degeneration in those individuals with a tissue prosthesis. All these factors lead to the conclusion that in many, if not most instances, valve surgery in a child provides only a palliative solution. The variable and frequently disappointing results with valve replacement surgery in the young underscore the importance of valve repair techniques, especially of the mitral valve, with replacement being an option of last resort.

Perioperative management in a paediatric patient undergoing open-heart surgery

The unique approach to an infant or a child undergoing cardiac surgery begins in the operating room. Surgery and, in particular, surgery involving the use of cardiopulmonary bypass (CPB) has a significantly more pronounced effect in a young patient, and early recognition of those individuals who are at an increased risk is the key to improved outcomes. Detrimental effects of the CPB are well documented. It is associated with complement activation, exaggerated sympathetic response, capillary leak, disturbance in fluid balance and abnormalities in the distribution of cardiac output.[1-6] In addition, whereas some procedures can be performed with CPB alone, other ones may require the use of hypothermia with low-flow or deep hypothermic circulatory arrest (DHCA). Whichever of these measures may be used and whatever associated sequelae a patient may face, a state of temporary low cardiac output is a predictable postoperative occurrence in all patients requiring cardiac arrest. This low cardiac output syndrome has been shown to be proportional to the length of myocardial ischaemic period and inversely proportional to the age of the patient.[7] Early recognition and aggressive treatment of this phenomenon is critical to improved survival and reduced morbidity in such an individual.[8] Therefore, every step in the care of an infant or a child after open-heart surgery entails meticulous monitoring of parameters of cardiac performance. This may include simple clinical assessment such as measurement of the capillary refill or a number of invasive steps such as monitoring lactate levels, mixed-venous O_2 saturation or central venous pressure.[7,8] Abnormality in any of these parameters should prompt immediate action aimed at optimising the underlying contributing factors: contractility, rhythm, rate, preload and afterload.[7]

Perioperative measures designed to improve outcomes in these patients include minimising CPB time and reducing the circuit priming volume, as well as routine use of high-dose steroids and aprotinin.[1,2] Intraoperative initiation of catecholamines or phosphodiesterase inhibitors may also be critical. Milrinone is a drug shown to be effective in improving cardiac performance in children after heart surgery. Its beneficial effects include increased cardiac index, as well as lowered systemic and pulmonary vascular resistance and pressure.[8-12] Pulmonary hypertension is a serious problem in a postoperative child after repair of many congenital heart defects. These patients will frequently require hyperventilation and an extended period of paralysis. Inhaled nitric oxide may be of some benefit in this group, but the results have been inconsistent.[13,14] More recently, the use of sildenafil has been encouraging.[15]

As noted previously, even if the surgical repair is perfect, cardiopulmonary bypass is associated with major morbidity when used in infants and children. It is generally agreed that many of the side-effects seen with CPB are reversed with the use of modified ultrafiltration (MUF).[1,8,16,17] It has been shown to improve pulmonary, cardiac and cerebral function by decreasing haemodilution and tissue oedema.

Judicious placement of temporary pacing wires may prove helpful as well. We have shown that the incidence of postoperative arrhythmias in a paediatric cardiac intensive care unit is high.[18,19] Appropriate pharmacological treatment of these arrhythmias, in particular the use of amiodarone, combined with A-V pacing, frequently promotes successful recovery in these patients.[8]

Finally, if the period of CPB is prolonged and significant tissue oedema is present, the cardiac and pulmonary function may be so marginal that the patient will not tolerate a closed chest, and delayed sternal closure may be the only alternative in these patients. Its use has been associated with acceptable outcomes.[20]

In conclusion, a number of advances in the recent past have led to a dramatic reduction in the immediate postoperative mortality and morbidity in infants and children undergoing open-heart surgery. Vigilant surveillance and early correction of any abnormalities as they present are the keys to successful outcomes.

Valve surgery in the paediatric patient

Valve replacement in a child should be considered even more of a palliative treatment. The size limitations of the available valves, the somatic growth of the patient, risk of anticoagulation associated with mechanical valves, as well as early degeneration seen with the tissue valves are just some of the underlying reasons. The inconsistent and frequently disappointing results observed with a variety of prostheses underscores the importance of valve repair as the first-line therapy. New valvuloplasty techniques are continuously being introduced and modified as alternatives to valve replacement.

Mechanical valves

The first paediatric valve replacements with mechanical valves were performed in the late 1960s and early 1970s using the caged-ball valves. Use of these valves was aban-

doned because of issues related to the poor haemodynamic profile of these valves as well as obstruction of the left ventricular outflow tract when placed in the mitral position. However, despite these concerns, recently published data have shown good long-term results associated with the use of these prostheses, with a low incidence of thromboembolic or coagulation-related complications.[21] Currently, several other mechanical prostheses are available for use in paediatric patients. The tilting-disc and bileaflet valves have superior flow characteristics and smaller diameters, allowing for implantation in younger individuals.[22] Notwithstanding significant improvements in design, these valves share some of the same problems. When used at an early age, the smaller-size valves inevitably require future replacements secondary to the somatic growth of the individual. In addition, patients are faced with the burden and risks of anticoagulation for life.

As a result of interest in the application of the Ross procedure in younger individuals, the most frequent location for the use of mechanical valves is currently in the mitral position. A number of centres have looked at their outcomes in this patient group, giving insight into long-term management issues facing individuals with mechanical mitral valve prosthesis.[23–34] Mitral valve replacement in a child is associated with very high perioperative mortality. Whether it is due to the underlying valve pathology, associated cardiac disease or complexity of the procedure, these patients are high operative risk candidates, with reported operative mortality of up to 20% in most series. The highest risk group was the very young patients with low weight and small valve size.

Mechanical valves in the aortic position have not been as widely used as in the mitral position since good results have been shown when the alternative prosthesis, such as a homograft or, in particular, pulmonary autografts are used for aortic valve replacement. Some have shown unfavourable results with the use of mechanical valves in the aortic position secondary to left ventricular outflow obstruction from pannus formation on the ventricular side of the valve.[35] Nonetheless, several series reported satisfactory results when mechanical valves were used in this position.[36–40] All these patients are still faced with the issues of anticoagulation, as discussed below, whereas somatic growth is a problem for the smaller individuals. Therefore, their follow-up does not differ from that for the patients with a mechanical valve in any other position.

Xenografts and homografts

The issues of thrombosis and anticoagulation-related bleeding complications are avoided by the use of xenografts or homografts. Unfortunately, experience with the use of these valves in the paediatric population does not mirror that of the adult patients. Despite early enthusiasm for these prostheses, in the late 1970s, their use on the systemic side of the circulation has been hampered by early calcification and tissue degeneration.

Experience with the use of homografts is by no means uniform. The results with the use of pulmonary allografts for the reconstruction of the left ventricular outflow are poor.[41,42] Some authors have reported favourable results with the use of an aortic homograft in the aortic position and recommend it as the prosthesis of choice second only to the pulmonary autograft.[36,43–47] With some of the data originating from the adult population and the obvious difficulty in extrapolating it to the paediatric patients, concerns of long-term durability remain. Other clinicians have noted less encouraging results with the use of these prostheses, with the data suggesting that immune function is responsible for the early graft failure.[48–53] Experience with mitral valve replacement with a homograft in young patients is very limited, and the results are poor.[54]

Whereas mixed results are reported with homograft use, uniformly disappointing findings are reported with the use of xenografts for left ventricular outflow tract reconstruction. However, with the growing popularity of the Ross procedure for reconstruction of the left ventricular outflow tract, a number of alternatives have been proposed for the pulmonary valve replacement. Homografts, both aortic and pulmonary, have shown good long-term durability when used to reconstruct the right ventricular outflow tract in children, particularly in the older age group.[55–57]

Unfortunately, limited availability of these grafts has led to a search for alternative conduits. One such conduit is a valve-containing bovine jugular vein (Contegra, Medtronic, Inc., Minneapolis, MN). Several reports have shown promising results, with freedom from calcification and good haemodynamic function during a mean follow-up of 10–26 months.[58–60] However, long-term results are not known, and several early complications, such as aneurysm formation at the proximal end of the graft, stenotic membrane formation at the distal anastomosis and valve thrombus formation, have been reported.[58,61,62]

Pulmonary autograft

First described in 1967, the Ross procedure involves replacement of the diseased aortic valve with a pulmonary autograft and the use of an alternative conduit to repair the right ventricular outflow tract.[63] It possesses a number of features that make it an attractive alternative to mechanical, xenograft or homograft valves in the treatment of aortic stenosis in children and young adults. It does not require anticoagulation and has been shown to grow in proportion to somatic growth.[64,65] The Ross procedure has been accepted by an increasing number of centres as the

method of choice for the repair of aortic valve disease in children and adults alike.[66–68] A number of series have shown very good mid- to long-term results, with satisfactory durability and lack of early degeneration of the pulmonary valve autografts.[66,69–73] Pulmonary autograft use has been associated with improvement in left ventricular dilatation and hypertrophy.[74] The Ross procedure may also be the best choice, when combined with Konno aortoventriculoplasty, for the repair of complex left ventricular outflow tract obstruction.[75–77] Finally, it has been suggested as the procedure of choice for the treatment of active aortic valve endocarditis in children.[78]

The Ross procedure is not without risk. It converts a one-valve surgery to a two-valve procedure, and lifetime surveillance of both valves is necessary. As described earlier, the conduits available for the right ventricular outflow tract reconstruction are not perfect, with patients requiring future surgery for their replacement. Increased incidence of perioperative as well as postoperative arrhythmias has been described with this procedure.[79,80]

Patient follow-up

Clearly, any young individual who has undergone a valve replacement, whether the valve is mechanical, a homograft/xenograft or an autograft, requires close observation. There is little difference in terms of frequency of follow-up between the patient groups. After the initial postoperative visit, most series report follow-up at 3, 6 and 12 months postoperatively and annually thereafter, but some patients, specifically those with poor preoperative ventricular function or a prolonged and complicated postoperative course, may need to be seen more frequently. Each visit includes a complete history and physical examination, and an echocardiogram evaluation is especially indicated in patients with allografts and xenografts for evidence of valve degeneration, whereas patients with a Ross procedure are examined specifically for the presence of autograft insufficiency or dilation of neoaortic root.

After a successful surgery, irrespective of the valve type, patients have few limitations. Most do not require any long-term medications and have no restrictions with regard to their activities, except avoidance of strong isometric exercise such as weightlifting. The exceptions are individuals with mechanical valves, requiring lifelong anticoagulation treatment and follow-up. They are also limited from the standpoint of their activities, where avoidance of any contact sports is clearly advisable.

Interestingly, with few exceptions, most of the series of mechanical prostheses, after the initial high perioperative mortality, report very good long-term results with high survival and low incidence of prosthetic valve endocarditis, thromboembolic events or bleeding complications secondary to anticoagulation. Even though the risk of such complications is usually less than 10%, enthusiasm for these results needs to be tempered by associated morbidity. A thromboembolic event can result in serious sequelae, as a stroke in any individual, particularly a young person, is a devastating event. Hence, emphasis is placed on the need for aggressive anticoagulation in those patients. Despite attempts at minimising anticoagulation regimens and control of thromboembolic events with antiplatelet agents alone,[81,82] most authorities recommend that patients with mechanical valves be maintained on a warfarin protocol.[83–86]

Anticoagulation with warfarin sodium is a part of daily routine for any patient with a mechanical valve. The American Heart Association recommends maintaining the international normalised ratio (INR) between 2.5 and 3.5 in patients with a mechanical valve in the mitral position and at least 2.0–2.5 in patients with a mechanical valve in the aortic position, depending on the type of implanted valve.[41] This level of anticoagulation carries with it a small, yet not insignificant, risk of bleeding. Most of the observed bleeding events can be considered minor, such as spontaneous nose or gum bleeds or bleeding episodes associated with dental procedures; however, even those at times may require blood transfusions.

Obvious activity limitations exist for patients on warfarin therapy. Interestingly, when one study looked at the quality of life in patients with mechanical mitral valves, surprisingly satisfactory results were reported.[24] Most patients tolerated anticoagulation well, with minimal impairment or limitations. Whereas daily medications were not a problem to any of the patients, the older individuals reported some disruption to their routine from the need for regular blood testing. Most recently, satisfactory results have been reported with the increased use of home self-test kits that should become more widely available in the future. In other respects, anticoagulation control in paediatric patients follows the same generic rules as in adult patients, as discussed in Chapter 8.

Patients with allografts or xenografts avoid warfarin and the risks associated with it, although, as seen with the Contegra graft, low-dose anticoagulation occasionally may be necessary. All patients require close follow-up, as calcification and early valve degeneration, particularly in the youngest patients, is of major concern. In addition, the use of these valves does not address the issue of somatic growth, with the smaller patients requiring future surgery.

With regards to the Ross procedure, concerns have been raised regarding durability of the repair when carried out for aortic insufficiency.[86] Most recent series have reported good autograft valve function, with 75–90% freedom from reoperation at 8–16 years.[87,88] Unfortunately, those reports frequently include adult patients as well as children. The results in children are promising, with freedom from autograft valve degeneration of up to 83% at 12 years.[89] In the majority of patients, the main indication for reoperation is severe neoaortic valve insufficiency, followed by dilatation of the neoaortic root. Other causes of autograft failure, such as endocarditis, false aneurysm or rheumatic fever, are rare.[90] For further discussion of the Ross procedure, see Chapter 6.

Finally, children who have been subjected to mitral valve repair require long-term vigilance of valve function, which depends essentially on the initial result and on the pathology. As discussed in Chapter 7, rheumatic valves show the worst results of all. In any case, special care must be taken to avoid the ventricular impact of residual or recurrent mitral valve dysfunction, especially regurgitation. Early reoperations and valve substitution may be necessary in some cases, although moderate degrees of dysfunction may be well tolerated in the long term, with appropriate medical therapy.

Conclusions

In summary, valve replacement surgery in a child is even more of a palliative treatment. Hence, valvuloplasty, especially of the mitral valve, is preferable in most situations. When a sufficiently large mechanical valve is used, the patient may avoid future surgery but will require anticoagulation for life. With the current homograft preservation techniques and the currently available xenografts, a young individual will almost certainly need future surgery. The Ross procedure, even though it appears to fix the left-sided pathology, has its own risks. Hence, with the currently available choices to address valve disease in children, even after the best procedure, the patient will require lifelong follow-up.

References

1. Shen I, Giacomuzzi C, Ungerleider RM. Current strategies for optimizing the use of cardiopulmonary bypass in neonates and infants. Ann Thorac Surg 2003; 75:S729–34.
2. Butler J, Pathi VL, Paton RD, et al. Acute-phase responses to cardiopulmonary bypass in children weighing less than 10 kilograms. Ann Thorac Surg 1996; 62:538–42.
3. Edmunds LH. Inflammatory response to cardiopulmonary bypass. Ann Thorac Surg 1998; 66:S12–16.
4. Kirklin JK, Westaby S, Blackston EH, et al. Complement and the damaging effects of cardiopulmonary bypass. J Thorac Cardiovasc Surg 1983; 86:845–57.
5. Downing SW, Edmunds LH. Release of vasoactive substances during cardiopulmonary bypass. Ann Thorac Surg 1992; 54:1236–43.
6. Wan S, LeClerc JL, Vincent JL. Inflammatory responses to cardiopulmonary bypass: mechanisms involved and possible therapeutic strategies. Chest 1997; 112:676–92.
7. Tweddell JS, Hoffman GM. Postoperative management in patients with complex congenital heart disease. Semin Thorac Cardiovasc Surg Pediatr Card Surg Annu 2002; 5:187–205.

8. Ravishankar C, Tabbutt S, Wernovsky G. Critical care in cardiovascular medicine. Curr Opin Pediatr 2003; 15:443–53.

9. Bailey JM, Miller BE, Wei L, et al. The pharmacokinetics of milrinone in pediatric patients after cardiac surgery. Anesthesiology 1999; 90:1012–18.

10. Chang AC, Atz AM, Wernovsky G, et al. Milrinone: systemic and pulmonary hemodynamic effects in neonates after cardiac surgery. Crit Care Med 1995; 23:1907–14.

11. Hoffman TM, Wernovsky G, Atz AM, et al. Prophylactic intravenous use of milrinone after cardiac operation in pediatrics (PRIMACORP) study. Am Heart J 2002; 143:15–21.

12. Hoffman TM, Wernovsky G, Atz AM, et al. Efficacy and safety of milrinone in preventing low cardiac output syndrome in infants and children after corrective surgery for congenital heart disease. Circulation 2003; 107:996–1002.

13. Atz AM, Munoz RA, Adatia I, Wessel DL. Diagnostic and therapeutic uses of inhaled nitric oxide in neonatal Ebstein's anomaly. Am J Cardiol 2003; 91:906–8.

14. Day RW, Hawkins JA, McGough EC, et al. Randomized controlled study of inhaled nitric oxide after operation for congenital heart disease. Ann Thorac Surg 2000; 69:1907–13.

15. Atz AM, Lefler AK, Fairbrother DL, Uber WE, Bradley SM. Sildenafil augments the effect of inhaled nitric oxide for postoperative pulmonary hypertensive crisis. J Thorac Cardiovasc Surg 2002; 124:628–9.

16. Koutlas TC, Gaynor JW, Nicolson SC, et al. Modified ultrafiltration reduces postoperative morbidity after cavopulmonary connection. Ann Thorac Surg 1997; 64:37–42.

17. Gaynor JW. The effect of modified ultrafiltration on the postoperative course in patients with congenital heart disease. Semin Thorac Cardiovasc Surg Pediatr Card Surg Annu 2003; 6:128–39.

18. Hoffman TM, Wernovsky G, Wieand TS, et al. The incidence of arrhythmias in a pediatric cardiac intensive care unit. Pediatr Cardiol 2002; 23:598–604.

19. Hoffman TM, Bush DM, Wernovsky G, et al. Postoperative junctional ectopic tachycardia in children: incidence, risk factors, and treatment. Ann Thorac Surg 2002; 74:1607–11.

20. Tabbutt S, Duncan BW, McLaughlin D, et al. Delayed sternal closure after cardiac operations in a pediatric population. J Thorac Cardiovasc Surg 1997; 113:886–93.

21. Higashita R, Ichikawa S, Niinami H, et al. Long-term results after Starr–Edwards mitral valve replacement in children aged 5 years or younger. Ann Thorac Surg 2003; 75:826–9.

22. Bottio T, Caprili L, Casarotto D, Gerosa G. Small aortic annulus: the hydrodynamic performance of 5 commercially available bileaflet mechanical valves. J Thorac Cardiovasc Surg 2004; 128:457–62.

23. van Doorn C, Yates R, Tsang V, de Level M, Elliott M. Mitral valve replacement in children: mortality, morbidity, and haemodynamic status up to medium term follow up. Heart 2000; 84:636–42.

24. van Doorn C, Yates R, Tunstill A, Elliott M. Quality of life in children following mitral valve replacement. Heart 2000; 84:643–7.

25. Daou L, Sidi D, Mauriat P, et al. Mitral valve replacement with mechanical valves in children under two years of age. J Thorac Cardiovasc Surg 2001; 121:994–6.

26. Yoshimura N, Yamaguchi M, Oshima Y, et al. Surgery for mitral valve disease in the pediatric age group. J Thorac Cardiovasc Surg 1999; 118:99–106.

27. Masuda M, Kado H, Tatewaki H, Shiokawa Y, Yasui H. Late results after mitral valve replacement with bileaflet mechanical prosthesis in children: evaluation of prosthesis–patient mismatch. Ann Thorac Surg 2004; 77:913–17.

28. Alexiou C, Galogavrou M, Chen Q, et al. Mitral valve replacement with mechanical prostheses in children: improved operative risk and survival. Eur J Cardiothorac Surg 2001; 20:105–13.

29. Caldarone CA, Raghuveer G, Hills CB, et al. Long-term survival after mitral valve replacement in children aged <5 years: a multi-institutional study. Circulation 2001; 104:I143–7.

30. Raghuveer G, Caldarone CA, Hills CB, et al. Predictors of prosthesis survival, growth, and functional status following mechanical mitral valve replacement in children aged <5 years, a multi-institutional study. Circulation 2003; 108:II174–9.

31. Erez E, Kanter KR, Isom E, Williams WH, Tam VK. Mitral valve replacement in children. J Heart Valve Dis 2003; 12:25–30.

32. Gunther T, Mazzitelli D, Schreiber C, et al. Mitral-valve replacement in children under 6 years of age. Eur J Cardiothorac Surg 2000; 17:426–30.

33. Eble BK, Fiser WP, Simpson P, et al. Mitral valve replacement in children: predictors of long-term outcome. Ann Thorac Surg 2003; 76:853–60.

34. Lupinetti FM, Duncan BW, Scifres AM, et al. Intermediate-term results in pediatric aortic valve replacement. Ann Thorac Surg 1999; 68:521–6.

35. Fiane AE, Lindberg HL, Saatvedt K, Svennevig JL. Mechanical valve replacement in congenital heart disease. J Heart Valve Dis 1996; 5:337–42.

36. Lubiszewska B, Rozanski J, Szufladowicz M, et al. Mechanical valve replacement in congenital heart disease in children. J Heart Valve Dis 1999; 8:74–9.

37. Alexiou C, McDonald A, Langley SM, et al. Aortic valve replacement in children: are mechanical prostheses a good option? Eur J Cardiothorac Surg 2000; 17:125–33.

38. Champsaur G, Robin J, Tronc F, et al. Mechanical valve in aortic position is a valid option in children and adolescents. Eur J Cardiothorac Surg 1997; 11:117–22.

39. Mazzitelli D, Guenther T, Schreiber C, et al. Aortic valve replacement in children: are we on the right track? Eur J Cardiothorac Surg 1998; 13:565–71.

40. Naegele H, Bohlmann M, Doring V, Kalmar P, Rodiger W. Results of aortic valve replacement with pulmonary and aortic homografts. J Heart Valve Dis 2000; 9:215–21.

41. Dacey LJ. Pulmonary homografts: current status. Curr Opin Cardiol 2000; 15:86–90.

42. Doty JR, Salazar JD, Liddicoat JR, Flores JH, Doty DB. Aortic valve replacement with cryopreserved aortic allograft: ten-year experience. J Thorac Cardiovasc Surg 1998; 115:371–80.

43. Lupinetti FM, Duncan BW, Lewin M, Dyamenahalli U, Rosenthal GL. Comparison of autograft and allograft aortic valve replacement in children. J Thorac Cardiovasc Surg 2003; 126:240–6.

44. Lupinetti FM, Warner J, Jones TK, Herndon SP. Comparison of human tissue and mechanical prostheses for aortic valve replacement in children. Circulation 1997; 96:321–5.

45. Alexiou C, Keeton BR, Salmon AP, Monro JL. Repair of truncus arteriosus in early infancy with antibiotic sterilized aortic homografts. Ann Thorac Surg 2001; 71:S371–4.

46. Clarke DR, Campbell DN, Hayward AR, Bishop DA. Degeneration of aortic valve allografts in young recipients. J Thorac Cardiovasc Surg 1993; 105:934–42.

47. Yankah AC, Alexi-Meskhishvili V, Weng Y, et al. Accelerated degeneration of allografts in the first two years of life. Ann Thorac Surg 1995; 60:S71–7.

48. Cattaneo SM, Bethea BT, Alejo DE, et al. Surgery for aortic root aneurysm in children: a 21-year experience in 50 patients. Ann Thorac Surg 2004; 77:168–76.

49. Shaddy RE, Hawkins JA. Immunology and failure of valved allografts in children. Ann Thorac Surg 2002; 74:1271–5.

50. Turrentine MW, Ruzmetov M, Vijay P, Bills RG, Brown JW. Biological versus mechanical aortic valve replacement in children. Ann Thorac Surg 2001; 71:S356–60.

51. Rajani B, Mee RB, Ratliff NB. Evidence for rejection of homograft cardiac valves in infants. J Thorac Cardiovasc Surg 1998; 115:111–17.

52. Ross DB, Hamilton GR, Wright JR Jr, Lee TD. Homograft valve failure in children. J Thorac Cardiovasc Surg 1999; 117:1044–5.

53. Chauvaud S, Waldmann T, d'Attellis N, et al. Homograft replacement of the mitral valve in young recipients: mid-term results. Eur J Cardiothorac Surg 2003; 23:560–6.

54. Homann M, Haehnel JC, Mendler N, et al. Reconstruction of the RVOT with valved biological conduits: 25 years experience with allografts and xenografts. Eur J Cardiothorac Surg 2000; 17:624–30.

55. Lange R, Weipert J, Homann M, et al. Performance of allografts and xenografts for right ventricular outflow tract reconstruction. Ann Thorac Surg 2001; 71:S365–7.

56. Dittrich S, Alexi-Meskishvili VV, Yankah AC, et al. Comparison of porcine xenografts and homografts for pulmonary valve replacement in children. Ann Thorac Surg 2000; 70:717–22.

57. Tiete AR, Sachweh JS, Roemer U, et al. Right ventricular outflow tract reconstruction with the contegra bovine jugular vein conduit: a word of caution. Ann Thorac Surg 2004; 77:2151–6.

58. Purohit M, Kitchiner D, Pozzi M. Contegra bovine jugular vein right ventricle to pulmonary artery conduit in Ross procedure. Ann Thorac Surg 2004; 77:1707–10.

59. Corno AF, Qanadli SD, Sekarski N, et al. Bovine valved xenograft in pulmonary position: medium-term follow-up with excellent hemodynamics and freedom from calcification. Ann Thorac Surg 2004; 78:1382–8.

60. Boudjemline Y, Bonnet D, Agnoletti G, Vouhe P. Aneurysm of the right ventricular outflow following bovine valved venous conduit insertion. Eur J Cardiothorac Surg 2003; 23:122–4.

61. Kadner A, Dave H, Stallmach T, Turina M, Pretre R. Formation of a stenotic fibrotic membrane at the distal anastomosis of bovine jugular vein grafts (contegra) after right ventricular outflow tract reconstruction. J Thorac Cardiovasc Surg 2004; 127:285–6.

62. Ross DN. Replacement of aortic and mitral valves with a pulmonary autograft. Lancet 1967; 2:956–8.

63. Elkins RC, Knott-Craig CJ, Ward KE, McCue C, Lane MM. Pulmonary autograft in children: realized growth potential. Ann Thorac Surg 1994; 57:1387–94.

64. Simon P, Aschauer C, Moidl R, et al. Growth of the pulmonary autograft after the Ross operation in childhood. Eur J Cardiothorac Surg 2001; 19:118–21.

65. Rubay JE, Buche M, El Khoury GA, et al. The Ross operation: mid-term results. Ann Thorac Surg 1999; 67:1355–8.

66. Savoye C, Auffray JL, Hubert E, et al. Echocardiographic follow-up after Ross procedure in 100 patients. Am J Cardiol 2000; 85:854–7.

67. Al-Halees Z, Pieters F, Qadoura F, et al. The Ross procedure is the procedure of choice for congenital aortic valve disease. J Thorac Cardiovasc Surg 2002; 123:437–42.

68. Oswalt JD. Acceptance and versatility of the Ross procedure. Curr Opin Cardiol 1999; 14:90–4.

69. Elkins RC, Lane MM, McCue C. Ross operation in children: late results. J Heart Valve Dis 2001; 10:736–41.

70. Brown JW, Ruzmetov M, Vijay P, Rodefeld MD, Turrentine MW. Surgery for aortic stenosis in children: a 40-year experience. Ann Thorac Surg 2003; 76:1398–411.

71. Hraska V, Krajci M, Haun CL, et al. Ross and Ross–Konno procedure in children and adolescents: mid-term results. Eur J Cardiothorac Surg 2004; 25:742–7.

72. Elkins RC, Knott-Craig CJ, Ward KE, Lane MM. The Ross operation in children: 10-year experience. Ann Thorac Surg 1998; 65:496–502.

73. Brown JW, Ruzmetov M, Vijay P, Bills RG, Turrentine MW. Clinical outcomes and indicators of normalization of left ventricular dimensions after Ross procedure in children. Semin Thorac Cardiovasc Surg 2001; 13:28–34.

74. Reddy VM, Rajasinghe HA, Teitel DF, Hass GS, Hanley FL. Aortoventriculoplasty with the pulmonary autograft: the 'Ross–Konno' procedure. J Thorac Cardiovasc Surg 1996; 111:158–67.

75. Erez E, Kanter KR, Tam VKH, Williams WH. Konno aortoventriculoplasty in children and adolescents: from prosthetic valves to the Ross operation. Ann Thor Surg 2002; 74:122–6.

76. Marino BS, Wernovsky G, Rychik J, et al. Early results of the Ross procedure in simple and complex left heart disease. Circulation 1999; 100:II162–6.

77. Birk E, Sharoni E, Dagan O, et al. The Ross procedure as the surgical treatment of active aortic valve endocarditis. J Heart Valve Dis 2004; 13:73–7.

78. Bockoven JR, Wernovsky G, Vetter V, et al. Perioperative conduction and rhythm disturbances after the Ross procedure in young patients. Ann Thorac Surg 1998; 66:1383–8.

79. Phillips JR, Daniels CJ, Orsinelli DA, et al. Valvular hemodynamics and arrhythmias with exercise following the Ross procedure. Am J Cardiol 2001; 87:577–83.

80. Masuda M, Kado H, Tatewaki H, Shiokawa Y, Yasui H. Late results after mitral valve replacement with bileaflet mechanical prosthesis in children: evaluation of prosthesis–patient mismatch. Ann Thorac Surg 2004; 77:913–7.

81. el Makhlouf A, Friedli B, Oberhansli I, Rouge JC, Faidutti B. Prosthetic heart valve replacement in children: results and follow-up of 273 patients. J Thorac Cardiovasc Surg 1987; 93:80–5.

82. Bradley SM, Sade RM, Crawford FA Jr, Stroud MR. Anticoagulation in children with mechanical valve prostheses. Ann Thorac Surg 1997; 64:30–6.

83. Edmunds LH. Thrombotic and bleeding complications of prosthetic heart valves. Ann Thorac Surg 1987; 44:430–45.

84. Schaffer MS, Clarke DR, Campbell DN, et al. The St. Jude medical cardiac valve in infants and children: role of anticoagulant therapy. J Am Coll Cardiol 1987; 9:235–9.

85. Robbins RC, Bowman FO, Malm JR. Cardiac valve replacement in children: a twenty-year series. Ann Thorac Surg 1988; 45:56–61.

86. Bonow RO, Carabello B, de Leon AC Jr, et al. Guidelines for the management of patients with valvular heart disease. A report of the American College of Cardiology/American Heart Association Task Force on Practice Guidelines (Committee on Management of Patients with Valvular Heart Disease). Circulation 1998; 98:1949–84.

87. Laudito A, Brook MM, Suleman S, et al. The Ross procedure in children and young adults: a word of caution. J Thorac Cardiovasc Surg 2001; 122:147–53.

88. Kouchoukos NT, Masetti P, Nickerson NJ, et al. The Ross procedure: long-term clinical and echocardiographic follow-up. Ann Thorac Surg 2004; 78:773–81.

89. Elkins RC, Elkins CC, Lane MM, et al. Ross operation – sixteen year experience. 85th Annual Meeting of the American Association for Thoracic Surgery, April 10–13, 2005, San Francisco, CA.

90. de Vries H, Bogers AJ, Schoof PH, et al. Pulmonary autograft failure caused by a relapse of rheumatic fever. Ann Thorac Surg 1994; 57:750–1.

19

Prosthetic valve complications: interpreting the literature

YingXing Wu and Gary L Grunkemeier

The American Association for Thoracic Surgery (AATS) and the Society of Thoracic Surgeons (STS) first proposed guidelines for reporting complications after cardiac valvular operations in 1988.[1] The guidelines provide the definitions and recommendations to facilitate the analysis and reporting of results after cardiac valvular surgeries. The guidelines were updated in 1996.[2] In 1994, the US Food and Drug Administration (FDA) issued a guidance document for pre-market evaluation of new heart valves.[3] The guidance lists the objective performance criteria (OPC) as the target values for complication rates (Table 19.1).

Prosthetic valve complications

There are six categories of morbidity defined in the AATS/STS guidelines: structural valvular deterioration (SVD), non-structural dysfunction, valve thrombosis, embolism, bleeding and endocarditis (Table 19.2). For

Table 19.1 FDA objective performance criteria (OPC) for mechanical and biological heart valve studies

Morbidity	OPC (% per patient-year)	
	Mechanical	Biological
Structural valvular deterioration	–	–
Thromboembolism	3.0	2.5
Valve thrombosis	0.8	0.2
Bleeding:		
All bleeding	3.5	1.4
Major bleeding	1.5	0.9
Non-structural dysfunction:		
All leaks	1.2	1.2
Major perivalvular leak	0.6	0.6
Endocarditis	1.2	1.2

Table 19.2 AATS/STS definitions for morbidities after cardiac valvular operations

Morbidity	Definition
Structural valvular deterioration	Valve dysfunction or deterioration, exclusive of infection or thrombosis, such as wear, fracture, poppet escape, calcification, leaflet tear, stent creep and suture line disruption of components
Non-structural dysfunction	Entrapment by pannus, tissure or suture; leak; inappropriate sizing or positioning; leak or obstruction from implantation; haemolytic anaemia; excludes thrombosis and infection
Thromboembolism	New temporary or permanent neurological deficit; peripheral arterial emboli; excludes acute myocardial infarction, septic emboli, bleeding and immediate surgical events
Valve thrombosis	Thrombosis proved by operation, autopsy or clinical investigation; excludes infection
Bleeding	Major bleeding that causes death, hospitalisation, permanent injury or requires transfusion regardless of whether the patient is receiving anticoagulants and/or antiplatelet drugs
Endocarditis	Any infection involving an operated valve; other morbidity associated with active infection is included under this category

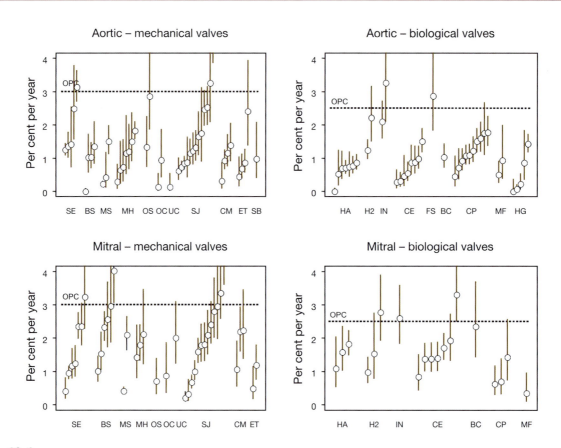

Figure 19.1

Thromboembolism rates for mechanical and biological valves in the aortic and mitral positions. The vertical axis is the linearised rate. Each circle represents one series. The height of the circles represents the point estimates of the linearised rates extracted from the literature, and the vertical lines show the 90% confidence intervals (which have the same endpoints as two *one-sided* 95% CIs). Different series of the same valve models are grouped together, and the 2-letter abbreviations of the valve models are indicated below the horizontal axis. SE = Starr–Edwards, BS = Björk–Shiley, MS = Monostrut, MH = Medtronic Hall, OS = Omniscience, OC = Omnicarbon, UC = Ultracor, SJ = St. Jude, CM = Carbomedics, ET = Edwards Tekna or Duromedics, SB = Sorin Bicarbon, HA = Hancock I and MO, H2 = Hancock II, IN = Medtronic Intact, CE = Carpentier–Edwards Porcine, FS = Medtronic Freestyle, BC = St Jude Medical Biocor, CP = Carpentier–Edwards Perimount, MF = Mitroflow, HG = homograft.

most morbidities except SVD, the complication rates are often assumed to be approximately constant after the first postoperative month. Thus, to facilitate calculation and comparison, a single statistic, the so-called 'linearised' rate, is commonly used to summarise these complications. Linearised rates can be easily calculated as the total number of events divided by the total number of late follow-up years (subtracting 30 days follow-up time for each operative survivor) and multiplying by 100 to convert to percentages. It is also suggested that linearised rates be reported with confidence intervals (CIs). The upper one-sided 95% CIs of the linearised rates being lower than two times the OPC is a standard for approval of new heart valves.

SVD is a special case where linearised rates are not applicable; therefore, there is no OPC. For biological valves, it has long been recognised that the risk of SVD increases over time. Freedom from SVD over time, usually

estimated by Kaplan–Meier curves, is used to describe the risk of SVD for biological valves. For mechanical valves, theoretically, the risk should be zero.

There are thousands of published reports of prosthetic valve complications. A PubMed search using the key words 'heart valve prosthesis' and 'follow-up study' produced 3338 hits through March 2005. These are either original studies of single or multiple valve series from the experiences of single or multiple centres, or meta-analyses that integrate the results of several independent studies. Figures 19.1 and 19.2 show the linearised rates of thromboembolism and bleeding for typical series published in the literature. The two upper panels of Figure 19.3 show the SVD-free curves of biological valves by fitting Weibull distributions to Kaplan–Meier curves extracted from the literature. Visually, it is clear that the reported results vary considerably.

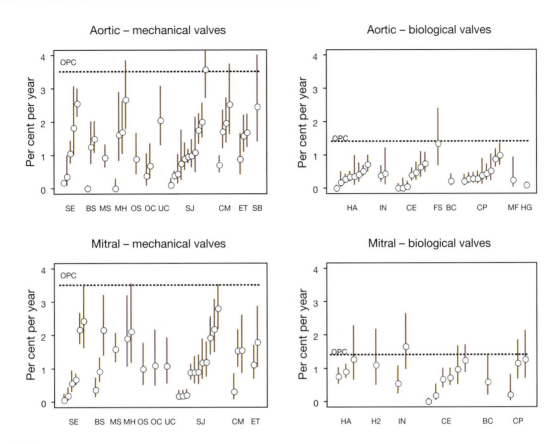

Figure 19.2
Bleeding rates for mechanical and biological valves in the aortic and mitral positions. See legend to Figure 19.1.

What would be the possible reasons for the variation? How should one interpret different reports with different or even contradictory findings for the same valve model? How should one interpret reports comparing different valve models?

Factors affecting reported complications

The OPCs for thromboembolism, valve thrombosis and bleeding are different between mechanical and biological valves (Table 19.1). Mechanical valves are believed to be more thrombogenic than biological valves and they are also considered to have higher bleeding rates because of the anticoagulation therapy. SVD is regarded to be exclusive to biological valves and SVD rates were observed to be higher in the mitral than in the aortic position. There are many factors other than the valves themselves that account for the variation of reported complication rates to a large extent.

Patient-related factors

Patient selection bias can greatly influence the results of a series of heart valve replacements, more so than the selection of the valve model itself (Figures 19.1–19.3). Patient characteristics such as age, gender and preoperative co-morbidities are major factors determining the outcomes after heart valve surgeries. Imbalance of critical patient characteristics, especially when strongly correlated with the outcome, will significantly affect the estimation of the effect due to the valve itself. An 80-year-old patient with diabetes, renal failure and atrial fibrillation is more prone to have postoperative thromboembolism than a 60-year-old patient with only isolated valve disease. For patients with biological valves, younger age is the most important predictor for SVD (Figure 19.3). Thus, direct comparison between series with different patient characteristics is invalid. For non-randomised studies, patients in different valve groups usually have different characteristics, and these differences sometimes arise by chance, but more often by patient selection. Many studies have overt or subtle inclusion and/or exclusion criteria, such as patient age, prior or concomitant cardiac procedures, etc.

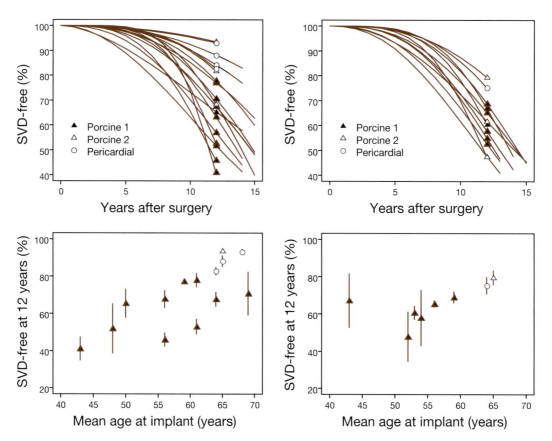

Figure 19.3
The two upper panels contain structural valvular deterioration (SVD)-free curves for aortic and mitral biological valves, produced by fitting Weibull distributions to Kaplan–Meier curves extracted from the literature. Each line represents one series. The lower two panels show the mean age of the patients in each series. The pericardial and the second generation of porcine valves had higher freedom from SVD than the first generation of porcine valves. But the first generation of porcine valves had younger mean ages, which partly accounts for the variation in observed SVD.

Surgeons and centres

In addition to different patient populations, the application of cardiac valvular surgery is not uniform between centres. Differences in surgical volumes and techniques should not be ignored. It has been demonstrated that there is a significant inverse relationship between surgical volume and adverse outcomes for both surgeons and hospitals.[4–6] Surgical techniques can also influence the results of valve replacement. For example, suturing techniques and the use of pledgets can influence the subsequent risk of paravalvular leak[7–9]

Event definitions

The FDA guidance document and the AATS/STS guidelines for reporting define the complications after cardiac valvular surgeries (Table 19.2), and most heart valve reports claim to adhere to the guidelines, but the event definitions actually being used still vary. The most common problems are:

- all events other than late events are used to calculate linearised rates
- categorisation of sudden or unknown deaths varies[10]
- thromboembolism and thrombosis rates are not reported separately
- only major leaks that result in explant are reported
- other complications associated with endocarditis, such as thrombosis and leak, are counted duplicately, and so on.

A composite end point called a major adverse cardiac event (MACE) has been used in analysing outcomes after coronary artery bypass grafting (CABG)[11] or percutaneous cardiac intervention (PCI).[12] Some researchers suggest amalgamating many or all valve-related events into one composite complication.[13–15] This might help to get around the problem of misclassification of events, e.g. thromboembolism being misclassified as intracerebral bleeding, or endocarditis as leak. This approach has been used in analysing MACEs after PCI. The drawback is that each of the events has a different level of severity and probably should not be given the same weight. Also, each event may have different risk factors and should be modelled by different mathematical models. On the other hand, some investigators advocate grading the same category of event according to its severity and reporting the complication rates separately.[16]

Study design

Randomised trials are considered to be the ideal study design, but they are rarely used in comparing prosthetic heart valves – a PubMed search found about 30 randomised studies which compared prosthetic heart valves – because they are extremely resource-intensive, requiring many valves and long-term follow-up to complete: e.g. the AVERT study of the St Jude Medical Silzone valve, designed to distinguish a 50% reduction in endocarditis rates, would have required 4400 valves and 4 years to complete.[17] Randomised studies also have their own limitations, and results from randomised studies are not necessarily representative of the results obtained outside of the specialised randomised controlled trial (RCT) environment.[18] There have been two major RCTs: the Veterans Administration[19-21] and the Edinburgh trials.[22-24] But these studies only confirmed information that was already known from observational studies, and the valves used were already discontinued by the time the studies were completed. A few other randomised studies[17,25-27] have compared heart valves, whereas others have compared anticoagulation management[28-31] or surgical techniques (i.e. minimal invasive vs conventional). Even though randomised studies are not necessary or even inappropriate for getting a new valve approved, they may be useful for determining optimal anticoagulation therapy or surgical techniques for valves that have already been approved and are being used in large numbers.

Postoperative management

Appropriate postoperative management is essential for patients undergoing heart valve replacement. For mechanical valves, lifelong anticoagulation is unavoidable; therefore, safe and efficient anticoagulation control can reduce the risk of bleeding and embolic events. Thromboembolic and bleeding rates may be substantially influenced by the levels of anticoagulation achieved, yet the anticoagulation

regimens vary between centres. The standardisation of anticoagulation measure has been changed from setting a common target range of international normalised ratio (INR), regardless of the position and type of the valves,[32,33] to prosthesis-specific and patient-specific anticoagulation.[15,34-36] The optimum INR should be determined according to the type of prosthesis and the thromboembolic risk for the individual patient.[37] Such an anticoagulation strategy has been shown to achieve low thromboembolism and bleeding rates as well as improve patient survival.[38,39] Also, the concept of anticoagulation is evolving over time: there has been a trend of lowering the target INR in recent years.[28,29,40] Patient self-monitoring anticoagulation therapy has been introduced and achieved better results than physician monitoring in several studies[30,41-43] (see also Chapter 8).

Follow-up strategies

The quality of the data depends largely on the follow-up strategies. Data collected prospectively are generally of higher quality than data collected retrospectively. For prospective follow-up, data to be collected are defined before patients are enrolled, and patients are contacted periodically thereafter. For retrospective follow-up, data are collected at one time long after the surgery, and events that happened years before may be unobtainable (patient died before being queried about complications) or underreported (patient's memory may be inadequate to recall long-past events). Some studies rely on a national 'death index' to reveal the outcome because it is much less labour-intensive. But by its very nature it cannot provide information for non-fatal complications. Most heart valve studies report completeness of follow-up as a measure of the quality of the data, but the completeness of follow-up should be considered together with the follow-up strategy (prospective or retrospective), follow-up intensity (whether the follow-up was performed semiannually, annually or biennially), follow-up technique (in-person office visit, telephone or mail), and so forth.[44,45]

Statistical analysis

Appropriate use of statistical methods is also important to the reliability of reported results.[46] Linearised rates and Kaplan–Meier event-free curves are most commonly used in summarising and comparing prosthetic valve complications. Other methods such as cumulative incidence, Cox regression and parametric regression are also used very often. Valid use of linearised rates is based on the assumption that the complication rates are approximately constant over time. For Cox regression, the assumption of proportional hazard should be tested. Compared with the Kaplan–Meier method, cumulative incidence provides an estimation of true event probabilities when analysing non-fatal complications.[47,48]

The majority of heart valve studies are observational studies. Propensity score analysis has recently been adopted in an attempt to compensate for the limitations of non-randomised comparison groups in heart valve studies: e.g. in comparing surgical techniques such as mitral valve replacement and repair.[49–51] Propensity score analysis tends to balance the distribution of baseline patient characteristics, as if patients were 'randomised' into different treatment groups. It may reduce patient selection bias to some extent, but unlike the real randomised trials, it may not balance unobserved factors that can also affect the outcome.[52,53] Also, many patients may not be used because of the inability to find propensity score-matched samples; propensity score stratification will end up with subgroups with unbalanced sample size. Grossi et al[54] tried to use the propensity score method as a supplementary analysis to compare mitral valve repair vs replacement, but no balance was achieved among propensity score quantiles. Propensity score analysis may be useful as a supplementary method in conjunction with traditional analysis but is not a substitute.[52,55]

Meta-analysis has been widely used to generate pooled results from separate literature reports.[56–59] Usually, meta-analysis is based on summary data extracted from the literature, where patient-level data are rarely available. Thus, the information that can be used is very limited. Patients in different studies are very likely to be heterogeneous, which makes data pooling technically difficult, so results derived from inappropriately conducted meta-analysis can be misleading.[60,61] There are different methods proposed to combine results from different studies, but no single method is absolutely superior.[62–64] Researchers even question the validity of using meta-analysis for comparing prosthetic valvular complications, because patients in different studies differ in characteristics and represent different practices, postoperative management and follow-up strategies.[65]

Publication bias

Bias can be introduced at any stage of the research, including patient selection bias in study design, procedure selection bias during conduct of the study, information bias in data collection, significance bias in data analysis and interpretation and bias in paper submission and publication.[66] Of these biases, publication bias is of special importance in interpreting prosthetic valve outcomes in the literature.

Publication bias has long been recognised to affect the results appearing in the literature significantly. It is introduced when the publication of research depends on the nature and the results of the study. For example, studies with significant results are more likely to get published than studies without significant results as a result of selective submission or selective acceptance of papers[67,68] and multicentre studies are more likely to be published than single-centre studies.[69] More attention to publication bias is needed for meta-analysis, particularly when only published papers are used.[70]

Interpreting prosthetic valve complications

Quality of the study (level of evidence)

The quality of the study should be considered when interpreting prosthetic valve complications. Results obtained from randomised studies are considered of the highest level of evidence.[71] Observational studies with larger sample size, longer follow-up time, intensive, prospective follow-up and rigorous statistical analysis also provide high levels of evidence.

Sources of variation

Examination of large numbers of published heart valve studies shows there appears to be more variability within series of the same model than between series of different models.[72,73] Since there are so many factors beside the valve model that affect the outcome of heart valve studies, it is impossible to completely separate the effect of valve, patient and other factors no matter how well the study was designed and conducted, and how rigorous the statistical analysis was. It is inappropriate to attribute all complications to the prosthetic valve; patient characteristics and other factors should always be considered. For example, thromboembolism has been said to be more patient-related than prosthesis-related, and age, hypertension, atrial fibrillation and other risk factors for stroke are the main predictors for thromboembolism.[15] Postoperative anticoagulation will affect the thromboembolism rate as well. Even among the general population without prosthetic heart valves, there is a 'background incidence' of thromboembolism, which in higher age groups actually exceeds the risk attributed to prosthetic valves.[15] The risk of bleeding is strongly related to the level of variability[15] of postoperative anticoagulation. Patient mortality, paravalvular leak and endocarditis are also in many cases related to patient risk factors, rather than (or in addition to) features of the valve itself.

Statistical significance vs clinical relevance (negative findings)

Sample size is crucial in detecting statistical difference. With small sample sizes, clinically important difference may not be shown to be statistically significant, whereas with large sample size, clinically insignificant difference may be shown as statistically significant. Moreover, small difference will eventually become statistically significant as the sample size increases. It is arbitrary to judge whether there is a difference by p-values only; the clinical relevance must also be taken into account.[74,75] Also, any complication rate should be reported with a CI. A point estimate by itself is meaningless without specifying the precision of the estimate.[76]

Conclusion

Although randomised studies are considered the gold standard for establishing valid conclusions about drugs, for medical devices in general, and for heart valves in particular, the large, prospective, carefully conducted observational studies comprise our main source of information. But these studies must be evaluated critically. There is more variability of published complication rates within series of the same model of prosthetic heart valve than between series of different models (Figures 19.1–19.3). Many factors besides valve model are influential to the outcomes, and contribute to the wide variation in reported complication rates. The results reported in the literature must not be interpreted literally, without consideration of these other factors.

References

1. Edmunds LH Jr, Cohn LH, Weisel RD. Guidelines for reporting morbidity and mortality after cardiac valvular operations. J Thorac Cardiovasc Surg 1988; 96:351–3.
2. Edmunds LH Jr, Clark RE, Cohn LH, et al. Guidelines for reporting morbidity and mortality after cardiac valvular operations. The American Association for Thoracic Surgery, Ad Hoc Liaison Committee for Standardizing Definitions of Prosthetic Heart Valve Morbidity. Ann Thorac Surg 1996; 62:932–5.
3. Division of Cardiovascular R, and Neurological Devices, Center for Devices and Radiological Health, Food and Drug Administration. Draft replacement heart valve guidance, version 4.1. 1994.
4. Carey JS, Robertson JM, Misbach GA, Fisher AL. Relationship of hospital volume to outcome in cardiac surgery programs in California. Am Surg 2003; 69:63–8.
5. Shahian DM. Improving cardiac surgery quality – volume, outcome, process? JAMA 2004; 291:246–8.
6. Hannan EL, Kilburn H Jr, Bernard H, et al. Coronary artery bypass surgery: the relationship between inhospital mortality rate and surgical volume after controlling for clinical risk factors. Med Care 1991; 29:1094–107.
7. Newton JR Jr, Glower DD, Davis JW, Rankin JS. Evaluation of suture techniques for mitral valve replacement. J Thorac Cardiovasc Surg 1984; 88:248–52.
8. Ionescu A, Payne N, Fraser AG, et al. Incidence of embolism and paravalvar leak after St Jude Silzone valve implantation: experience from the Cardiff Embolic Risk Factor Study. Heart 2003; 89:1055–61.
9. Schaff HV, Carrel TP, Jamieson WR, et al. Paravalvular leak and other events in silzone-coated mechanical heart valves: a report from AVERT. Ann Thorac Surg 2002; 73:785–92.
10. Butchart EG. The significance of sudden and unwitnessed death after heart valve replacement. J Heart Valve Dis 1994; 3:1–4.
11. Lenzen MJ, Boersma E, Bertrand ME, et al. Management and outcome of patients with established coronary artery disease: the Euro Heart Survey on coronary revascularization. Eur Heart J 2005; 26:1169–79.
12. Schuhlen H, Kastrati A, Dirschinger J, et al. Intracoronary stenting and risk for major adverse cardiac events during the first month. Circulation 1998; 98:104–11.
13. Akins CW. Results with mechanical cardiac valvular prostheses. Ann Thorac Surg 1995; 60:1836–44.
14. Cannegieter SC, Rosendaal FR, Wintzen AR, et al. Optimal oral anticoagulant therapy in patients with mechanical heart valves. N Engl J Med 1995; 333:11–17.
15. Butchart EG, Bodnar E, eds. Current issues in heart valve disease: thrombosis, embolism and bleeding. London: ICR Publishers, 1992.
16. Horstkotte D, Schulte HD, Bircks W, Strauer BE. Lower intensity anticoagulation therapy results in lower complication rates with the St. Jude Medical prosthesis. J Thorac Cardiovasc Surg 1994; 107:1136–45.
17. Schaff H, Carrel T, Steckelberg JM, Grunkemeier GL, Holubkov R. Artificial Valve Endocarditis Reduction Trial (AVERT): protocol of a multicenter randomized trial. J Heart Valve Dis 1999; 8:131–9.
18. Grunkemeier GL, Starr A. Alternatives to randomization in surgical studies. J Heart Valve Dis 1992; 1:142–51.
19. Hammermeister K, Sethi GK, Henderson WG, et al. Outcomes 15 years after valve replacement with a mechanical versus a bioprosthetic valve: final report of the Veterans Affairs randomized trial. J Am Coll Cardiol 2000; 36:1152–8.
20. Hammermeister KE, Sethi GK, Henderson WG, et al. A comparison of outcomes in men 11 years after heart-valve replacement with a mechanical valve or bioprosthesis. Veterans Affairs Cooperative Study on Valvular Heart Disease. N Engl J Med 1993; 328:1289–96.
21. Hammermeister KE, Henderson WG, Burchfiel CM, et al. Comparison of outcome after valve replacement with a bioprosthesis versus a mechanical prosthesis: initial 5 year results of a randomized trial. J Am Coll Cardiol 1987; 10:719–32.
22. Oxenham H, Bloomfield P, Wheatley DJ, et al. Twenty year comparison of a Björk–Shiley mechanical heart valve with porcine bioprostheses. Heart 2003; 89:715–21.
23. Bloomfield P, Wheatley DJ, Prescott RJ, Miller HC. Twelve-year comparison of a Björk–Shiley mechanical heart valve with porcine bioprostheses. N Engl J Med 1991; 324:573–9.
24. Bloomfield P, Kitchin AH, Wheatley DJ, et al. A prospective evaluation of the Björk–Shiley, Hancock, and Carpentier–Edwards heart valve prostheses. Circulation 1986; 73:1213–22.
25. Lim KH, Caputo M, Ascione R, et al. Prospective randomized com-

parison of CarboMedics and St Jude Medical bileaflet mechanical heart valve prostheses: an interim report. J Thorac Cardiovasc Surg 2002; 123:21–32.

26. Kuntze CE, Blackstone EH, Ebels T. Thromboembolism and mechanical heart valves: a randomized study revisited. Ann Thorac Surg 1998; 66:101–7.

27. Kim YI, Lesaffre E, Scheys I, et al. The Monostrut versus Medtronic Hall prosthesis: a prospective randomized study. J Heart Valve Dis 1994; 3:254–9.

28. Acar J, Iung B, Boissel JP, et al. AREVA: multicenter randomized comparison of low-dose versus standard-dose anticoagulation in patients with mechanical prosthetic heart valves. Circulation 1996; 94:2107–12.

29. Saour JN, Sieck JO, Mamo LA, Gallus AS. Trial of different intensities of anticoagulation in patients with prosthetic heart valves. N Engl J Med 1990; 322:428–32.

30. Huth C, Friedl A, Rost A. Intensity of oral anticoagulation after implantation of St. Jude Medical aortic prosthesis: analysis of the GELIA Database. Eur Heart J Suppl 2001; 3:Q33–8.

31. Koertke H, Minami K, Boethig D, et al. INR self-management permits lower anticoagulation levels after mechanical heart valve replacement. Circulation 2003; 108:II75–8.

32. Stein PD, Collins JJ Jr, Kantrowitz A. Antithrombotic therapy in mechanical and biological prosthetic heart valves and saphenous vein bypass grafts. Chest 1986; 89:46–53S.

33. Hirsh J, Deykin D, Poller L. "Therapeutic range" for oral anticoagulant therapy. Chest 1986; 89:11–15S.

34. ACC/AHA guidelines for the management of patients with valvular heart disease. A report of the American College of Cardiology/American Heart Association. Task Force on Practice Guidelines (Committee on Management of Patients with Valvular Heart Disease). J Am Coll Cardiol 1998; 32:1486–588.

35. Stein PD, Alpert JS, Dalen JE, Horstkotte D, Turpie AG. Antithrombotic therapy in patients with mechanical and biological prosthetic heart valves. Chest 1998; 114:602–10S.

36. Gohlke-Bärwolf C, Acar J, Oakley C, et al. Guidelines for prevention of thromboembolic events in valvular heart disease. Study Group of the Working Group on Valvular Heart Disease of the European Society of Cardiology. Eur Heart J 1995; 16:1320–30.

37. Stein PD, Alpert JS, Bussey HI, Dalen JE, Turpie AG. Antithrombotic therapy in patients with mechanical and biological prosthetic heart valves. Chest 2001; 119:220–7S.

38. Butchart EG, Li HH, Payne N, Buchan K, Grunkemeier GL. Twenty years' experience with the Medtronic Hall valve. J Thorac Cardiovasc Surg 2001; 121:1090–100.

39. Butchart EG, Payne N, Li HH, et al. Better anticoagulation control improves survival after valve replacement. J Thorac Cardiovasc Surg 2002; 123:715–23.

40. Altman R, Rouvier J, Gurfinkel E, et al. Comparison of two levels of anticoagulant therapy in patients with substitute heart valves. J Thorac Cardiovasc Surg 1991; 101:427–31.

41. Bernardo A. Experience with patient self-management of oral anticoagulation. J Thromb Thrombolysis 1996; 2:321–5.

42. Kortke H, Korfer R. International normalized ratio self-management after mechanical heart valve replacement: is an early start advantageous? Ann Thorac Surg 2001; 72:44–8.

43. Horstkotte D, Piper C. Improvement of oral anticoagulation therapy by INR self-management. J Heart Valve Dis 2004; 13:335–8.

44. Horstkotte D, Trampisch HJ. [Long-term studies following heart valve replacement]. Z Kardiol 1986; 75:641–5 [in German].

45. Wouters CW, Noyez L. Is no news good news? Organized follow-up, an absolute necessity for the evaluation of myocardial revascularization. Eur J Cardiothorac Surg 2004; 26:667–70.

46. Wu Y, Grunkemeier GL. Statistical analysis of the results of heart valve replacement. Expert Rev Cardiovasc Ther 2003; 1:559–68.

47. Grunkemeier GL, Jamieson WR, Miller DC, Starr A. Actuarial ver-

sus actual risk of porcine structural valve deterioration. J Thorac Cardiovasc Surg 1994; 108:709–18.

48. Grunkemeier GL, Wu Y. Interpretation of nonfatal events after cardiac surgery: actual versus actuarial reporting. J Thorac Cardiovasc Surg 2001; 122:216–19.

49. Moss RR, Humphries KH, Gao M, et al. Outcome of mitral valve repair or replacement: a comparison by propensity score analysis. Circulation 2003; 108:II90–7.

50. Yau TM, El-Ghoneimi YA, Armstrong S, Ivanov J, David TE. Mitral valve repair and replacement for rheumatic disease. J Thorac Cardiovasc Surg 2000; 119:53–60.

51. Gillinov AM, Wierup PN, Blackstone EH, et al. Is repair preferable to replacement for ischemic mitral regurgitation? J Thorac Cardiovasc Surg 2001; 122:1125–41.

52. Joffe MM, Rosenbaum PR. Invited commentary: propensity scores. Am J Epidemiol 1999; 150:327–33.

53. Blackstone EH. Comparing apples and oranges. J Thorac Cardiovasc Surg 2002; 123:8–15.

54. Grossi EA, Goldberg JD, LaPietra A, et al. Ischemic mitral valve reconstruction and replacement: comparison of long-term survival and complications. J Thorac Cardiovasc Surg 2001; 122:1107–24.

55. D'Agostino RB Jr. Propensity score methods for bias reduction in the comparison of a treatment to a non-randomized control group. Stat Med 1998; 17:2265–81.

56. Puvimanasinghe JP, Steyerberg EW, Takkenberg JJ, et al. Prognosis after aortic valve replacement with a bioprosthesis: predictions based on meta-analysis and microsimulation. Circulation 2001; 103:1535–41.

57. Massel D, Little SH. Risks and benefits of adding anti-platelet therapy to warfarin among patients with prosthetic heart valves: a meta-analysis. J Am Coll Cardiol 2001; 37:569–78.

58. Kassai B, Gueyffier F, Cucherat M, Boissel JP. Comparison of bioprosthesis and mechanical valves, a meta-analysis of randomised clinical trials. Cardiovasc Surg 2000; 8:477–83.

59. Vink R, Kraaijenhagen RA, Hutten BA, et al. The optimal intensity of vitamin K antagonists in patients with mechanical heart valves: a meta-analysis. J Am Coll Cardiol 2003; 42:2042–8.

60. Egger M, Schneider M, Davey Smith G. Spurious precision? Meta-analysis of observational studies. BMJ 1998; 316:140–4.

61. Butchart EG, Gohlke-Bärwolf C. Anticoagulation management of patients with prosthetic valves. J Am Coll Cardiol 2004; 44:1143–4; author reply 1144–5.

62. Brockwell SE, Gordon IR. A comparison of statistical methods for meta-analysis. Stat Med 2001; 20:825–40.

63. Berlin JA, Laird NM, Sacks HS, Chalmers TC. A comparison of statistical methods for combining event rates from clinical trials. Stat Med 1989; 8:141–51.

64. Egger M, Smith GD, Phillips AN. Meta-analysis: principles and procedures. BMJ 1997; 315:1533–7.

65. Butchart EG, Ionescu A, Payne N, et al. A new scoring system to determine thromboembolic risk after heart valve replacement. Circulation 2003; 108:II68–74.

66. Sackett DL. Bias in analytic research. J Chronic Dis 1979; 32:51–63.

67. Stern JM, Simes RJ. Publication bias: evidence of delayed publication in a cohort study of clinical research projects. BMJ 1997; 315:640–5.

68. Easterbrook PJ, Berlin JA, Gopalan R, Matthews DR. Publication bias in clinical research. Lancet 1991; 337:867–72.

69. Dickersin K, Min YI, Meinert CL. Factors influencing publication of research results. Follow-up of applications submitted to two institutional review boards. JAMA 1992; 267:374–8.

70. Egger M, Smith GD. Bias in location and selection of studies. BMJ 1998; 316:61–6.

71. Hadorn DC, Baker D, Hodges JS, Hicks N. Rating the quality of evidence for clinical practice guidelines. J Clin Epidemiol 1996; 49:749–54.

72. Grunkemeier GL, Li HH, Naftel DC, Starr A, Rahimtoola SH. Long-term performance of heart valve prostheses. Curr Probl Cardiol 2000; 25:73–154.

73. Grunkemeier GL, Wu Y. "Our complication rates are lower than theirs": statistical critique of heart valve comparisons. J Thorac Cardiovasc Surg 2003; 125:290–300.

74. Kieser M, Rohmel J, Friede T. Power and sample size determination when assessing the clinical relevance of trial results by 'responder analyses'. Stat Med 2004; 23:3287–305.

75. Hojat M, Xu G. A visitor's guide to effect sizes: statistical significance versus practical (clinical) importance of research findings. Adv Health Sci Educ Theory Pract 2004; 9:241–9.

76. Poole C. Low P-values or narrow confidence intervals: which are more durable? Epidemiology 2001; 12:291–4.

Index

Page numbers in *italics* refer to tables, figures and boxes.